Dr Podcast Scripts for the Primary FRCA

Dr Podcast Scripts for the Primary FRCA

Edited by

Rebecca A. Leslie
Speciality Registrar in Anaesthesia
Severn Deanery, Bristol, UK

Emily K. Johnson
Speciality Registrar in Anaesthesia
West Midlands Deanery, Birmingham, UK

Alexander P.L. Goodwin
Consultant in Anaesthesia and Intensive Care
Royal United Hospital, Bath, UK

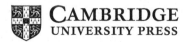

CAMBRIDGE
UNIVERSITY PRESS

CAMBRIDGE
UNIVERSITY PRESS

University Printing House, Cambridge CB2 8BS, United Kingdom

One Liberty Plaza, 20th Floor, New York, NY 10006, USA

477 Williamstown Road, Port Melbourne, VIC 3207, Australia

314-321, 3rd Floor, Plot 3, Splendor Forum, Jasola District Centre, New Delhi - 110025, India

79 Anson Road, #06-04/06, Singapore 079906

Cambridge University Press is part of the University of Cambridge.

It furthers the University's mission by disseminating knowledge in the pursuit of education, learning and research at the highest international levels of excellence.

www.cambridge.org
Information on this title: www.cambridge.org/9781107401013

First published 2011
14th printing 2018

A catalogue record for this publication is available from the British Library

ISBN 978-1-107-40101-3 Paperback

Cambridge University Press has no responsibility for the persistence or accuracy of URLs for external or third-party internet websites referred to in this publication, and does not guarantee that any content on such websites is, or will remain, accurate or appropriate.

. . . .

Every effort has been made in preparing this book to provide accurate and up-to-date information which is in accord with accepted standards and practice at the time of publication. Although case histories are drawn from actual cases, every effort has been made to disguise the identities of the individuals involved. Nevertheless, the authors, editors and publishers can make no warranties that the information contained herein is totally free from error, not least because clinical standards are constantly changing through research and regulation. The authors, editors and publishers therefore disclaim all liability for direct or consequential damages resulting from the use of material contained in this book. Readers are strongly advised to pay careful attention to information provided by the manufacturer of any drugs or equipment that they plan to use.

To Reston,
For his unfailing support, patience and voice.

RL

To Alan and my parents,
For their help and understanding through my exams
and again through the busy times with Dr Podcast,
and the editing of this book.

EJ

To Juliette, William, Tiggy and Chorlie,
Ma raison d'aitre.

APLG

Contents

2 – Pharmacology

3 – Physics

Contributors

Sarah F Bell
Speciality Registrar in Anaesthesia
Wales Deanery, Cardiff, Wales, UK

Adrian Clarke
Speciality Registrar in Anaesthesia
Wales Deanery, Cardiff, Wales, UK

Caroline SG Janes
Specialist Registrar in Anaesthesia
Oxford Deanery, Oxford, UK

Emily K Johnson
Speciality Registrar in Anaesthesia
West Midlands Deanery, Birmingham, UK

Natasha A Joshi
Speciality Registrar in Anaesthesia
Severn Deanery, Bristol, UK

Dana L Kelly
Speciality Registrar in Anaesthesia
Oxford Deanery, Oxford, UK

Rebecca A Leslie
Speciality Registrar in Anaesthesia
Severn Deanery, Bristol, UK

Henry Murdoch
Speciality Registrar in Anaesthesia
Severn Deanery, Bristol, UK

Archana Panickar
Speciality Registrar in Anaesthesia
South Yorkshire and Humber Deanery, UK

Caroline V Sampson
Speciality Registrar in Anaesthesia
East Midlands Deanery, Nottingham, UK

Joy M Sanders
Speciality Registrar in Anaesthesia
Wessex Deanery, Winchester, UK

Matthew C Thomas
Consultant in Anaesthesia and
Intensive Care Medicine Frenchay
Hospital, Bristol, UK

Consultant Reviewing Panel

Alexander PL Goodwin
Consultant in Anaesthesia and Intensive Care Medicine
Royal United Hospital, Bath, UK

Jeffrey Handel
Consultant in Anaesthesia and Perioperative Medicine
Royal United Hospital, Bath, UK

Patrick Magee
Consultant in Anaesthesia and Perioperative Medicine, Royal United Hospital, Bath, UK
Senior Visiting Lecturer, Dept Mechanical Engineering, University of Bath, Bath, UK

Mike Wilkinson
Consultant in Anaesthesia and Perioperative Medicine
Northampton General Hospital, Northampton, UK

Preface

Students learn in many different ways. Over the last 2 years Rebecca Leslie and Emily Johnson of Dr Podcast have developed a genre of education to assist doctors in training to achieve educational goals. To date, over 200 000 podcasts have been downloaded. Trainees particularly use these innovative podcasts to learn and revise prior to examinations where they are assessed in structured oral examinations and where they might be asked to express their understanding verbally. Having examined trainees in the primary FRCA for 10 years, I am convinced that those candidates who were well prepared and rehearsed fared better in oral examinations. The podcasts for Primary FRCA undoubtedly assist in that preparation and are a great success. Now this book satisfies the demand for the podcast scripts accompanied by relevant diagrams.

This book, *Dr Podcast Scripts for the Primary FRCA*, presents podcasts in the written word as the voices recording the podcasts would have read them. They are enhanced by simple diagrams which illuminate the scripts in a way not possible in the spoken versions. They have also been reviewed by the original authors. It is hoped that students might use the written versions with their illustrations to complement the spoken form.

The scripts have been written by those who have recently passed the primary FRCA examination. All the scripts have been reviewed by senior anaesthetists involved in education. The level of knowledge is specifically aimed at those approaching the exam. It must be emphasised that the scripts should form part of a multifaceted preparation to sit, and be successful in, a Fellowship exam. In themselves they present a different take on each topic, compared to a conventional textbook. Questions are asked, answered, and then tips on understanding or answering a verbal question are given. Those not sitting exams will find them useful for revising topics and help them to prepare teaching material.

This book demonstrates the overlap between traditional methods of presenting facts and knowledge with those teaching techniques available in the twenty-first century. The book is an excellent example of how well the old and new complement each other. It will undoubtedly add another tool to a student's toolbox, allowing them to be best prepared for the daunting hurdles of professional examinations.

Dr A.P.L. Goodwin

Acknowledgements

When we first started Dr Podcast it was an untried and untested formula, and we had no idea if it would be a success. We would like to thank all our authors, voices and especially our consultant reviewers, Alex, Jeff, Patrick and Mike who committed endless time and effort to turn our idea into a popular revision aid.

We thank Cambridge University Press for permission to use diagrams from *Fundamentals of Anaesthesia* 3rd Edition and *Physics, Pharmacology and Physiology for Anaesthetists* Key Concepts for the FRCA 1st Edition. We also thank the original providers of these diagrams: Tim Smith, Colin Pinnock, Ted Lin, Robert Jones, Matthew Cross and Emma Plunkett.

Respiratory physiology

1.1.1. Lung volumes and control of breathing – Emily K Johnson

Can you draw and explain the volumes and capacities of the lung?

You should be able to draw, label and add values to the spirometer trace. You should practice doing this until you are confident with it and can talk it through as you draw it.

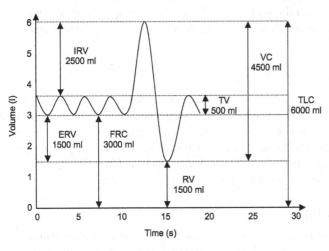

Figure 1.1.1a. Lung volumes. Reproduced with permission from Cross, M. and Plunkett, E. 2008. *Physics, Pharmacology and Physiology for Anaesthetists: Key Concepts for the FRCA.* Cambridge: Cambridge University Press. © M. Cross and E. Plunkett 2008.

Lung volumes can be measured using a spirometer. The tidal volume is the volume of a normal breath and in an adult is around 500 ml (Figure 1.1.1a). The functional residual capacity (FRC) is the volume of air in the lungs at the end of normal expiration with the subject in the standing position and is around 3000 ml in a normal adult. It can be considered as the volume of air in the lungs when the elastic recoil of the lungs is equal to the outward force of the chest wall and diaphragm tone. This is an important volume as it acts as an oxygen reserve, maintaining oxygenation of blood passing through pulmonary capillaries during expiration or breath-holding. FRC increases with subject height and in males. It is important to realise that it decreases approximately 1000 ml in the supine position due to the upward force of the abdominal contents.

Dr Podcast Scripts for the Primary FRCA, ed. Rebecca A. Leslie, Emily K. Johnson and Alexander P. L. Goodwin.   Published by Cambridge University Press. © R. A. Leslie, E. K. Johnson and A. P. L. Goodwin 2011.

Inspiratory reserve volume is the volume that can be inspired over and above the normal tidal volume and equals approximately 2500 ml. Inspiratory capacity is the total volume that can be inspired above FRC and equals around 3000 ml.

Vital capacity is the maximal volume that can be expired after a maximal inspiration and is around 4500 ml.

Expiratory reserve volume is the additional volume that can be expired at the end of expiration and is approximately 1500 ml. Residual volume is the volume of air remaining in the lungs at the end of maximal expiration and is approximately 1000 to 1500 ml.

Which volumes cannot be measured using simple spirometry?

The residual volume cannot be measured and therefore any lung capacity which includes this volume can also not be measured. These are the total lung capacity and the functional residual capacity.

What is the difference between a volume and a capacity?

A capacity is the sum of two or more volumes. Therefore a volume is directly measured whereas a capacity is deduced from the measured volumes. For example the vital capacity is the sum of the expiratory reserve volume, the tidal volume and the inspiratory reserve volume.

What is closing capacity?

Closing capacity is the lung volume at which airways close. It is equal to the residual volume plus the closing volume. In healthy young subjects the closing capacity is less than the FRC so airway closure does not occur in normal breathing. Closing capacity increases with age, increased intra-thoracic pressure and smoking. In neonates, infants, the supine person aged 40 and the standing person aged 65 the closing capacity is equal to FRC. Once closing capacity exceeds FRC there is airway closure and gas trapping in normal breathing.

What is the work of breathing?

The work of breathing is the work required to move the lung and chest wall. In normal breathing the muscles of inspiration do all the work and expiration is passive. The forces that have to be overcome to expand the lung are divided into elastic forces and non-elastic forces. The non-elastic forces are also called frictional forces and encompass airway and tissue resistance. Half of the work of the inspiratory muscles is in overcoming the non-elastic forces. The other half is in overcoming the elastic forces, which is then stored as potential energy in the lung tissue. This potential energy is released on expiration as the elastic tissue returns to its resting state, and it is used to overcome frictional forces. In increased airways resistance or increased respiratory rate the work of expiration may exceed the potential energy stored so expiratory muscles are recruited and expiration becomes active. When the lung is inflated to larger volumes or compliance is low there will be more work required to overcome the elastic forces, and so more energy stored at end inspiration. The work done to overcome the non-elastic forces is lost as heat. This is increased in rapid respiratory rates or high airways resistance.

The work of breathing can be demonstrated using pressure–volume curves of the lung on inspiration and expiration (Figure 1.1.1b).

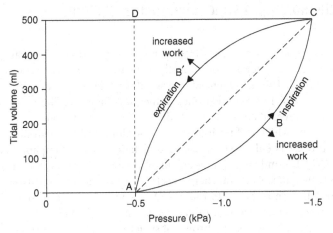

Figure 1.1.1b. Work of breathing. Modified with permission from Cross, M. and Plunkett, E. 2008. *Physics, Pharmacology and Physiology for Anaesthetists: Key Concepts for the FRCA.* Cambridge: Cambridge University Press. © M. Cross and E. Plunkett 2008.

Inspiratory work:
- ACDA area = work to overcome elastic tissues
- ABCA area = work to overcome viscous resistance and friction

Expiratory work:
- CB′AC area = work to overcome airways resistance (within area ACDA therefore supplied from stored energy UNLESS increased work causes curve to bow to the left).
- Difference between CB′AC and CDAC areas = lost as heat energy.

You should learn these pressure–volume curves and the areas relevant to the work of breathing. Practice drawing and explaining them.

How is alveolar ventilation controlled?

Alveolar ventilation is controlled by feedback loops. The system of control has three main components:

- A control centre, which is the medullary respiratory centre
- Effectors, which are the respiratory muscles
- Sensors feeding information to the central control, which are chemoreceptors and other types of receptors.

The respiratory centre lies in the pons and medulla and consists of three groups of neurones. The medullary centre is in the reticular formation below the floor of the fourth ventricle. It has a dorsal respiratory group, thought to be responsible for inspiration, and a largely dormant ventral group, thought to be responsible for expiration. The other two groups of neurones make up the apneustic centre in the lower pons and the pneumotaxic centre in the upper pons. Their exact involvement in respiration is not clear.

When the respiratory centre is appropriately stimulated it coordinates synchronised activity from the muscles of respiration, which are the diaphragm, the intercostal muscles, the abdominal muscles, and the accessory muscles, such as sternocleidomastoid. These muscle groups increase their work, and ventilation is increased appropriately.

Tell me more about the chemoreceptors and other sources of input to the respiratory centre

The afferent input into the respiratory centre comes from a number of sources. Central chemoreceptors play an important role. They respond mostly to hydrogen ion (H^+) concentration in brain extra-cellular fluid. This is influenced by arterial partial pressure of CO_2. These chemoreceptors are situated near the ventral surface of the medulla. If ventilation is decreased $PaCO_2$ will rise and an increased amount of CO_2 diffuses across the blood–brain barrier. This liberates more H^+ ions which diffuse into the extra-cellular fluid and stimulate the chemoreceptors. This process is enhanced by the vasodilatation that accompanies increased arterial pressures of CO_2. H^+ and HCO_3^- ions are unable to cross the blood–brain barrier, so it is increased $PaCO_2$ that affects central chemoreceptors. This is a very sensitive mechanism for increasing ventilation in response to raised CO_2 because the pH of CSF is usually 7.32 and there is less protein buffering than in plasma, so smaller pH changes are detected. In a chronically raised $PaCO_2$ such as in chronic obstructive pulmonary disease (COPD) compensatory changes occur and HCO_3^- ions are actively transported across the blood–brain barrier.

Peripheral chemoreceptors are situated in the carotid bodies and the aortic arch. The carotid bodies contain two types of glomus cells. Type 1 cells are rich in dopamine and are close to the end of the carotid sinus nerve. The glomus cells are affected by raised $PaCO_2$ and decreased pH, although pH has no effect on the aortic arch chemoreceptors. Peripheral chemoreceptors also mount a response to low PaO_2 and are the only receptors responsible for this response. Overall the peripheral chemoreceptors are only responsible for 20% of the body's response to a raised $PaCO_2$, with the rest being due to the central chemoreceptors; however, it is the peripheral chemoreceptors that act fastest.

Other receptors that feed information to the respiratory centre include lung stretch receptors in bronchial smooth muscle, which transmit signals in the vagus with large amounts of distension causing an increased expiratory time and reduced respiratory rate. This is the Hering–Breuer reflex. Irritant receptors lie between airway epithelial cells and cause bronchoconstriction and hyperventilation in response to noxious gases. J, or juxtacapillary, receptors are non-myelinated C fibres in the alveolar walls that respond to circulatory changes and can cause shallow fast breathing and apnoea. There are other receptors in the nose and upper airways that respond to mechanical and chemical stimuli. Joint and muscle receptors are also thought to influence ventilation by stimulation of the respiratory centre when limbs move, such as in exercise. Arterial baroreceptors decrease ventilation when they increase blood pressure, and pain and temperature receptors can also influence ventilation. To a certain degree ventilation is under voluntary control from higher centres and cortical input can override brainstem control centres. The limbic system and hypothalamus also have input in extreme emotional states.

1.1.2. Respiratory compliance and surface tension – Rebecca A Leslie

What is the normal intra-pleural pressure?

The intra-pleural pressure is normally negative due to the lungs natural tendency to collapse inwards and the chest walls tendency to spring outwards. When standing and at normal

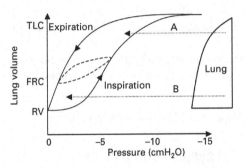

Figure 1.1.2. Whole lung pressure–volume loop. Modified with permission from Cross, M. and Plunkett, E. 2008. *Physics, Pharmacology and Physiology for Anaesthetists: Key Concepts for the FRCA.* Cambridge: Cambridge University Press. © M. Cross and E. Plunkett 2008.

resting volume the intra-pleural pressure at the apex is -10 cmH$_2$O and at the base it is -2.5 cmH$_2$O.

The intra-pleural pressure becomes more negative during normal ventilation. It normally changes by 3–4 cmH$_2$O unless the inspiration is particularly forceful or the airway resistance increases. During expiration the intra-pleural pressure returns back to normal unless expiration is forced or resistance increased. During forced expiration the intra-pleural pressure may even exceed zero, and hence airway pressure.

What is compliance?

To answer this question you should draw a pressure–volume curve. You should practice drawing this curve so you can draw it quickly and easily when answering any question on respiratory compliance.

Compliance is the change in volume for a pressure change across the lung (Figure 1.1.2). Therefore compliance is how easily the lungs expand, and it represents the slope of the pressure–volume curve.

The normal expanding pressures of the lung are between -5 and -10 cmH$_2$O. At these pressures the slope of the pressure–volume curve is steep, so for a small change in pressure there is a large change in volume. Therefore it can be said at these pressures that the lung is remarkably compliant. The compliance of the normal lung is approximately 200 ml/cmH$_2$O.

At higher expanding pressures, the lung is stiffer, and much less compliant, as demonstrated by the flatter part of the curve.

What are the components that influence respiratory compliance?

The two main components to respiratory compliance are lung compliance and thoracic wall compliance.

The lung compliance is determined by the elastic recoil properties of the pulmonary connective tissue and the surface tension at the fluid/air interface within the alveoli. The lungs expand in response to the pressure gradient across their surface. This is called the transpulmonary pressure, and it is produced by the respiratory muscles. Transpulmonary pressure is the difference between alveolar pressure and intra-pleural pressure. Alveolar pressures during quiet ventilation can be approximated to atmospheric pressure, so transpulmonary pressure equates to intra-pleural pressure. The lung compliance at FRC is 200 ml/cmH$_2$O. At high transmural pressures the lung compliance drops. This is because the elastic fibres are fully stretched close to their elastic limit.

The compliance of the chest wall at FRC is also found to be 200 ml/cmH$_2$O. The chest wall compliance is reduced by diseases such as ankylosing spondylitis where the chest wall becomes virtually rigid.

In the respiratory system the lungs and thoracic cage work together during inspiration and expiration. The respiratory compliance is therefore the combination of the lung and chest wall compliances.

1/Total respiratory compliance = 1/Lung compliance + 1/Chest wall compliance.

Describe the difference between static and dynamic compliance

Static and dynamic compliance represent two different methods of determining compliance.

Static compliance is the volume change per unit change in distending pressure when there is no airflow. The distending pressure is the transpulmonary pressure, which during quiet breathing is equal to the intra-pleural pressure because alveolar pressure is the same as atmospheric pressure. Therefore to determine the compliance we need to know the intra-pleural pressure. We can estimate intra-pleural pressure by measuring oesophageal pressure. This is done by asking the subject to swallow a small balloon on the end of a catheter.

The subject takes a maximal inspiration, and then breathes out into a spirometer in steps of 500 ml. The lungs are given a few seconds to stabilise after each exhalation and then the oesophageal pressure is recorded. This process is repeated until the patient has breathed out their total lung capacity. These measurements can then be used to produce a static pressure–volume curve. The lung compliance at specific lung volumes can be calculated by the slope of the curve.

In dynamic compliance the pressure–volume curve is plotted continuously throughout the respiratory cycle during spontaneous breathing or mechanical ventilation.

The pressures recorded in dynamic compliance for a given volume are always higher than those recorded in static compliance, and as a consequence the lung compliance is found to be lower.

What factors influence compliance?

Remember always to first classify your answer.

Compliance is influenced by physiological and pathological factors.
Physiological factors:

- Posture – the lungs are more compliant when the patient is upright, and compliance declines when the patient becomes supine
- Age – compliance is reduced at the extremes of age
- Pregnancy – the FRC is reduced and the lungs become less compliant.

Pathological factors can both increase and decrease lung compliance.
Diseases that decrease the compliance of the lung include:

- Pulmonary fibrosis – due to an increase in lung fibrous tissue
- Acute respiratory distress syndrome and pulmonary oedema – by preventing the inflation of alveoli

- Atelectasis – decreases lung compliance as greater pressure is required to recruit alveoli
- Increased pulmonary venous pressure – decreases lung compliance because the lungs become engorged with blood.

A disease that increases lung compliance is pulmonary emphysema where there is an alteration in the elastic tissue in the lung.

What is hysteresis?

Hysteresis is where a measurement differs according to whether the value is increasing or decreasing. For example in the pressure–volume curve the inspiration and expiration curves are not identical but form a loop where the expiration curve differs from the inspiration curve, see Figure 1.1.2. This loop is known as hysteresis.

Hysteresis normally results from the absorption of energy, often as friction. The area of the loop represents the amount of energy expended or wasted as heat. In the pressure–volume curve the lung loses energy when the elastic tissues stretch and then recoil and in order to overcome airway resistance. A factor that reduces this wasted energy and thus improves the efficiency of the breathing cycle is the reduction of alveolar surface tension by surfactant.

What causes surface tension in the alveoli?

First demonstrate your understanding of what surface tension is by defining it and then move on to what causes it in the alveoli.

The definition of surface tension is the force acting across an imaginary line 1 cm long in the surface of a liquid. Surface tension is measured in dynes.

The alveoli are lined by a thin layer of fluid. This fluid contributes to the surface tension acting on the alveoli because the attractive forces between these water molecules are greater than the attractive forces at the air–fluid interface. This results in the liquid surface area becoming as small as possible, and tending to collapse the alveolus.

This behaviour can be seen when blowing a soap bubble on the end of a tube. The liquid molecules in the surface of the bubble have much stronger attractive forces than the forces between the liquid and the air at the liquid–air interface. This means that the surface of the bubble contracts as much as possible which creates a sphere that has the smallest surface area for a given volume of air and generates a pressure within the bubble.

How can you predict the pressure inside a bubble or alveoli?

With this question they are testing your knowledge and understanding of Laplace's law. First state Laplace's law and then explain how this equates to the lung.

Laplace's law states that the pressure in a bubble or alveoli is proportional to four times the surface tension divided by the radius of the bubble. Therefore $P = 4T/r$. This means that internal pressure is proportional to 1/radius.

From this law it can be seen that an alveolus with a small radius will have a greater pressure inside it than a larger alveolus. Now imagine these alveoli are connected together. Because the smaller alveolus has a higher pressure inside it, it will tend to collapse into the larger alveolus. In addition the inward force created by this surface tension will also tend to suck fluid into the alveoli, this is called transudation.

How are these problems minimised in the lung?

In the lung the problems of surface tension are overcome by the production of surfactant by type 2 pneumocytes. Surfactant is a mixture of phospholipids, of which dipalmitoyl phosphatidylcholine (DPPC) is the most important constituent. The molecules of DPPC are hydrophobic at one end and hydrophilic at the other end. As a result they align themselves over the surface of the liquid which lines the alveoli. Their intermolecular repulsive forces oppose the normal attractive forces between the liquid molecules so reduce the surface tension.

If the alveoli shrink, the molecules of surfactant become closer together and consequently repel each other more. This further reduces the surface tension and helps prevent the alveoli from collapsing.

What are the advantages of surfactant?

Surfactant lowers the surface tension in the alveoli and as a result increases the compliance of the lung and reduces the work required to expand the alveoli.

In addition surfactant prevents the transudation of fluid into the alveoli from the surrounding capillaries. We previously mentioned how the surface tension forces in the alveoli not only tend to collapse the alveoli but also tend to suck fluid into the alveolar spaces from the capillaries. Surfactant reduces these surface tension forces and therefore helps to keep the alveoli dry.

Surfactant also increases the stability of the alveoli. We know that the pressure generated by the surface forces of the alveolus is inversely proportional to the radius, so if the surface tensions are the same then the pressure in the small alveolus is greater than the pressure in the large alveolus. However if surfactant is present the surface tension in a small alveolus is much smaller than the surface tension in a large alveolus. This reduces the tendency for the small alveoli to empty into the large alveoli, and overall the alveoli are more stable.

What happens if there is no surfactant?

Base your answer to this question on the three functions of surfactant that you have already mentioned. It is also worth mentioning infant respiratory distress syndrome in your answer.

Without surfactant your lungs would be non-compliant, with areas of atelectasis and a tendency to pulmonary oedema because the alveoli would become filled with transudate. These are the pathophysiological features of infant respiratory distress syndrome. Infant respiratory distress syndrome is a syndrome which occurs when babies are born prematurely before adequate levels of surfactant are produced. Ideally this condition is prevented by giving maternal steroids prior to delivery which induces the production of foetal surfactant, however this is not always achievable and it is now possible to treat these infants by instilling synthesised surfactant into their lungs.

1.1.3. Ventilation, perfusion and dead-space – Rebecca A Leslie

How is the blood flow distributed within the lungs?

When answering this question it is a good idea to draw a graph, with the region of the lung on the x axis and blood flow in litres per minute on the y axis. Remember always label your axes and add on an appropriate scale. See Figure 1.1.3a.

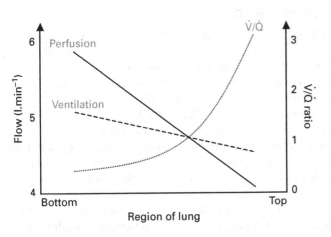

Figure 1.1.3a. Ventilation/ perfusion. Reproduced with permission from Cross, M. and Plunkett, E. 2008. *Physics, Pharmacology and Physiology for Anaesthetists: Key Concepts for the FRCA.* Cambridge: Cambridge University Press. © M. Cross and E. Plunkett 2008.

In the upright lung the blood flow decreases linearly from the bottom to the top. At the apex of the lung the blood flow is very low. This effect is mainly determined by gravity and the hydrostatic pressures within the blood vessels. The pressure difference between the bottom and the top of the lung could be as high as 30 cmH$_2$O which is a large pressure difference for the low pressure pulmonary circulation.

What will happen to the blood flow if the patient lies down?

The pulmonary blood flow is very dependent on posture. If the patient lies down the blood flow to the posterior regions of the lungs will become greater than to the anterior regions of the lungs. The difference between the apex and base of the lung will diminish in a supine patient.

How can you measure the distribution of blood flow in the lungs?

Radioactive xenon can be used to determine the distribution of blood flow in the lungs. The radioactive xenon is dissolved in normal saline and then injected into a peripheral vein. Xenon has a very low solubility, so when it reaches the pulmonary capillaries it will quickly move from the blood into the alveolar gas. If the patient breath-holds the distribution of the radioactive xenon can be measured by counters over the chest wall.

Tell me about the distribution of ventilation within the lungs

It has been found that there are significant differences in the ventilation of different regions of the lungs. The bases of the lung ventilate better than the upper zones.

How can you demonstrate this difference in ventilation?

Remember to keep it simple. This is the sort of question where they are expecting some lateral thinking; they do not necessarily expect you to have learnt this. Just think logically about how this could be done, and mention principles without worrying about the specifics.

The regional variations in ventilation can be demonstrated by asking the patient to inhale radioactive xenon gas. A radiation camera can then determine the volume of radioactive xenon throughout the chest cavity.

What causes this variation in ventilation?

To explain this concept it will be beneficial to draw a graph with intra-pleural pressure (with values becoming more negative to the right) on the x axis, and lung volume on the y axis, see Figure 1.1.2, page 5. This curve is an upward sloping sigmoid curve and helps to explain why more ventilation occurs at the bases of the lungs compared to the top. Remember always label your axes and draw diagrams big enough for the examiners to see easily.

The intra-pleural pressure is less negative, and therefore greater at the bases of the lung when compared to the apex. The reason for this difference in intra-pleural pressure has to do with the weight of the lung. In order to balance out the downward acting force due to the weight of the lung, the pressure below the lung must be greater than the pressure above it. As a result the pressure near the bases is $-2.5\,cmH_2O$ compared to the pressure at the apex which is $-10\,cmH_2O$.

If lung volume is plotted on a graph against intra-pleural pressure, with values becoming more negative towards the right, an upward sloping sigmoid curve is formed. From this curve it is evident that at resting state pressures of $-2.5\,cmH_2O$, like those at the bases of the lung, there is only a small volume of gas. However for a small decrease in intra-pleural pressure, for example when a patient takes a breath, there is a large increase in lung volume (indicated by the steep part of the sigmoid curve).

At the apex of the lung, where pressure at resting state is approximately $-10\,cmH_2O$, from the graph you can see that there is already a large volume of gas in the alveoli. When the patient takes a breath and the pressure becomes more negative there is very little change in volume of gas in this area of the lung because the alveoli are already fully expanded. This is why the curve flattens out at this point.

So in summary the bases of the lung have a small resting volume, but a large changing volume, so ventilation is good. In contrast at the apex the resting volume is large and a change in pressure results in only a small change in volume with inspiration.

Therefore, like the blood flow, ventilation decreases from bottom to top of the lung. However it is worth mentioning that the regional differences in blood flow from the bottom to the top of the lungs vary more than the regional changes in ventilation.

This can be shown on another graph, with the rib number on the x axis, starting with the bottom and moving to the top of the lung (remembering that the bottom of the lungs is indicated by rib number 12, so the numbers decrease as you move to the right) and the blood flow in L/min and the percentage of lung volume on the y axis. A straight downward sloping line can be drawn for blood flow indicating a better blood flow at the bottom compared to the top of the lungs. Another straight downward sloping line can be drawn for the ventilation, however this line has a smaller gradient than for blood flow showing that although there are regional differences in ventilation, these are less noticeable than for blood flow, see Figure 1.1.3a.

What happens to the distribution of ventilation at very low lung volumes?

The main principle behind this question is that at low lung volumes the intra-pleural pressure increases, i.e. becomes more positive. If you remember this by using the graph that you drew for the last question showing intra-pleural pressure on the x axis and lung volume on the y axis you will be able to work out the answer.

At low lung volumes, for example at the reserve volume after a maximal expiration, the intra-pleural pressures become more positive because the lung is not so well expanded and the elastic recoil forces are smaller.

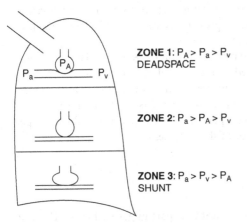

Figure 1.1.3b. West zones of the lung.

ZONE 1: $P_A > P_a > P_v$
DEADSPACE

ZONE 2: $P_a > P_A > P_v$

ZONE 3: $P_a > P_v > P_A$
SHUNT

There is still a difference in intra-pleural pressure between the apex and the base of the lung. At reserve volume, the intra-pleural pressure in the bases is approximately $+2.5$ cmH$_2$O, while the pressure at the apex is approximately -4 cmH$_2$O.

A pressure of $+2.5$ cmH$_2$O at the base of the lung is higher than the airway pressure, which is equal to atmospheric pressure. In this situation the alveoli are not being expanded but compressed, and as a result ventilation is not possible until the intra-pleural pressure falls below atmospheric pressure.

By contrast, at the apex of the lung the pressure is now -4 cmH$_2$O. This is on the favourable part of the curve and ventilates well when the patient takes a breath.

So at low lung volumes, the normal distribution of ventilation is reversed, with the upper regions ventilating better than the bases.

Explain the significance of the West zones

You must know the difference between the three West zones, and it commonly comes up in the exam. Draw a quick diagram of one lung, mark on the three West zones and write down the difference between alveolar, arterial and venous partial pressures for each zone, see Figure 1.1.3b.

There are three West zones described.

Zone 1 occurs at the apex of the lung. It describes a situation where the pulmonary artery (P_a) pressure falls below alveolar pressure (P_A). If this occurs the higher pressure in the alveoli squashes the blood vessels flat, and no blood flow is possible. When zone 1 occurs, the lung is ventilated but not perfused therefore no gas exchange can take place, and is known as alveolar dead-space. This zone does not normally occur as pulmonary arterial pressure is normally just sufficient to pump blood to the top of the lungs. However, if there is a reduction in pulmonary artery pressure, for example with severe haemorrhage or if there is an increase in alveolar pressure with positive pressure ventilation, zone 1 will occur. In summary in zone 1, the alveolar partial pressure exceeds arterial partial pressure which in turn is higher than venous partial pressure (P_v).

Zone 2 describes the situation where there is optimal ventilation–perfusion matching. The arterial pressure is higher than at the apex due to the effect of gravity and as a result it now exceeds alveolar pressure. However the alveolar pressure is still greater than the venous partial pressure, which results in a characteristic pressure–flow relationship which is often called Starling's resistor or the waterfall effect. Under these conditions blood flow is determined by the difference between arterial and alveolar pressures, rather than the normal arterial–venous pressure difference. So in zone 2 the arterial partial pressure exceeds the alveolar partial pressure which in turn exceeds venous partial pressure.

In zone 3, at the lung bases, the venous partial pressure now exceeds alveolar partial pressure. This means blood flow is now determined by the arterial–venous pressure difference. The pressure within the vessels increases down this zone whilst the pressure in the alveoli remains constant. In summary in zone 3, arterial partial pressure is greater than venous partial pressure which in turn is greater than alveolar partial pressure. Because in this zone perfusion is better than ventilation there is a degree of shunt present.

What is dead-space ventilation?

Remember define then classify.

It is the volume of fresh inspired gas that does not take part in gas exchange. There are two types of dead-space: anatomical and alveolar.

Anatomical dead-space corresponds to the volume of gas in the conducting airways. The normal value is approximately 150 ml, however, it increases with large inspirations because of the traction exerted on the bronchi by the surrounding lung parenchyma.

The alveolar dead-space corresponds to the part of the lung which is ventilated but not perfused.

Physiological dead-space is the sum of anatomical and alveolar dead-space.

How can you measure anatomical dead-space?

Whilst describing Fowler's technique draw the two key graphs. The first one with nitrogen concentration in percent against time in seconds, showing the three different phases, phase 1, 2 and 3 (the plateau phase). The second graph shows nitrogen concentration in percent against expired volume in millilitres. Remember that the anatomical dead-space is normally approximately 150 ml so make sure the scale on your graph is appropriate.

You can measure anatomical dead-space using Fowler's method. The patient takes a maximal breath of 100% oxygen at the end of a normal expiration. The patient then slowly exhales through a nitrogen analyser and the nitrogen concentration is plotted against time. In the first phase there is no nitrogen expired as this is the gas from the conducting airways (anatomical dead-space). In phase 2 the gas from the alveoli starts to mix with the gas in the airways, so the concentration of nitrogen slowly rises. A plateau phase is reached by phase 3 which is where the alveolar gas which contains nitrogen present in the alveoli prior to the oxygen breath is exhaled. It has a slight upwards slope. A second graph is then created which plots the nitrogen concentration against the volume of expired gas. This curve is sigmoid in shape. The anatomical dead-space is determined by drawing a vertical line through the curve so that the area on either side of the line is equal. The anatomical dead-space is the volume up to this line. See Figure 1.1.3c.

How can you measure physiological dead-space?

The Bohr equation is much loved by examiners. Do not just learn the formula, you will find it much easier to understand if you take the time to understand the principles behind the equation. Expect to be asked to derive the equation.

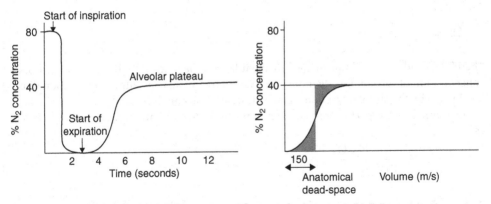

Figure 1.1.3c. Fowler's method for measuring anatomical dead-space.

To measure physiological dead-space Bohr's method is used. The principle behind this equation is that expired carbon dioxide comes only from alveolar gas and not from the dead-space. Therefore, expired carbon dioxide is equal to inspired carbon dioxide plus alveolar carbon dioxide. Since inspired carbon dioxide is negligible it may be ignored, thus expired carbon dioxide is equal to alveolar carbon dioxide. From this we can say that the expired fractional concentration of carbon dioxide (F_E) multiplied by tidal volume (T_V) is equal to the alveolar fractional concentration of carbon dioxide (F_A) times the alveolar ventilation (V_A). Let's call this equation A.

Equation A:

$$F_E \times V_T = F_A \times V_A.$$

We also know that tidal volume is equal to the sum of dead-space volume (V_D) and alveolar volume:

$$V_T = V_A + V_D.$$

By rearranging we can say that alveolar volume is equal to tidal volume minus dead-space volume, let's call this equation B.

Equation B:

$$V_A = V_T - V_D.$$

We can then substitute equation B into equation A, thus substituting ($V_T - V_D$) for V_A in equation A.

Therefore:

$$F_E \times V_T = F_A(V_T - V_D).$$

Next expand the equation:

$$F_E \times V_T = (F_A \times V_T) - (F_A \times V_D).$$

Then rearrange:

$$(F_A \times V_D) = (F_A \times V_T) - (F_E \times V_T).$$

And again:

$$(F_A \times V_D) = V_T(F_A - F_E).$$

And finally:

$$\frac{V_D}{V_T} = \frac{F_A - F_E}{F_A}.$$

Therefore, dead-space volume divided by the tidal volume is equal to the alveolar fractional concentration of carbon dioxide minus the expired fractional concentration of carbon dioxide divided by the alveolar fractional concentration of carbon dioxide.

However, because partial pressures are proportional to concentrations, it can be rewritten as;

$$\frac{V_D}{V_T} = \frac{P_A CO_2 - P_E CO_2}{P_A CO_2}.$$

1.1.4. Alveolar gas equation and shunt – Rebecca A Leslie

What does the body use oxygen for?

Cells need energy to enable them to work. The source of cellular energy is adenosine triphosphate (ATP) which can lose one phosphate group to produce usable energy and adenosine diphosphate (ADP). Thus cells rely on processes that produce ATP in order to keep working. ATP is produced from metabolic fuels such as carbohydrates, fatty acids and proteins that are oxidised to produce energy. Oxidation involves removing electrons at a high potential from the fuel molecule and transferring them to a lower potential, thus releasing energy. In mammalian cells oxygen is the electron acceptor used via intermediate molecules to produce energy.

Let's look at this process in further detail. Glucose is first converted in a series of 10 steps to pyruvate in the cytoplasm of the cell by a process called glycolysis. During this process two ATP molecules are used but four ATP molecules are produced, so there is a net production of two ATP molecules. Oxygen is not required for this process and carbon dioxide is not produced.

Pyruvate then passes into the inner matrix of the mitochondria where it enters the tricyclic acid cycle. Through a number of stages this cycle produces carbon dioxide, ATP, and reduced nicotinamide adenine dinucleotide (NADH) and flavin adenine dinucleotide ($FADH_2$). NADH and $FADH_2$ carry electrons to the electron transfer chain in the inner membrane of the mitochondria. In the electron transfer chain the electrons are transferred through a series of carriers from high to lower potentials until they combine with oxygen to produce water. In this process energy is released and ATP is produced from ADP and phosphate ions by a process called oxidative phosphorylation.

Can you tell me about the alveolar gas equation?

The alveolar oxygen tension is less than the inspired oxygen concentration because as soon as air enters the alveoli some oxygen is absorbed in exchange for carbon dioxide which is excreted. Therefore the alveolar oxygen tension is determined by the rate at which the oxygen is introduced to the alveoli, which in turn is dependent on alveolar ventilation and inspired oxygen concentration. The alveolar oxygen tension is also dependent on the rate of oxygen removal by pulmonary capillaries and the rate of carbon dioxide delivery to the alveoli. The decrease in oxygen tension caused by oxygen being absorbed is estimated by the tension of carbon dioxide excreted.

The alveolar gas equation states that alveolar partial pressure of oxygen (P_AO_2) is equal to the inspired partial pressure of oxygen (P_iO_2) minus the alveolar partial pressure of carbon dioxide (P_ACO_2) divided by the respiratory quotient (RQ).

$$P_AO_2 = P_iO_2 - P_ACO_2/RQ$$

The partial pressure of oxygen can be calculated by multiplying the fraction of inspired oxygen by the atmospheric pressure (P_{ATM}) minus the saturated vapour pressure (SVP):

$$P_iO_2 = F_iO_2(P_{ATM} - SVP)$$

Therefore the alveolar gas equation can be rewritten as:

$$P_AO_2 = F_iO_2(P_{ATM} - SVP) - P_ACO_2/RQ$$

The importance of the alveolar oxygen tension is that it determines the partial pressure gradient driving oxygen across the alveolar–capillary membrane. The alveolar oxygen tension can also be used to determine the alveolar–arterial oxygen difference which is a useful index of gas exchange efficiency in the lungs.

What is the respiratory quotient?

The respiratory quotient is the amount of carbon dioxide produced divided by the amount of oxygen consumed. It is dependent on the metabolic substrate that is used for metabolism, it is normally assumed to be 0.8.

$$RQ = \frac{CO_2 \text{ produced}}{O_2 \text{ consumed}}.$$

What will affect the alveolar oxygen tension?

The easiest way to think about this answer is to think about each of the components of the alveolar gas equation and then think about what factors could affect them.

The alveolar partial pressure of oxygen is affected by the inspired oxygen fraction. Increasing the inspired oxygen fraction will increase the alveolar partial pressure of oxygen.

Hypermetabolic states such as sepsis, malignancy and hyperthermia will significantly increase the oxygen consumption and carbon dioxide production. In these cases the respiratory quotient will be lower than normal. A lower respiratory quotient will cause a reduction in the alveolar partial pressure of oxygen. As a result these patients may require a higher inspired oxygen fraction and alveolar ventilation to maintain oxygenation.

Iatrogenic sodium bicarbonate infusions will increase arterial carbon dioxide levels, and hence carbon dioxide delivery to the lungs, which will again decrease your alveolar oxygen partial pressure.

What do you understand by the oxygen cascade?

Try and draw a diagram of the oxygen cascade as you are explaining it, see Figure 1.1.4a. Remember to label each of the axes, and remember to try and make the scale realistic.

The oxygen cascade describes the stepwise reduction in oxygen partial pressure starting at inspired air until the oxygen reaches the tissues. This allows a gradient to be produced and oxygen can move down this gradient.

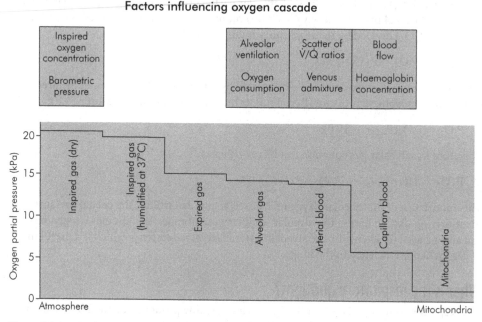

Figure 1.1.4a. Oxygen cascade. Reproduced with permission from Smith, T., Pinnock, C. and Lin, T. 2009. *Fundamentals of Anaesthesia.* Cambridge: Cambridge University Press. © Cambridge University Press 2009.

At sea level, the atmospheric pressure is 101.3 kPa and oxygen makes up roughly 21% of inspired air, so oxygen exerts a partial pressure of $101.3 \times 0.21 = 21.3$ kPa. This is the starting point of the oxygen cascade.

The first obstacle that oxygen encounters is water vapour, which under normal circumstances humidifies inspired air. The water vapour dilutes the amount of oxygen by reducing the partial pressure of oxygen by the saturated vapour pressure which is 6.3 kPa. This will affect the partial pressure of inspired oxygen, which is recalculated as $(101.3 - 6.3) \times 0.21 = 19.9$ kPa.

By the time the oxygen has reached the alveoli the partial pressure has reduced significantly, this is because the alveolar gas is determined by the balance of oxygen removal by the pulmonary capillaries, carbon dioxide excretion, and by alveolar ventilation. Hence by using the alveolar gas equation the alveolar partial pressure of oxygen is found to be 13.3 kPa.

The next step is the movement of oxygen from the alveolus to the arterial blood, and as you would expect there is a small downward gradient, usually 0.5–1 kPa. This is explained by small ventilation–perfusion abnormalities and venous admixture.

As arterial blood moves through the body to the tissues the partial pressure of oxygen reduces dramatically as oxygen moves down its gradient into the mitochondria. The oxygen concentration in the mitochondria is at its lowest, normally approximately 1.5 kPa.

What is the Pasteur point?

The Pasteur point is the oxygen concentration below which oxidative phosphorylation cannot occur.

If a healthy person breathes 100% oxygen for 10 minutes and an arterial blood gas is taken what would the PaO_2 be?

Use the principles that we have just discussed to help you answer this question.

By assuming the person is fit and healthy you can make certain assumptions which would allow you to use the alveolar gas equation in order to estimate the arterial partial pressure of oxygen.

It is known that when blood passes through the pulmonary capillaries it equilibrates with the alveolar oxygen and carbon dioxide partial pressures provided that there is no significant shunt or VQ mismatch. Therefore first we must assume that there is no shunt or VQ mismatch and that arterial partial pressure of carbon dioxide is the same as the alveolar partial pressure of carbon dioxide, which is 5.3 kPa. We must also assume that the patient has a normal diet and that their respiratory quotient is 0.8 (remember a purely carbohydrate diet produces a respiratory quotient of 1.0).

Therefore, using the alveolar gas equation:

$$P_AO_2 = F_iO_2(P_{ATM} - SVP) - P_ACO_2/RQ$$
$$P_AO_2 = 1 \times (101.3 - 6.3) - 5.3/0.8$$
$$P_AO_2 = 88.4 \text{ kPa.}$$

Therefore a patient breathing 100% oxygen for 10 minutes will have an alveolar partial pressure of oxygen of 88.4 kPa. The normal alveolar–arterial oxygen tension gradient is 0.5–1 kPa due to shunt and venous admixture. As a result we would expect the arterial partial pressure of oxygen to approximately 87–88 kPa.

What do you mean by shunt?

Shunt refers to the blood that enters the arterial system without taking part in gas exchange.

What causes physiological shunting?

In the normal lung, the blood supply to the bronchial tree is via the bronchial artery which comes off the aorta. The partly deoxygenated blood is then returned to the left side of the heart in the pulmonary veins, reducing the partial pressure of oxygen in the arterial system.

The coronary venous blood also adds to physiological shunt, as it drains directly into the left ventricle via the Thebesian veins. The effect of the addition of this poorly oxygenated blood is to depress the arterial oxygen partial pressure. The normal shunt fraction is between 2 and 5%.

What are the pathological causes of shunt?

Remember to first classify your answer, then move on a describe each in more detail.

The pathological causes of shunt can be divided into cardiovascular causes and respiratory causes.

Some patients have an abnormal connection between their pulmonary artery and vein, called a pulmonary arterio-venous fistula, which causes shunting of blood. In other patients there may be a direct communication between the right and left side of the heart, for example through a patent foramen ovale, which shunts deoxygenated blood from the right to the left side of the heart.

Respiratory causes of a shunt include anything that prevents oxygen passing through the airways to the alveoli. Examples include pneumonia, acute respiratory distress syndrome, bronchial obstruction and one-lung ventilation.

If a patient has a pathological shunt, what would happen if you increase the inspired oxygen concentration?

The significance of a shunt is that the hypoxia cannot be overcome by giving the patient 100% oxygen to breathe. This is because the blood which is shunted and therefore bypasses the alveoli is never exposed to the higher alveolar partial pressures of oxygen. However, there is a small rise in arterial oxygen tension because more oxygen becomes dissolved in the blood at higher partial pressures.

Why is there not normally an increase in carbon dioxide when a patient has a respiratory shunt?

A shunt does not normally cause an increase in carbon dioxide partial pressure because the higher concentration of carbon dioxide is sensed by the central chemoreceptors which respond by increasing the ventilation. The ventilation is increased until the arterial carbon dioxide level returns back to normal.

At this point to show good understanding of the principles involved you should mention the carbon dioxide dissociation curve.

The relationship between the partial pressure of carbon dioxide and the total carbon dioxide concentration can be shown in the carbon dioxide dissociation curve. The partial pressure of carbon dioxide is displayed on the x axis whilst the total carbon dioxide content is plotted on the y axis. The curve produced, unlike the sigmoid curve of the oxygen dissociation curve, is a more linear curve. So a reduction in the partial pressure of carbon dioxide, due to increased ventilation, causes a decrease in the total carbon dioxide content.

Derive the shunt equation

It is important you really understand the principles of the shunt equation rather than just reproducing the equation. First draw a simplified diagram to show you have a good understanding of the concepts behind the shunt equation, see Figure 1.1.4b. If you show this broad understanding it is unlikely the examiners will then expect you to go through all the steps to derive the formula.

With each heart beat, the cardiac output, denoted as Q_T, is pumped into the pulmonary circulation. After passing through the pulmonary circulation, this blood is pumped via the heart into the systemic circulation. From the diagram you can see that the cardiac output is made up from blood which is shunted away from the pulmonary alveoli (Q_S) and blood that passes directly through the pulmonary circulation ($Q_T - Q_S$).

The oxygen content of the shunted blood is the same as the oxygen content of the venous blood (CvO_2) because it has no way of becoming oxygenated as it passes through the lungs. In contrast the blood which is not shunted but adjacent to ventilated alveoli becomes oxygenated to a concentration known as the capillary oxygen content (CcO_2). The shunted blood and the non-shunted blood are then combined together in the arterial system, producing the arterial oxygen content (CaO_2). The bigger the respiratory shunt the lower the arterial oxygen content.

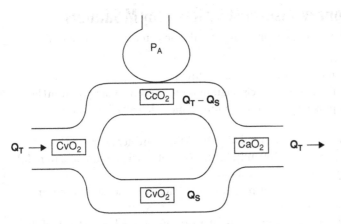

Figure 1.1.4b. A diagram to explain the shunt equation.

From our discussion so far, we can now say that the total oxygen content of the blood leaving the system is equal to the partial pressure of arterial oxygen multiplied by the cardiac output ($Q_T \times CaO_2$).

We also know that this is equal to the sum of the amount of shunted blood multiplied by the venous oxygen content ($Q_S \times CvO_2$) plus the capillary oxygen content multiplied by the remainder of the blood ($[Q_T - Q_S] \times CcO_2$).

So in summary:

$$Q_T \times CaO_2 = (Q_S \times CvO_2) + ([Q_T - Q_S] \times CcO_2).$$

This formula can then be simplified through a number of steps to produce the final equation.

First expand:

$$Q_T \times CaO_2 = (Q_S \times CvO_2) + (Q_T \times CcO_2) - (Q_S \times CcO_2).$$

Move the Q_S to the left side, as you are aiming for Q_S/Q_T in the final equation:

$$(Q_S \times CcO_2) - (Q_S \times CvO_2) = (Q_T \times CcO_2) - (Q_T \times CaO_2).$$

Then simplify:

$$Q_S(CcO_2 - CvO_2) = Q_T(CcO_2 - CaO_2).$$

Then divide both sides by Q_T and by ($CcO_2 - CvO_2$):

$$\frac{Q_S}{Q_T} = \frac{(CcO_2 - CaO_2)}{(CcO_2 - CvO_2)}.$$

The shunt equation is used to calculate the proportion of the cardiac output which is being shunted. The normal shunt fraction is 2–5%.

The capillary oxygen concentration (CcO_2) is generally assumed to be the same as the alveolar oxygen concentration, which can be calculated by the alveolar gas equation. The arterial oxygen concentration (CaO_2) can be measured from a sample taken from an arterial cannula and the mixed venous oxygen concentration (CvO_2) can be determined from a sample taken from a central line.

1.1.5. Hypoxic pulmonary vasoconstriction – Joy M Sanders

How does the vascular resistance in the pulmonary circulation compare with that in the systemic circulation?

- The pulmonary circulation is a very low resistance circuit.
- The pressure drop across the pulmonary circulation is only approximately 10 mmHg (mean pulmonary artery pressure of 15 mmHg minus mean left atrial pressure of 5 mmHg).
- The pressure drop across the systemic circulation is 10 times greater at around 100 mmHg (mean aortic pressure of 100 mmHg minus right atrial pressure of 2 mmHg).
- The flow is the same as in the systemic circulation.
- Applying Ohm's law: $V = IR$, where V is pressure difference across a vascular system, I is total flow and R is vascular resistance.
- It can therefore be seen that the pulmonary vascular resistance is only one-tenth of the systemic vascular resistance.

What are the major factors that affect pulmonary vascular resistance (PVR)?

The three major factors are hypoxic pulmonary vasoconstriction, lung volume and pulmonary artery pressure.

What do you mean by hypoxic pulmonary vasoconstriction (HPV)?

- HPV is a protective physiological mechanism that diverts blood flow away from hypoxic/collapsed areas of the lung, shunting it to better ventilated zones.
- Low alveolar oxygen tension (of less than around 11–13 kPa) is detected and results in reflex vasoconstriction of the smaller pulmonary arterioles in adjacent alveoli.
- This local mechanism acts rapidly to help match ventilation and perfusion which is advantageous in maintaining oxygen uptake. It starts within seconds of the reduction in PO_2 of alveolar gas, and within minutes lobar blood flow may be halved.
- It is a biphasic response, suggesting that HPV involves multifactorial mechanisms. There is an initial transient increase in PVR followed by a second, more sustained phase of vasoconstriction.
- This is an unusual response, as elsewhere in the systemic circulation localised hypoxia results in vasodilatation of vascular beds.

What is the significance of HPV?

There are some specific situations, both pathological and physiological, where HPV is of clinical importance.

- Early left ventricular failure: HPV is responsible for the upper lobe diversion seen in the lungs, where blood in the hypoxic and congested lower zones is diverted to the upper zones.
- Chronic lung disease: HPV may cause pulmonary hypertension with ensuing cor pulmonale and right ventricular failure.
- Cardiac shunts: Hypoxaemia may cause a global rise in PVR, which increases the work of the right ventricle and encourages shunting from right to left.

- Foetal pulmonary circulation: Low P_AO_2 levels are responsible for generalised HPV in the pulmonary vessels, increasing PVR and reducing blood flow through the pulmonary vascular bed. When oxygen enters the lungs at the first breath, the PVR falls dramatically (due to vascular smooth muscle relaxation) and the pulmonary blood flow increases.
- Altitude: At high altitude, generalised HPV causes a significant increase in PVR.

What is the mechanism for HPV?

The exact mechanism for HPV is unknown, but it does occur in excised isolated lung so is not thought to be neurally mediated.

It is likely to involve nitric oxide (NO), a potent vasodilator synthesised by the pulmonary artery endothelium when the alveolar PO_2 is normal. If the alveolar PO_2 falls below 9.3 kPa, less NO is synthesised, resulting in pulmonary vasoconstriction.

It may also involve inhibition of oxygen-sensitive potassium channels in pulmonary blood vessels, leading to membrane depolarisation, increased cytoplasmic calcium ion concentrations and smooth muscle contraction. This effect is not seen systemically.

What factors modify HPV?

- HPV is potentiated or increased by acidosis, hypercarbia and drugs such as cyclo-oxygenase inhibitors, propranolol and the respiratory stimulant almitrine.
- It is attenuated or reduced by alkalosis, hypocapnia, vasodilators (e.g., nitrates, nitroprusside, NO, calcium channel blockers and dobutamine), bronchodilators and volatile anaesthetic agents.

What is the importance of HPV to an anaesthetist?

Maintaining higher alveolar partial pressure of oxygen by using a high F_iO_2 may prevent HPV, even in those alveoli that are under-ventilated. HPV is also inhibited by all volatile agents, with a dose-dependent effect. Nitrous oxide, however, has a less potent action, and intra-venous induction agents have minimal effect. HPV may be potentiated by factors which reduce cardiac output as this will cause a reduction in mixed venous PO_2.

HPV is of importance in one-lung anaesthesia, where it should improve oxygenation. During thoracic surgery when the surgical side is uppermost, HPV is responsible for 50% of the reduction in flow to this non-ventilated non-dependent lung and may further reduce the shunt by 20%. The compressed dependent lung may lose lung volume, and HPV may help to redirect some blood to the non-dependent lung.

What is the relationship between PVR and lung volume?

See Figure 1.1.5.

- The PVR is high at both high and low lung volumes, which is due to different mechanisms. The lowest PVR is at functional residual capacity (FRC).
- At low lung volumes, the extra-alveolar vessels are compressed and narrow, with high resistance. With lung expansion, the walls of these vessels are pulled by the elastic fibres in the lung, their diameter increases and resistance decreases.
- At high volumes, increased stretching distorts and decreases the diameter of the pulmonary capillaries, causing an increase in resistance.

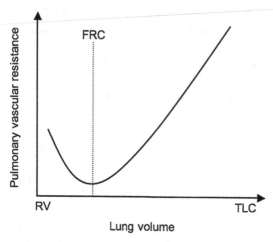

Figure 1.1.5. Lung volume versus PVR. Reproduced with permission from Cross, M. and Plunkett, E. 2008. *Physics, Pharmacology and Physiology for Anaesthetists: Key Concepts for the FRCA.* Cambridge: Cambridge University Press. © M. Cross and E. Plunkett 2008.

How does pulmonary artery pressure affect PVR?

- An increase in pulmonary artery pressure causes a significant reduction in PVR. This is due to recruitment and distension of pulmonary capillaries. Recruitment describes the opening of previously closed pulmonary capillaries. This is the most important mechanism if pulmonary pressure is low initially.
- As pulmonary pressure increases further, the open capillaries now distend even more, which causes further lowering of PVR.

How do you calculate PVR?

$$PVR = \frac{(MPAP - PCWP)}{CO} \times 80 \text{ dynes/sec/cm}^{-5}$$

Where MPAP is mean pulmonary artery pressure (in mmHg), PCWP is mean pulmonary capillary wedge pressure (in mmHg) and CO is cardiac output (in L/min). A conversion factor of 80 is used to convert from base units (mmHg and L/min) to the commonly used units of the result (dynes/sec/cm^5).

All three of these variables can be determined using a Swan–Ganz catheter. The normal value is 50–150 dynes/sec/cm^5 which is approximately one-tenth of the systemic vascular resistance (1000–1500 dynes/sec/cm^5).

1.1.6. Oxyhaemoglobin dissociation curve – Caroline SG Janes

Understanding oxygen delivery and consumption is an integral part of anaesthesia. This is therefore a pass/fail question – examiners will expect you to know this topic very well so make sure you do.

How is oxygen transported in the body?

A total of 99% of oxygen is transported by binding to haemoglobin and 1% is dissolved in solution. The oxygen content of blood is approximately 200 ml/L for arterial blood at 97% saturation.

What is oxygen flux?

The partial pressure of oxygen reduces gradually during the transfer through the lungs, into the vascular system and finally to the tissues – this is termed the oxygen flux. The oxygen cascade is used to describe this journey from atmospheric pressure to the mitochondria.

For more information see Figure 1.1.4a.

What equation is used to calculate the oxygen content of blood?

This is a crucial equation which you must know – practice writing it is as you talk about it.

$$CaO_2 = (PaO_2 \times 0.03) + (Hb \times Sats \times 1.34).$$

This equation states that the oxygen content of blood is the sum of the partial pressure of oxygen in the blood multiplied by 0.03 (if PaO_2 is measured in kilopascals) added to the haemoglobin concentration multiplied by the percentage saturation multiplied by 1.34, which is Huffner's constant.

What is a haemoglobin molecule composed of?

Haemoglobin is composed of a globin molecule with a haem moiety. The globin molecule is made up of four polypeptide subunits in pairs. The haem moiety contains iron in the ferrous state and a protoporphyrin ring. One haem moiety containing one iron atom is conjugated to each polypeptide and each haem moiety can bind one molecule of oxygen – thus a molecule of haemoglobin can bind four molecules of oxygen.

What different types of Hb molecules do you know of?

The structure of the globin chains can vary. In HbA, or adult haemoglobin, the globin portion contains two α and two β chains. Foetal haemoglobin, HbF, contains two α and two γ chains. HbA2 is present in 2–3% of the population and contains two α and two δ. In health HbF is replaced by HbA within 6 months of birth.

What disorders of Hb synthesis can occur?

There can be reduced production of normal globin chains such as thalassaemia or production of abnormal globin chains such as sickle cell anaemia.

Tell me more about thalassaemia

Thalassaemia results from reduced synthesis of α or β chains. In thalassaemia major the patient is a homozygote and there is no production of HbA. This results in severe anaemia and is usually fatal before adulthood. In thalassaemia minor there is usually only mild anaemia as the patient is heterozygous and can produce some HbA. Thalassaemia most commonly originates from Mediterranean, Indian or Southeast Asian populations.

What do you know about sickle cell anaemia?

Sickle cell anaemia occurs when abnormal β chains are produced. The abnormal β chain contains valine instead of glutamic acid. This substitution causes the deoxygenated Hb chains to polymerise and precipitate within the red blood cell (RBC) which results in the structure of the RBC being distorted and more rigid. These distorted RBCs impede blood flow and increase blood viscosity, this can result in capillary and venous thrombosis and organ infarction. It can also cause gallstones due to increased bilirubin concentration and bony deformity due to increased erythropoiesis. Sickle cell crises occur following vascular occlusion and can be extremely painful.

Homozygotes possess only HbS and are said to have sickle cell disease. Heterozygotes have both normal and abnormal haemoglobin and are said to have sickle cell trait. Sickle cell trait is mostly asymptomatic. Sickle cell disease is most common in west central Africa and parts of India and Saudi Arabia. The incidence of sickle cell disease in the black UK population is 1% and the incidence of sickle cell trait is 10%.

What are the anaesthetic implications of sickle cell disease?

Pre-operatively all the races mentioned above should be screened for sickle cell with the Sickledex test and electrophoresis. Patients with severe disease with end-organ failure should be investigated appropriately and optimised in cases of renal and respiratory impairment. Exchange transfusion is sometimes performed before major surgery to reduce the amount of HbS. During anaesthesia hypoxaemia, hypothermia, dehydration and acidosis should be prevented at all times. Frequent arterial blood gases should be performed. Tourniquets should be avoided in HbS. Post-operatively patients should ideally be nursed in a high dependency area and oxygen should be administered for 24 hours. It is imperative that sickle cell patients should be kept well hydrated and warm throughout, this may involve using body warmers and administering intra-venous fluids pre-operatively. Day case surgery is usually not appropriate. Post-operative analgesia can sometimes be difficult to manage as frequent sicklers can be very tolerant to opiates. The acute pain team should therefore be involved early and regional anaesthesia used where appropriate.

What is the oxyhaemoglobin dissociation curve (OHDC)?

You should be able to draw the OHDC effortlessly so make sure you practice (Figure 1.1.6). Label the axes accurately and always begin the curve by plotting the key points – if the examiners see you know it well they will be less likely to ask you sticky questions about Huffner's constant! The units for PO2 should preferably be in kPa but you would not fail for using mmHg.

The OHDC is a plot of the oxygen saturation of haemoglobin against the partial pressure of oxygen for normal Hb at 37°C at a normal partial pressure of carbon dioxide.

What is the shape of the OHDC, and what is its significance?

The OHDC is sigmoid in shape. This reflects the increased affinity of haemoglobin for oxygen as each successive oxygen molecule binds to it, this is termed cooperative binding. In arterial blood oxygen saturations are usually above 97%. This corresponds to a PO_2 of 13.3 kPa and is on the flat part of the curve. In venous blood the saturations are approximately 75% – this corresponds to the start of the steep part of the curve and a PO_2 of approximately 5.3 kPa.

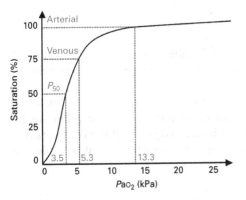

Draw and label the axes as shown; O_2 content can also be used on the y axis with a range of 0–21 ml.100 ml^{-1}. Your graph should accurately demonstrate three key points. The arterial point is plotted at 100% saturation and 13.3 kPa. The venous point is plotted at 75% saturation and 5.3 kPa. The P_{50} is plotted at 50% saturation (definition) and 3.5 kPa. Only when these three point are plotted should you draw in a smooth sigmoid curve that passes through all three. The curve is sigmoid because of the cooperative binding exhibited by Hb. In the deoxygenated state (deoxy-Hb), the Hb molecule is described as 'tense' and it is difficult for the first molecule of O_2 to bind. As O_2 binds to Hb the molecule relaxes (a conformational change occurs) and it become progressively easier for further molecules to bind. If asked to compare your curve with that of a different O_2 carrier such as myoglobin, draw a hyperbolic curve to the left of the original line. Myoglobin can only carry one O_2 molecule and so the curve does not have a sigmoid shape.

Figure 1.1.6. Oxyhaemoglobin dissociation curve. Reproduced with permission from Cross, M. and Plunkett, E. 2008. *Physics, Pharmacology and Physiology for Anaesthetists: Key Concepts for the FRCA.* Cambridge: Cambridge University Press. © M. Cross and E. Plunkett 2008.

Clinically the sigmoid shape is important because a small drop in PO_2 at normal oxygen levels causes only a slight fall in arterial saturation of oxygen because the curve is flat at this point. However, where oxygen levels are already low, and on the steep part of the curve, the same small fall in PO_2 will cause a sharp fall in SaO_2.

What is the *P50*?

The *P50* is the point on the OHDC where the Hb is 50% saturated and corresponds to a PO_2 of 3.5 kPa. The *P50* is the point which best describes the position of the curve.

The examiners will expect you to continue to talk about the P50 and what shifts the OHDC to the right and left. You should practice talking and drawing at the same time to make best use of time. If you know this topic you should be able to answer everything quickly allowing the examiners to move on to other things and collect as many points as possible.

The curve will shift to the right in:

- Acidosis
- Hypoxia
- High levels of 2,3-diphosphoglycerate (2,3-DPG)

- Hyperthermia
- Hypercapnia.

This causes lower saturation levels for the same PO_2 resulting in oxygen being off-loaded more easily to surrounding tissues. Physiologically this ensures greater tissue oxygenation in states of reduced tissue perfusion.

The curve will shift to the left in the opposite situations, i.e., alkalosis and hypothermia. In addition to the curve for HbF, carboxyhaemoglobin and methaemoglobin will move the curve to the left because they all have a higher affinity for oxygen. In HbF this ensures that oxygen is readily transferred from the maternal blood to the foetal blood. It also enables the foetus to tolerate greater levels of acidosis.

What is the Bohr effect?

The Bohr effect is the resultant shift in the OHDC to the right following a rise in PCO_2 and/or a fall in the pH.

What is 2,3-diphosphoglycerate?

2,3-DPG is a molecule formed by red blood cells during glycolysis which binds strongly to the β chains of deoxygenated Hb. It reduces oxygen binding and shifts the OHDC to the right. Levels are increased by anaemia, alkalosis, chronic hypoxaemia, high altitude, exercise, pregnancy and hyperthyroidism. Levels are reduced in stored blood due to the acidosis, and following transfusion of packed red cells it takes up to 24 hours to restore 2,3-DPG levels.

What is carboxyhaemoglobin?

Carbon monoxide (CO) bound to haemoglobin is called carboxyhaemoglobin. Carbon monoxide has an affinity for haemoglobin 250 times that of oxygen for haemoglobin.

Tell me more about carbon monoxide poisoning

Carbon monoxide poisoning results from inhaling fumes from car exhausts, and coal and gas fires. It is an odourless and colourless gas. It is not directly toxic but when present in large amounts it causes tissue ischaemia by reducing oxygen carriage and offloading in the blood. To make matters worse the aortic and carotid bodies do not respond to the hypoxia because the pO_2 remains normal.

CO values in the blood are normally less than 2% in non-smokers and 5–6% in smokers. At 10–30% mild symptoms start to occur and above 60% symptoms are very severe. Mild symptoms include headache, weakness, dizziness and gastrointestinal (GI) tract disturbance. In severe cases convulsions, coma and death can result. Patients with CO poisoning are sometimes said to have a cherry red appearance. Pulse oximetry in CO poisoning is misleading as it will still give a high reading despite profound hypoxia as carboxyhaemoglobin is interpreted as oxygenated haemoglobin.

CO poisoning is treated with oxygen therapy. Its half-life in air is 4 hours and with 100% oxygen it is reduced to 1 hour. Hyperbaric oxygen can be used to reduce the half-life to less than 30 minutes and is recommended in patients with convulsions, arrhythmias, in pregnancy and where levels are above 40%. Neurological problems can persist in severe cases.

What is methaemoglobinaemia?

Methaemoglobinaemia is the presence of circulating Hb in which the iron atom is in the ferric state, i.e., Fe^{3+}. Normally levels are less than 1%. These levels can rise due to congenital defects or following administration of certain drugs. Congenital methaemoglobinaemia is caused by a deficiency in the enzymes that normally convert methaemoglobin back into haemoglobin. Drugs which cause methaemoglobinaemia include prilocaine, quinolones, nitrites and sulphonamides.

Methaemoglobin is dark and gives patients a cyanosed look. It causes pulse oximetry to be inaccurate, and readings trend towards 85%. It is less able to bind oxygen but is then also less likely to offload hence shifting the OHDC to the left. At levels over 20% symptoms start to occur, these include headache and shortness of breath. Methaemoglobinaemia is treated with reducing agents such as methylene blue or ascorbic acid.

1.1.7. Altitude physiology – Caroline SG Janes

The composition and temperature of the atmosphere at high altitude is substantially different to that at sea level. This produces a cascade of altered physiological and psychological responses. Understanding these responses will suggest to an examiner that you have a thorough appreciation of cardiovascular and respiratory physiology.

What effects does altitude have on the air that we breathe?

Barometric pressure decreases almost exponentially as the distance from the earth's surface increases. This does not affect the composition of the air so the F_iO_2 will still be 0.21 but the partial pressure of oxygen will fall accordingly. High altitude is sometimes referred to as being 1500 m above sea level.

What compensatory changes occur to maintain tissue oxygenation at high altitude?

As with all structured oral examination answers try to classify your answers.

Compensatory changes can be divided into acute which happen immediately and chronic which develop over a period of weeks to months. Initially the shape of the OHDC maintains oxygen saturations above 90% up to 10 000 feet, but acute desaturation starts to occur thereafter triggering compensatory mechanisms.

The aortic and carotid bodies detect the fall in partial pressure of oxygen and stimulate both the respiratory and cardiovascular systems. Hyperventilation is the most important response initially. For the first couple of days the increased ventilation and subsequent fall in carbon dioxide cause an alkalaemia and transiently shifts the OHDC to the left. This is gradually corrected by increased loss of renal bicarbonate. Once the pH is normalised ventilation is able to increase further.

Sinus tachycardia also occurs along with a small reduction in stroke volume. There is increased fluid loss and circulating volume falls slightly. The 2,3-DPG production increases causing the OHDC to then shift to the right thus improving offloading of oxygen to surrounding tissues.

In the long-term high altitude causes polycythaemia and a higher haematocrit due to chronic hypoxia stimulating erythropoietin production. Red blood cell mass also increases, and 2,3-DPG levels remain high. Hypoxic pulmonary vasoconstriction occurs which can cause right ventricular hypertrophy. Myoglobin concentration increases and peripheral capillary proliferation occurs. At the mitochondrial level there is an increase in aerobic enzyme concentration and an increase in the size of the mitochondria.

What are the signs and symptoms of acute mountain sickness (AMS)?

AMS is a spectrum of signs and symptoms resulting from a maladaptive response to altitude. It usually occurs above 2500 m. It is caused by reduced partial pressure of oxygen, and it is characterised by nausea, headache, fatigue, loss of appetite, dizziness, and sleep disturbance. In extreme cases AMS can result in either high altitude pulmonary oedema known as HAPE or high altitude cerebral oedema known as HACE. Both these conditions can progress rapidly and are often fatal without treatment and descent to lower altitude, preferably sea level.

HAPE is characterised by a persistent dry cough, fever and severe dyspnoea at rest. As the disease process progresses the cough becomes productive of pink, frothy sputum. The mechanism for HAPE is uncertain; one hypothesis is that hypoxic pulmonary vasoconstriction causes increased pulmonary arterial and capillary pressures. Another hypothesis suggests an idiopathic non-inflammatory increase in the permeability of the vascular endothelium. Higher pulmonary arterial pressures are associated with the development of HAPE but it is not sufficient to explain the formation of pulmonary oedema and severe pulmonary hypertension can exist in the absence of clinical HAPE in subjects at high altitude.

HACE generally occurs after a week or more at high altitude. Its aetiology is also uncertain but it is thought to be caused by local vasodilatation of cerebral blood vessels in response to hypoxia, resulting in greater blood flow and, consequently, greater capillary pressures. Symptoms include headache, dizziness, and disturbance in vision, mood, memory, coordination, reasoning, neuromuscular control and concentration. In severe cases it results in convulsions, decreased consciousness, coma and death.

It is unknown what makes people susceptible to AMS, HAPE or HACE and is not thought to be related to athletic ability.

What is chronic mountain sickness?

This is also known as Monge's disease and occurs after prolonged exposure to high altitude despite acclimatisation. It is characterised by excessive polycythaemia, hypoxaemia, fatigue, and in severe cases pulmonary hypertension and congestive heart failure.

What is the treatment of AMS?

The only definitive treatment of AMS is immediate evacuation to lower altitude or sea level. Other treatments and therapies are only useful to buy time until this is possible. Supplementary oxygen can counteract the effects of hypoxia, and the most effective equipment to supply oxygen at high altitude is an oxygen concentrator that uses vacuum swing adsorption technology. For serious cases of AMS, a Gamow bag can be used to reduce the effective altitude by as much as 1500 meters (5000 feet). It is a portable plastic pressure bag inflated with a foot pump.

Drug treatments that may be useful include nifedipine, acetazolamide, sumatriptan, dexamethasone, salmeterol and sildenafil. In Peru and Bolivia the indigenous populations have used coca leaves for centuries to treat mild altitude sickness.

What other problems can occur at altitude?

There is a high risk of hypothermia at high altitude. The lower pressure causes the air to expand as it rises, this results in cooling and thus a drop in ambient temperature.

Another consideration at high altitude is the expansion of gas-containing cavities; this would be a particular problem if ascending with a pneumothorax or in individuals with inner ear problems.

Is there any effect on anaesthetic equipment at high altitude?

Vaporisers and flowmeters are affected by high altitude. Saturated vapour pressure and partial pressure of the volatile agent remains the same, however, an increase in attitude and hence a decrease in atmospheric pressure causes a higher concentration of agent to be delivered. This does not matter clinically though because the anaesthetic effect of the volatile agent is determined by the alveolar partial pressure of the agent not its concentration. Therefore the same settings can be used at high altitude as at sea level providing the temperature is not considerably lower. However this is not the case with the desflurane vaporiser which is electrically heated to 39°C. This causes there to be a vapour pressure of 2 atmospheres within the vaporiser regardless of ambient pressure. Therefore, in order to deliver a sufficient partial pressure of desflurane within the alveoli at altitude the concentration of desflurane has to be increased.

Flowmeters are affected by altitude because gases have a lower density. They therefore under-read at high altitude. However since it is the number of molecules that matter clinically and not the volume of gas they can be used as normal.

What effect does altitude have on athletic performance?

It is thought that acclimatisation from living and training at high altitudes enhances performance compared to living and training at sea level. However, this may not always be the case. Any positive acclimatisation effects may be negated by a de-training effect as athletes are usually not able to exercise with as much intensity at high altitudes compared to sea level. Therefore it is thought that the best compromise is to "Live-High and Train-Low", although this is a much debated issue and there is a lot of ongoing research in this area.

Cardiovascular physiology

1.2.1. Cardiac cycle – Rebecca A Leslie

This is always a difficult topic and one which many candidates fear; however, it is incredibly important you know it so take the time to learn it well. In particular spend time practising drawing the cardiac cycle so you can do it quickly and slickly in the exam.

Describe the cardiac cycle

Remember be logical. Start at the beginning and move through the cycle in a well-structured, logical manner. It is imperative that you draw a diagram as you talk through the cycle, see Figure 1.2.1a. Remember to make your diagram big enough to be clear and easily interpreted, always label the axes, and include an appropriate scale.

The cardiac cycle describes the events that occur during one heartbeat. There are two phases: diastole and systole.

Diastole can be further divided into four stages:

- Isovolumetric relaxation
- Rapid ventricular filling
- Slow ventricular filling
- Atrial contraction.

Systole has two stages:

- Isovolumetric contraction
- Ejection.

The start of the cycle is generally accepted to be towards the end of diastole, when the atrial and ventricular pressures are both low, and the whole heart is relaxed. The atrial pressures are slightly higher than ventricular pressure so the atrio-ventricular valves are open and blood flows slowly from the atria to the ventricle. This is called the slow ventricular filling phase. During diastole the pressure in the aorta and pulmonary vessels slowly decreases as blood moves into the vascular system.

In late diastole the sino-atrial node discharges and initiates atrial contraction, this is shown as the P wave on the ECG. During atrial systole the atria contracts and forces the

Dr Podcast Scripts for the Primary FRCA, ed. Rebecca A. Leslie, Emily K. Johnson and Alexander P. L. Goodwin.   Published by Cambridge University Press. © R. A. Leslie, E. K. Johnson and A. P. L. Goodwin 2011.

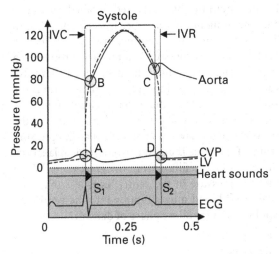

Figure 1.2.1a. Cardiac cycle. Reproduced with permission from Cross, M. and Plunkett, E. 2008. *Physics, Pharmacology and Physiology for Anaesthetists: Key Concepts for the FRCA.* Cambridge: Cambridge University Press. © M. Cross and E. Plunkett 2008.

remainder of the blood from the atria into the ventricle, producing a small rise in ventricular pressure. At rest, atrial contraction only contributes to one-fifth of ventricular filling because 80% has already passed into the ventricle due to venous pressure. There are no valves in the superior or inferior vena cava so when the atrium contracts there is a small pressure wave in the great veins, this is called the a wave on the CVP trace. End-diastolic ventricular volume is 130 ml when standing and 160 ml when lying. The end-diastolic pressure is less than 10 mmHg and is higher in the left than the right ventricle.

At the beginning of systole the ventricles contract and ventricular pressure rises dramatically, causing the atrio-ventricular valves to close producing the first heart sound. The onset of ventricular systole is at the same time as the R wave of the ECG. Whilst the pressure within the ventricle is still developing there is a period when the atrio-ventricular and the aortic and pulmonary valves are closed, as the pressure in the aorta and pulmonary arteries is still greater than that of the ventricles. This is called the isovolumetric contraction, as the volume of blood in the ventricle does not change. During this phase blood is forced against the atrio-ventricular valve and it bulges back into the atria. This produces the c wave in the atrial pressure wave form.

Eventually the pressure in the ventricles exceeds the pressure in the aorta and the pulmonary artery, so the aortic and pulmonary valves open, and blood is ejected. In a healthy patient the aortic pressure rises from a diastolic low of 80 mmHg to 120 mmHg during left ventricular systole. Pulmonary artery pressures rise from 8 mmHg during diastole to 25 mmHg at systole during right ventricular ejection. The flow from the ventricles is initially very rapid, but as the contraction wanes ejection is reduced.

In late systole the ventricles repolarise and begin to relax, this forms the T wave on the ECG. The pressure in the ventricle is soon less than that in the aorta and pulmonary arteries, but the blood continues to flow out of the ventricle because of the momentum created during the rapid ejection phase. Eventually the flow briefly reverses forcing the aortic and pulmonary valves to close and producing the second heartbeat. At this point there is a slight increase in aortic pressure, called the dicrotic notch. The amount of blood ejected is called the stroke volume, this is normally 70 ml, with 60 ml remaining in the ventricle. The ejection fraction is the stroke volume divided by the end-diastolic ventricular volume, in this case 70/130. During the rapid ejection phase of ventricular systole the pressures in the atria drop to zero or negative values. This is because the ventricular contraction pulls the atrio-ventricular valve downwards, and consequently lengthens and increases the volume of the atria. After this the pressures in the atria gradually rise as blood is returned from the systemic circulation.

Closure of the aortic and pulmonary valves marks the end of ventricular systole, and the ventricle rapidly relaxes. Initially the atrio-ventricular valves remain closed as the pressure in the ventricles is still higher than the atrium. This phase is called isovolumetric relaxation. Meanwhile the atrial pressure gradually increases due to filling from the great veins. When the ventricles have relaxed sufficiently that the pressure in the ventricles is less than that of the atria the atrio-ventricular valves open, and blood moves rapidly into the ventricles, down the pressure gradient. This is the rapid ventricular filling phase of diastole.

Describe the left ventricular pressure curve

This is a similar question, but we have included it as it is often asked and candidates can get confused between pressure–time curves and pressure–volume loops. Remember always listen carefully to the question you have been asked.

During diastole the pressure in the ventricle is low. When the atrial contraction occurs there is small rise in ventricular pressure as blood is forced from the atria into the ventricle. At the onset of systole when the ventricles start to contract the pressure in the ventricles rises rapidly, although the pressure is still less than the aortic pressure, so the aortic valve remains closed. This phase of the cycle is called the isovolumetric ventricular contraction. Before long, the pressure in the ventricle exceeds that of the aorta so the aortic valve opens, and blood is ejected into the aorta. Ventricular ejection consists of a rapid ejection phase followed by a prolonged reduced ejection phase. In late systole the ventricle repolarises and begins to relax so the pressure drops. When the pressure drops below the aortic pressure, initially blood continues to flow from the ventricle due to the momentum of the rapid ventricular ejection phase. Before long the blood briefly changes direction and forces the aortic valve closed, this symbolises the end of systole. The pressure in the ventricle continues to fall during the isovolumetric ventricular relaxation phase of diastole. When the pressure in the ventricle falls below that of the atria the atrio-ventricular valve opens. The pressure in the ventricle then rises alongside the rapid refilling of the ventricle. This is assisted by elastic recoil of the ventricle, virtually sucking the blood from the atrium into the ventricle.

How does the left ventricular pressure curve compare to the aortic pressure curve?

During diastole the aortic pressures slowly decline as blood flows from the aorta into the systemic vascular system. At the end of diastole the pressure in the aorta is at its lowest at 80 mmHg. When the aortic valve opens at the beginning of the ventricular ejection phase the aortic pressure rapidly increases to a pressure of approximately 120 mmHg as blood flows from the ventricle into the aorta. In late systole when the ventricle repolarises and begins to relax the pressure in the aorta also declines but is maintained by the elasticity of the stretched arterial walls and the presence of peripheral resistance to flow by the arterioles. When the pressure in the left ventricle drops below that of the aorta the aortic valve closes. The incisura is produced in the aortic wave form by the closure of the aortic valve.

When do the aortic and mitral valves open and close?

The atrio-ventricular valve closes at the end of diastole when the pressure in the ventricle exceeds the pressure in the atrium. There is then a short period called the isovolumetric ventricular contraction when the atrio-ventricular and the aortic and pulmonary valves are all closed. When the pressure in the ventricle exceeds that of the aorta the aortic valve opens, and blood is ejected from the ventricle into the aorta. When the pressure in the aorta exceeds the pressure in the ventricle the aortic valve will subsequently close. Again there is a short period when both the mitral and aortic valves are closed. This is called the isovolumetric relaxation phase. When the ventricle has relaxed to the extent that the pressure in the atria is higher than that of the ventricle the atrio-ventricular valve will again open. This induces atrial systole.

Describe the pressure–volume loop for the ventricle?

If the ventricular pressure is plotted against the volume a loop is generated, the area of which represents the work performed, often called stroke work (Figure 1.2.1b). In addition, the pressure–volume relationship at the end of systole reflects the contractile properties of the

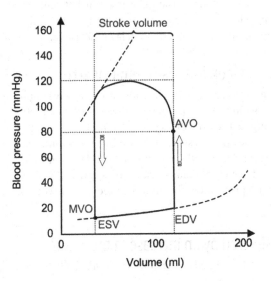

AVO = aortic valve opens, MVO = mitral valve opens, EOV = end diastoric volume, ESV = end systolic volume.

Figure 1.2.1b. Pressure–volume relationship. Reproduced with permission from Cross, M. and Plunkett, E. 2008. *Physics, Pharmacology and Physiology for Anaesthetists: Key Concepts for the FRCA.* Cambridge: Cambridge University Press. © M. Cross and E. Plunkett 2008.

ventricle, whilst the pressure–volume relationship at the end of diastole depends on passive properties or the stiffness of the ventricle.

The ventricular pressure–volume curves have four segments:

- The isovolumetric contraction
- Ventricular ejection
- Isovolumetric relaxation
- Diastolic ventricular filling.

In a normal heart the left ventricular pressure–volume loop is roughly rectangular. At the end-diastolic point the atrio-ventricular and aortic valves are closed, so blood can neither enter nor leave the ventricle. The ventricle begins to contract in the phase called the isovolumetric contraction, increasing the pressure within the ventricle. When the aortic valve opens blood is ejected from the ventricle into the aorta accompanied by a fall in volume in the ventricle, and initially a rise then fall in pressure. Maximum pressure in the left ventricle in a healthy heart is approximately 120 mmHg. After the aortic valve closes, the isovolumetric relaxation phase occurs, when the pressure in the ventricle dramatically falls. The flatter portion at the base of the loop represents the rest of diastole, the rapid ventricular filling phase when the atrio-ventricular valves open, followed by the slow ventricular filling phase which causes a slow and steady increase in pressure and volume, and then atrial contraction which causes a further increase in volume and pressure. Diastole ends in the end-diastolic point with the closure of the atrio-ventricular valve.

The pressure–volume loop in the right ventricle is more triangular than the left ventricle. This is because contraction of the right ventricle is not synchronised, starting at the inflow tract, and in a peristaltic manners reaching the outflow tract after a delay of 50 msec.

What happens to the pressure–volume loop in an ischaemic heart?

In ischaemia the pressure–volume loop appears to lean to the right. This is due to early lengthening of the ventricular fibres during the isovolumetric contraction phase of systole that is not normally seen. This is caused by bulging of the area of ischaemic muscle. Hence during the isovolumetric contraction not only does the pressure increase but the volume too is increased, making the loop lean to the right. During the isovolumetric relaxation phase of diastole there is post-systolic shortening of the ventricular muscle fibres caused by active shortening or elastic recoil of the ventricle with profound ischaemia. This reduces the volume as well as the pressure within the ventricle.

How is the pressure–volume loop affected by an increase in pre-load?

First define pre-load to show the examiner you have a good level of understanding, then move on to describe how it affects the pressure–volume loop.

In the heart pre-load is defined as the end-diastolic volume, which is the volume that produces the initial stretch of the myocardium prior to the contraction. An increase in preload increases the end-diastolic volume, which increases the end-diastolic fibre length of the ventricular muscle. This increases the velocity of the muscle shortening for a given after-load and ejects more blood from the ventricle. Thus for a constant contractility and after-load, increasing the pre-load increases the stroke volume. This makes the pressure–volume loop wider than normal. The end-systolic ventricular volume is the same.

How does after-load affect the pressure–volume loop?

After-load is the force that opposes the contraction of cardiac muscle and the ejection of blood from the ventricle. Increasing after-load increases the end-systolic ventricular volume, and hence a reduction in stroke volume. The end-diastolic volume does not alter. The pressure–volume loop is consequently taller and thinner.

How is the pressure–volume loop affected by contractility?

Contractility is defined as the intrinsic ability of the cardiac fibres to shorten independent of pre-load and after-load.

When after-load is altered and the pressure–volume loop is moved, a line can be drawn between the end-systolic points of both loops. This line is called the end-systolic pressure–volume line or the ESPV line and the gradient represents the contractility.

An increase in myocardial contractility increases the gradient of the slope of the ESPV and is associated with a widening of the pressure–volume loop. Unlike the widening of the pressure–volume loop caused by increasing pre-load, which moves the end-diastolic point to the right, and hence widens the pressure–volume loop by increasing the right border, increasing the contractility widens the pressure–volume loop by shifting the end-systolic point to the left.

1.2.2. Coronary circulation – Sarah F Bell

This subject might appear in the MCQ, the structured oral examination or the OSCE as a diagram to label. An understanding of the anatomy and physiology of the coronary circulation is vital to all anaesthetists.

What is the blood flow to the myocardium?

The heart receives a total of 5% of the cardiac output which equates to 250 ml/min. During exercise blood flow may increase by up to five times.

Can you describe the anatomy of the coronary arterial circulation?

In a structured oral examination this question is probably best answered verbally unless you have practiced drawing a diagram that is easy to produce quickly, see Figure 1.2.2a. In an OSCE this might present as a diagram or coronary angiogram to label.

The coronary arteries arise from the ascending aorta just superior to the aortic valve.

The left coronary artery arises from the posterior aortic sinus and passes lateral to the pulmonary trunk to reach the left atrio-ventricular groove. It soon divides into two branches, the left anterior descending and the circumflex. The left anterior descending branch continues along the inter-ventricular groove to the apex of the heart. It then turns around the inferior border of the heart to anastomose with the posterior inter-ventricular branch of the right coronary artery. In many patients the anterior descending branch has a diagonal branch that descends on the sterno-costal surface of the heart. The smaller circumflex branch of the left coronary artery follows the atrio-ventricular groove around to the posterior surface of the heart and commonly anastomoses with the terminal end of the right coronary artery. The circumflex has a marginal branch that follows the left margin of the heart.

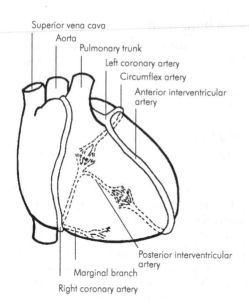

Superior vena cava
Aorta
Pulmonary trunk
Left coronary artery
Circumflex artery
Anterior interventricular artery
Posterior interventricular artery
Marginal branch
Right coronary artery

Figure 1.2.2a. The coronary arteries. Reproduced with permission from Smith, T., Pinnock, C. and Lin, T. 2009. *Fundamentals of Anaesthesia.* Cambridge: Cambridge University Press. © Cambridge University Press 2009.

The left coronary artery supplies most of the left ventricle, atrium and atrio-ventricular septum. It also supplies some of the right atrium and may supply the sino-atrial node.

The right coronary artery arises from the anterior aortic sinus and passes between the pulmonary trunk and the right atrium to descend in the atrio-ventricular groove. At the inferior border of the heart the right marginal artery branches towards the apex of the heart. The right coronary artery then turns to follow the posterior inter-ventricular groove on the posterior aspect of the heart. Its largest branch, the posterior inter-ventricular artery then heads towards the apex of the heart and anastomoses with the left anterior descending artery. The continuation of the right coronary artery continues to anastomose with the circumflex artery. The right coronary artery supplies the sino-atrial node in 60% of people and the atrio-ventricular node in 90% of people. It also supplies the right atrium and ventricle and the posterior–inferior portion of the left ventricle. In addition it supplies variable parts of the left atrium and inter-ventricular septum.

Can you describe the venous drainage of the heart?

The venous drainage of the heart is complex (Figure 1.2.2b). One-third of the drainage is via small veins, called the anterior cardiac veins, that flow directly into the right atrium. Nearly all the remaining drainage is via the coronary sinus which is located in the right atrium, by the opening of the inferior vena cava. Tributaries of this sinus include the great and left marginal veins which follow the course of the left coronary artery and the right marginal, middle and small veins that follow the course of the right coronary artery. A small proportion of the venous drainage is via the Thebesian veins which drain directly into the left side of the heart.

Does all of the heart muscle obtain its blood supply from the coronary arteries?

No, the inner 1 mm of the ventricles obtains blood via diffusion.

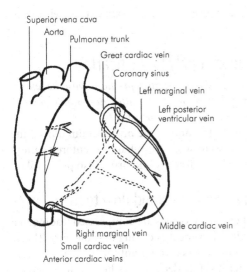

Figure 1.2.2b. Venous drainage of the heart. Reproduced with permission from Smith, T., Pinnock, C. and Lin, T. 2009. *Fundamentals of Anaesthesia.* Cambridge: Cambridge University Press. © Cambridge University Press 2009.

What are the sinuses of Valsalva?

You are doing well if this is asked!

The sinuses of Valsalva are small out-pockets of the aortic wall in close proximity to the coronary sinuses. These produce eddy currents that prevent the aortic valve cusps from obscuring the coronary sinuses.

Can you link the coronary circulation to the leads of an ECG?

This question is testing your ability to link your theoretical knowledge to an investigation we use every day. Try and answer it concisely and showing that you are confident with the anatomy and use of the investigation.

The leads of an ECG view different surfaces of the heart which are supplied by different arteries. Leads II, III and aVF view the inferior surface of the heart; leads V1 to V4 view the anterior surface; leads I, aVL, V5 and V6 view the lateral surface; and V1 and aVR view the right atrium and cavity of left ventricle.

For example:

- Antero-septal changes indicate disease of the left anterior descending artery.
- Isolated inferior infarcts (changes in leads II, III and aVF) are usually associated with disease in the right coronary or distal circumflex artery.
- Disease in the proximal circumflex artery is often associated with a lateral infarct pattern (leads I, aVL, V5 and V6).
- Right ventricular infarction is indicated by signs of inferior infarction, associated with ST segment elevation in lead V1.

How does oxygen consumption in the heart differ from skeletal muscle?

Myocardial oxygen consumption is high. In fact, 65% of arterial oxygen is extracted at rest compared to 25% in skeletal muscle. Therefore any increased myocardial metabolic demand must be matched by an increased blood flow. Oxygen consumption of the heart at rest is equal to 35 ml/min. This can rise to up to 150 ml/min during exercise and is almost entirely due to an increase in blood flow.

What are the factors that control the blood supply to the heart?

This question can be answered in a similar format to all blood supply questions with the following structure: specific factors to the organ, autoregulation and metabolites, autonomic nervous system, drugs. Try and list the factors before then continuing in more depth.

The blood flow to the heart is dependent on contraction of the myocardium during the cardiac cycle and the patency of the coronary vessels; it is also reliant on autoregulation, metabolites and the autonomic nervous system. Blood viscosity and drugs also play a role.

Can you explain the effects of the cardiac cycle on blood flow to the heart?

During contraction of the myocardium the left coronary vessels are compressed leading to a cessation of blood flow. It is important to note that flow occurs during diastole only. This is in contrast to the right coronary vessels where flow occurs throughout the cardiac cycle due to the lower transmural pressure gradients. Since diastole decreases as heart rate increases, coronary blood flow may be compromised by tachycardia.

What other mechanisms are important in controlling the blood supply to the heart?

The patency of the coronary arteries and collateral vessels is vital to the blood flow to the heart and may be affected by embolism, spasm or stenosis.

Autoregulation operates to maintain coronary perfusion pressure. Coronary perfusion pressure can be described as the difference between the aortic end-diastolic pressure and the left ventricular end-diastolic pressure. Sudden changes in coronary perfusion pressure between 60 and 180 mmHg will be counteracted by vasodilatation or constriction to maintain flow.

Furthermore, metabolites including adenine nucleotides, potassium, prostaglandins, hydrogen ions, lactic acid or carbon dioxide released from myocardial cells have been suggested to play a role in autoregulation and matching the delivery of oxygen to the demands of the myocardium.

The autonomic nervous system has some effect on the coronary blood flow. Activation of the sympathetic nervous system leads to chronotropy and inotropy, therefore increasing the metabolic demands of the heart. Vasodilatation mediated by β-adrenoceptors allows an increase in blood flow to meet these requirements. In contrast, α-adrenoceptors can cause vasoconstriction. Stimulation of the parasympathetic nervous system causes vasodilatation and bradycardia.

An increase in blood viscosity will reduce blood flow to the myocardium.

Can you suggest methods of increasing coronary blood flow in patients with ischaemic heart disease?

Drugs such as glyceryl trinitrate are known to cause coronary vasodilatation. β-Blockers act to slow the heart rate and will therefore increase the time allowed for diastole. In a situation of coronary embolism and myocardial infarction, anti-thrombotic agents including streptokinase will break down thrombus thus improving flow. Coronary angioplasty and bypass grafting may act to improve or bypass areas of inadequate flow.

What methods do you know of to measure coronary blood flow?

Questions concerning measurement of blood flow to an organ are common and it is important to have an answer ready. The Fick principle can often be applied.

The Fick principle can be applied to measure coronary blood flow. The principle describes the fact that the amount of tracer substance taken up by organ is equal to the product of the blood flow through it and the concentration difference of the substance across it. Thus the flow is equal to the uptake of a substance divided by the arterio-venous difference. This method can be performed using nitrous oxide or argon and requires coronary sinus catheterisation for estimation of venous concentration.

Thermodilution techniques allow estimation of coronary sinus flow.

Thallium scanning may indicate differences in regional flow, as may coronary angiography.

1.2.3. Pacemaker cells – Natasha A Joshi

What are pacemaker cells?

Pacemaker cells are specialised cardiac muscle cells that undergo slow spontaneous depolarisation, leading to the initiation of an action potential. This property is known as automaticity. Spontaneous depolarisation results from a slow increase in the permeability of the pacemaker cell membrane to sodium ions, accompanied by a reduction in potassium permeability. As a result, the intra-cellular concentration of sodium ions gradually increases, bringing the membrane potential towards the threshold potential for depolarisation. Pacemaker cells also exhibit a property known as rhythmicity: the ability to maintain a regular discharge rate of action potentials.

Where are pacemaker cells found?

Pacemaker cells are found in the conducting system of the heart. This is composed of the sino-atrial node, the atrio-ventricular node, the bundle of His and the bundle branch system of Purkinje fibres.

Describe the anatomy of the conducting system of the heart

It will be very helpful if you can draw a diagram (Figure 1.2.3a). This will convey lots of information in a short space of time and it demonstrates understanding.

The sino-atrial node is situated at the junction of the superior vena cava and the right atrium. Pacemaker cells in this area normally discharge more rapidly than the rest of the heart, thus setting the rate of contraction.

From here, action potentials are conducted to the atrio-ventricular node, via three bundles of atrial fibres; the anterior (Bachmann), the middle (Wenkebach) and the posterior (Thorel) tracts.

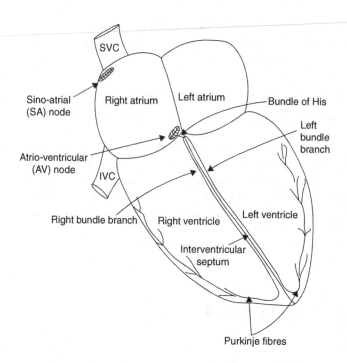

Figure 1.2.3a. Anatomy of the conducting system of the heart.

The atrio-ventricular node lies in the atrial septum, just above the opening of the coronary sinus. Normally, it is the only means of conduction between the atria and the ventricles. The atrio-ventricular node also gives rise to the bundle of His, which descends across the inter-ventricular septum and then divides into right and left bundle branches. Purkinje fibres spread from the ends of the bundle branches to the rest of the ventricles. The action potential is conducted from the atrio-ventricular node, down the route described.

Discuss the autonomic innervation of the heart

The autonomic innervation of the heart arises from the vagus nerve (providing parasympathetic fibres) and sympathetic nerves from the cervical and upper thoracic sympathetic ganglia. These autonomic nerve fibres are arranged in the superficial and deep cardiac plexi.

The sino-atrial and atrio-ventricular nodes receive both vagal and sympathetic innervation. Vagal fibres are "cardio-inhibitory", slowing the rate of conduction of action potentials through the atrio-ventricular node. Sympathetic fibres are "cardio-acceleratory", increasing the rate of conduction of action potentials through the atrio-ventricular node.

Can you describe the pacemaker action potential?

Draw a diagram as it will allow you to convey lots of information in a short space of time (Figure 1.2.3b). When drawing a graph remember to label the axes and include units. As you talk around the diagram, start in a logical place, so that events follow through. When describing the pacemaker action potential, a logical place to start is phase 4.

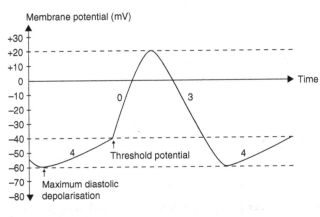

Figure 1.2.3b. Pacemaker action potential.

The pacemaker action potential can be described as a "slow response action potential". It has three distinct phases:

- Phase 4 (the resting phase)
- Phase 0 (rapid depolarisation)
- Phase 3 (repolarisation).

Unlike neurones and the rest of the myocardium, pacemaker cells do not have a stable resting membrane potential, rather they have a slowly decaying membrane potential and demonstrate "spontaneous diastolic depolarisation". This is due to the fact that during phase 4, the resting phase of the action potential, there is an increased permeability of the pacemaker cell membrane to sodium and calcium ions. Sodium ions and to a lesser extent calcium ions therefore diffuse across the cell membrane and into the cell, down a concentration gradient. This has been called the inward sodium "funny current". As a result, the pacemaker cell membrane potential slowly increases, with the inside of the cell becoming more positive with respect to the outside.

The membrane potential is most negative, –60 mV, at "maximum diastolic depolarisation", at the beginning of phase 4. From this point the membrane potential slowly increases to reach a threshold potential at –40 mV, when depolarisation is triggered and phase 0 begins.

At threshold potential, T-type calcium channels open in the pacemaker cell membrane. This leads to a rapid influx of calcium ions into the cell, resulting in depolarisation. The membrane potential rises to reach a peak of +20 mV.

Repolarisation, phase 3, then occurs due to potassium ion efflux, slowly returning the membrane potential down to –60 mV. At the beginning of phase 4 membrane pumps exchange sodium and calcium ions for potassium ions, which move back into the cell. The distribution of ions across the cell membrane is hence reset so that the whole process can begin again.

Describe the action potential in cardiac muscle

You should draw a diagram whilst describing the action potential, see Figure 1.2.3c.

There are five distinct phases in the cardiac muscle action potential.

Phase 4 is the resting potential which is mainly governed by potassium ions, and is approximately –90 mV. An action potential is initiated when the myocyte is depolarised to

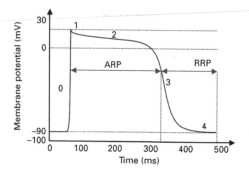

Phase 0 Rapid depolarization occurs after threshold potential is reached owing to fast Na^+ influx. The gradient of this line should be almost vertical as shown.

Phase 1 Repolarization begins to occur as Na^+ channels close and K^+ channels open. Phase 1 is short in duration and does not cause repolarization below 0 mV.

Phase 2 A plateau occurs owing to the opening of L-type Ca^{2+} channels, which off-set the action of K^+ channels and maintain depolarization. During this phase, no further depolarization is possible. This is an important point to demonstrate and explains why tetany is not possible in cardiac muscle. This time period is the absolute refractory period (ARP). The plateau should not be drawn completely horizontal as repolarization is slowed by Ca^{2+} channels but not halted altogether.

Phase 3 The L-type Ca^{2+} channels close and K^+ efflux now causes repolarization as seen before. The relative refractory period (RRP) occurs during phases 3 and 4.

Phase 4 The Na^+/K^+ pump restores the ionic gradients by pumping $3Na^+$ out of the cell in exchange for $2K^+$. The overall effect is, therefore, the slow loss of positive ionic charge from within the cell.

Figure 1.2.3c. Cardiac conduction system action potential. Reproduced with permission from Cross, M. and Plunkett, E. 2008. *Physics, Pharmacology and Physiology for Anaesthetists: Key Concepts for the FRCA.* Cambridge: Cambridge University Press. © M. Cross and E. Plunkett 2008.

a threshold potential of −65 mV. This is normally caused by transmission from an adjacent myocyte. At the threshold potential, fast voltage-gated sodium channels open, leading to an inward current which depolarises the membrane rapidly to +30 mV. This initial upstroke is called phase 0, and is similar to that of a normal nerve cell.

Phase 1, called partial repolarisation, is due to closure of the sodium channels and a sudden reduction in permeability of the cell to sodium. However, during the initial depolarisation at a threshold of −40 mV voltage-gated L-type calcium channels are activated, allowing positively charged calcium ions to flood into the cell. This positive influx of ions prevents the cell from repolarising and causes the plateau phase, also called phase 2. Phase 2 is maintained for approximately 200 msec until the L-type channels close. At this point repolarisation occurs due to outward movement of potassium ions, this is called phase 3.

The absolute refractory period starts when the sodium channels open at the beginning of phase 0, and lasts for 250 msec. The relative refractory period then lasts for a further 50 msec.

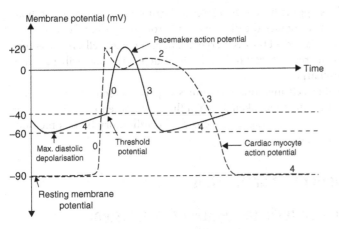

Figure 1.2.3d. Pacemaker and cardiac action potentials.

As the action potential of a cardiac muscle cell lasts almost as long as muscle contraction, its refractory period prevents another action potential being initiated until the muscle relaxes. This is important as it prevents cardiac muscle exhibiting tetanus.

How does the pacemaker action potential differ from that in cardiac myocytes?

In order to answer this question you should draw one graph with both action potentials on it, see Figure 1.2.3d.

There are a number of differences between the pacemaker and the cardiac action potential.

Firstly pacemaker cells demonstrate spontaneous diastolic depolarisation, whereas cardiac myocytes do not.

In addition, in phase 4 the membrane potential is less negative in pacemaker cells (–60 mV) compared with cardiac myocytes, which have a resting membrane potential of –90 mV. The threshold potential is also less negative in pacemaker cells.

Another difference is that the slope of phase 0 (depolarisation) is less steep in pacemaker cells than in cardiac myocytes. Depolarisation in cardiac myocytes results from the opening of "fast sodium channels" and rapid influx of sodium ions into the cell. The influx of sodium ions, and hence depolarisartion, is more rapid than that observed with the influx of calcium ions through T-type calcium channels in pacemaker cells.

Pacemaker action potential repolarisation is a single phase (phase 3). Cardiac myocytes display early rapid repolarisation in phase 1, a plateau phase in phase 2 and final rapid depolarisation in phase 3.

What factors affect the discharge rate of pacemaker cells?

The discharge rate of pacemaker cells is predominantly controlled by the autonomic nervous system. This control is affected by changes in the characteristics of the action potential.

An increase in the slope of phase 4 will reduce the time taken to reach threshold potential and hence depolarisation. This will therefore increase the discharge rate from the pacemaker cell. Likewise, a decrease in the slope of phase 4 will increase the time taken to reach threshold potential, depolarisation and hence reduce the discharge rate from the pacemaker cell.

The threshold potential may also affect the discharge rate of pacemaker cells. If it becomes less negative, the time taken to reach threshold and hence depolarisation will increase, thereby slowing the rate of discharge.

In addition if the pacemaker cell membrane becomes hyperpolarised, the membrane potential becomes more negative, the time taken to reach threshold potential will be longer and the discharge rate will decrease. The vagus nerve is cardio-inhibitory by this method, through the actions of acetylcholine.

1.2.4. Valsalva manoeuvre – Sarah F Bell

Where are the vasomotor centres in the central nervous system?
This question is mainly anatomical. Your answer may be brief.

The vasomotor centres are located in the reticular formation in the medulla and bulbar parts of the pons. They consist of a presser area in the ventrolateral medulla and a depressor area region in the ventromedial medulla. The balance between pressor-mediated sympathetic stimulation (vasoconstriction, tachycardia and inotropy) and the depressor-mediated inhibition of the sympathetic outflow produces the vasomotor tone.

What influences the vasomotor centres?
You can now indicate your more advanced knowledge.

Higher centres including the hypothalamus, cerebral cortex and limbic system exert influence on the vasomotor centres. Furthermore, inhibitory connections travel from the nucleus tractus solitarius in the medulla to the pressor centre. The nucleus tractus solitarius is the sensory nucleus for both the glossopharyngeal and vagus nerves. The glossopharyngeal nerve transmits afferent impulses from the carotid sinus baroreceptors and the carotid body chemoreceptors, whilst the vagus nerve carries afferent signals from the aortic arch chemoreceptors and baroreceptors.

How does the body sense acute changes in blood pressure?
This question probably needs you to focus on the carotid and aortic body baroreceptors, but it is worth mentioning the other receptors involved to convince the examiner of your extended knowledge.

Specialised groups of nerve endings called baroreceptors sense changes in blood pressure. They consist of stretch receptors located in the walls of blood vessels and the heart and are stimulated by distension. When the intra-luminal pressure increases, the frequency of the impulses discharged by the baroreceptors increases. Baroreceptors not only respond to changes in the pressure magnitude but also the rate of change of the pressure. When stimulated, the baroreceptors exert an inhibitory influence on the pressor centre thus leading to vasodilatation and bradycardia.

The location of the baroreceptors determines whether they are high or low pressure stretch receptors. The high pressure receptors are located in the aortic arch and the carotid sinus (those in the carotid sinus are more sensitive). Baroreceptors are also located in the atria, ventricles and pulmonary vessels. Chemoreceptors, both central and peripheral also have a small impact on the regulation of blood pressure.

How do the baroreceptors work?

Sometimes you many need to reiterate an important point!

The baroreceptors in the aortic arch and carotid sinus are progressively stimulated above a mean arterial pressure of 60 mmHg with a maximum effect at 180 mmHg. Increases in blood pressure lead to increased afferent firing via the vagus nerve for the aortic arch baroreceptors and the glossopharyngeal nerve for the carotid sinus baroreceptors. This leads to an increased inhibition of the vasomotor centre in the medulla, causing reduced sympathetic activity and increased excitation of the cardio inhibitory centre, increasing vagal tone. These act to reduce blood pressure (via systemic vasodilatation) and heart rate, thus regulating blood pressure.

How does the action of the baroreceptor reflex change in patients with chronic hypertension?

In patients with chronic hypertension, the baroreceptors reset their working range and sensitivity thus shifting the response curve to the right.

What is the Valsalva manoeuvre?

This is a common question and so you need to have an easily reproducible answer.

The Valsalva manoeuvre is the action of forced expiration against the closed glottis after full inspiration. A pressure of 40 mmHg should be achieved and held for 10 seconds.

Why is the Valsalva manoeuvre named and when was it first used?

The Valsalva manoeuvre is named after Antonio Valsalva, an Italian anatomist (1666–1723). It was first described when used to expel pus from the middle ear.

Can you describe the changes in blood pressure and heart rate that would be observed in a normal person performing the Valsalva?

This question would be best answered with a diagram of the phases and a description of the physiological principles underlying the changes in heart rate and blood pressure, see Figure 1.2.4.

The observations of arterial blood pressure and heart rate show four phases:

Firstly on commencing the manoeuvre, there is a sharp increase in the intra-thoracic pressure. This expels blood from thoracic vessels leading to an increase in cardiac output and therefore a transient increase in blood pressure.

Secondly, as the patient maintains the manoeuvre the positive intra-thoracic pressure is sustained. This leads to a reduction in the venous return to the heart and so a fall in blood pressure. This is sensed by the baroreceptors in the aortic arch and carotid sinus. Reduced afferent discharge is stimulatory to the vasomotor centre leading to a reflex tachycardia and vasoconstriction acting to return the blood pressure to near normal values.

In the third phase, the pressure is released. The venous return pools in the pulmonary vessels due to the fall in intra-thoracic pressure, thus left ventricular pre-load falls, cardiac output drops and the blood pressure decreases.

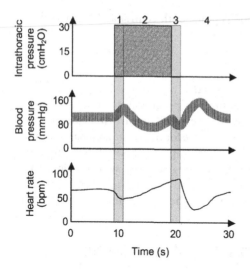

Draw and label all three axes. The uppermost trace shows the sustained rise in intrathoracic pressure during the 10 s of the manoeuvre. Mark the four phases on as vertical lines covering all three plot areas, so that your diagram can be drawn accurately.

Curves Draw normal heart rate and BP lines on the remaining two axes. Note that the BP line is thick so as to represent SBP at its upper border and DBP at its lower border.

Phase 1 During phase 1, the increased thoracoabdominal pressure transiently increases venous return, thereby raising BP and reflexly lowering heart rate.

Phase 2 During phase 2, the sustained rise in intrathoracic pressure reduces venous return VR and so BP falls until a compensatory tachycardia restores it.

Phase 3 The release of pressure in phase 3 creates a large empty venous reservoir, causing BP to fall. Show that the heart rate remains elevated.

Phase 4 The last phase shows how the raised heart rate then initially leads to a raised BP as venous return is restored. This is followed by a reflex bradycardia before both parameters eventually return to normal.

Figure 1.2.4. Valsalva manoeuvre. Reproduced with permission from Cross, M. and Plunkett, E. 2008. *Physics, Pharmacology and Physiology for Anaesthetists: Key Concepts for the FRCA.* Cambridge: Cambridge University Press. © M. Cross and E. Plunkett 2008.

Finally, the baroreceptors respond to the fall in blood pressure by reducing their inhibitory effect on the pressor centre. Vasoconstriction and tachycardia ensue. Once venous return is restored, there is an overshoot, as compensatory mechanisms continue to operate. The increased blood pressure causes a baroreceptor-mediated bradycardia.

Why might we use the Valsalva manoeuvre in clinical practice?

The Valsalva manoeuvre can be used as a test of autonomic function. It may also help terminate a supra-ventricular tachycardia due to the increased vagal tone during the fourth phase of the manoeuvre.

What abnormal responses may be seen when the Valsalva manoeuvre is performed?

The response may show a square waveform. This is seen in cases of congestive cardiac failure, constrictive pericarditis, cardiac tamponade and valvular heart disease, when the central venous pressure is markedly raised. The blood pressure remains high throughout the manoeuvre and returns to the previous level at the end.

In patients with autonomic dysfunction the blood pressure falls and remains low until the intra-thoracic pressure is released. The changes in pulse rate and overshoot are absent.

Patients who are ventilated or hypovolaemic will show an exaggerated fall in blood pressure during the Valsalva manoeuvre.

1.2.5. Exercise physiology – Emily K Johnson

What is the basal metabolic rate?

The basal metabolic rate is the amount of energy liberated by breakdown of food per unit time under standardised conditions. These conditions include a relaxed subject at comfortable temperature, 12 hours after a meal, and the basal metabolic rate must be corrected for age, sex and surface area. It is determined either by measuring the heat produced by a subject or their oxygen consumption knowing that per litre of oxygen consumed an average of 20.1 kJ energy is liberated.

The normal basal metabolic rate in adult males is 197 kJ/m^2/hr or 40 Cal/m^2/hr.

What factors increase the basal metabolic rate?

The basal metabolic rate is increased by muscle activity, raised catecholamines and stress, raised temperature, hyperthyroidism, pregnancy, a recent meal and in children and males.

What is a MET?

MET stands for metabolic equivalent. It is a measure of the metabolic demands of an activity in multiples of basal energy expenditure. For example resting, awake and fasted would be 1 MET, sleeping would be 0.9 MET, walking 3.5 MET, jogging 10–12 MET and marathon running 18–20 MET.

What is isometric and isotonic exercise?

Isometric, also known as static exercise, is when muscles contract against a resistance but they do not shorten or lengthen. Isotonic, also known as dynamic exercise, is when muscles shorten and lengthen and move joints. The same or similar muscles may be involved in both types of exercise but the pattern of contraction, blood flow and energy consumption may differ.

What are the types of muscle fibres in skeletal muscle?

There are two main types of muscle fibre in skeletal muscle. There are slow twitch, otherwise known as type I oxidative fibres or red fibres. They are red in colour, rich in myoglobin and obtain their energy from oxidative metabolism. The second type is fast twitch or type II glycolytic fibres that contract rapidly. They obtain their energy from anaerobic, glycolytic sources.

Type I slow twitch fibres are found in the back muscles, whereas type II fast twitch fibres are found in the small muscles of the hand. Most muscles of the body have roughly equal proportions of fast and slow twitch fibres.

Tell me about the metabolic features of exercise

During exercise the body can expend up to 20 times the amount of energy it does at rest, so the metabolic equivalent is 20 times the basal metabolic rate. Exercise can be aerobic or anaerobic.

In aerobic exercise the oxygen supply keeps up with demand. In anaerobic exercise the oxygen supply is unable to keep up with demand, such as in a fast sprint or in isometric exercise when muscle contraction compresses vessels and cuts off the blood and therefore the oxygen supply.

The efficiency of the body during external exercise is roughly 25%. Seventy-five percent of the energy used on external exercise is released as heat energy. The energy the body uses to carry out external exercise ultimately is from the oxidation of carbohydrate, fat and protein. However the immediate supply of energy is from the hydrolysis of ATP to ADP and inorganic phosphate. This occurs when the actin and myosin form cross-bridges. In skeletal muscle the ATP stores support around 2 seconds of vigorous exercise. Once exhausted the ATP is replenished by creatine phosphate which is present in muscle in concentrations roughly 4 times that of ATP. It rephosphorylates ADP to ATP.

The initial use of these two energy sources allows time for other, more long-term methods of energy production to commence. These include glycogen breakdown and glycolysis. This is an anaerobic process in which glucose is converted to pyruvate, producing two ATP molecules. Pyruvate is reduced to lactate which enters the blood and circulates to the liver where it is converted back to pyruvate. Glycogen stores release glucose-6-phosphate which enters the glycolytic pathway increasing activity 1000-fold. Glycogen phosphorylase is the enzyme responsible for releasing the glucose-6-phosphate from stores and this enzyme is activated by the increased calcium concentrations that occur in exercise. Some energy is obtained from gluconeogenesis, particularly from recycling lactate; however, this contribution is restricted due to the hepatic vasoconstriction that occurs in exercise.

In exercise the rate of glycolysis initially exceeds the oxygen supply so lactate accumulates, until the cardiovascular system responds and makes the necessary adjustments to increase oxygen supply.

During exercise the energy supplies are obtained predominantly from muscle glycogen and fat stores. Glucose from the liver and free fatty acids from adipose tissue makes negligible contributions compared to the stores in muscle.

Can you summarise the amounts of energy produced per glucose molecule in aerobic and anaerobic conditions?

In aerobic conditions a molecule of glucose will yield 38 ATPs, or 39 per glucose-6-phosphate obtained from glycogen stores.

In anaerobic conditions a molecule of glucose will yield only three ATP molecules.

What is an oxygen debt?

The oxygen debt refers to the period of increased oxygen consumption that continues after exercise ceases. It is this period of higher oxygen consumption post-exercise that is used to repay the oxygen deficit incurred at the start of exercise when the period of anaerobic energy production resulted in lactate accumulation.

What are the partial pressures of oxygen at the level of the mitochondria at rest compared to in extreme exercise?

Remember if you are asked a specific question like this in your structured oral examination and you do not know the answer, do not guess and do not start to waffle to avoid answering the question. It is acceptable to say "I don't know" without automatically failing.

At rest the partial pressure of oxygen in mitochondria is close to that in venous blood, around 2.7–4 kPa or 20–30 mmHg. During exercise the partial pressure of oxygen at the mitochondrial level can fall as low as 0.13 kPa or 1 mmHg before mitochondrial activity is impaired, this is called the Pasteur point.

Tell me about VO_2 max and the "anabolic threshold"?

VO_2 max is the maximal oxygen uptake achievable for an individual. It is limited by cardiovascular rather than metabolic or respiratory factors and it increases for an individual as they become fitter. It is calculated by exercising a subject gradually to a maximum level over 15 minutes. Levels of exercise can be expressed as a percentage of VO_2 max. For example low intensity exercise involving VO_2 at around 20% of VO_2 max are associated with greater fat oxidation than carbohydrate oxidation. With higher intensities of exercise more of the energy is obtained from oxidation of carbohydrates. At around 50 to 70% of the VO_2 max the "anabolic threshold" is reached. This is the point that oxygen delivery can no longer match demand and lactic acid accumulates. Metabolism shifts from aerobic to anaerobic.

What is the normal resting blood flow to skeletal muscle?

The normal resting blood flow to skeletal muscles is 1200 ml/min, which is equivalent to 20.5% of the cardiac output.

How does this change during exercise?

During exercise the blood flow to skeletal muscles can increase up to 20-fold. In light exercise it may increase to around 4500 ml/min which is 47% of the cardiac output, and as much as 22 000 ml/min in heavy exercise which would be 88% of the cardiac output.

How do these changes come about?

These changes in skeletal muscle blood flow are brought about as in resting musclearterioles are constricted by sympathetic tone to maintain the blood flow. The pre-capillary sphincters are closed and larger vessels maintain the circulation. During exercise the partial pressure of oxygen decreases, and that of carbon dioxide increases, as do temperature, hydrogen ion and potassium ion concentrations and ADP. All these factors cause the pre-capillary sphincters to relax and increase the total muscle blood flow by up to 20-fold.

What happens to regional blood flow during exercise?

Coronary blood flow increases during exercise to meet the extra oxygen requirement associated with increased cardiac work. The resting coronary blood flow of 250 ml/min increases to 1000 ml/min in heavy exercise. Renal blood flow decreases from resting flows of 1100 ml/min to 250 ml/min in heavy exercise. Blood flow to the GI tract also decreases from 1400 ml/min to 300 ml/min. Blood flow to the skin increases to aid with heat loss.

Overall in exercise, blood flow to skeletal muscle, coronary vessels and the skin increases at the expense of blood flow to the kidneys and GI tract. Cerebral blood flow does not alter at any level of exercise. It is skeletal muscle blood flow that shows the greatest proportional increase, up to 20-fold in very heavy exercise, compared to coronary flow which increases approximately 4-fold in heavy exercise.

What are the cardiovascular changes that occur during exercise?

The cardiac output can increase five-fold during exercise. There are many factors that contribute to this increase. Venous return to the heart is increased by compression of the veins in contracting muscle. It is also increased by the effect of abdominal contraction that occurs during inspiration and pushes blood out of abdominal veins, in coordination with a drop in intra-thoracic pressure. Deeper breathing with an increased rate further enhances this effect. Sympathetic stimulation results in venoconstriction, also improving venous return to the heart. Peripheral vascular resistance falls due to the action of local metabolites in muscle. This sustains the increased cardiac output. Heart rate increases, initially due to decreased vagal tone, in proportion with the severity of exercise to around a maximum of 200 beats per minute. Stroke volume also rises with severity of exercise, up to a point between medium and severe exercise. After this point it shows only a small further increase before it begins to fall in very extreme exercise as the heart rate exceeds 200. Such tachycardia will restrict diastolic filling time, limiting stroke volume.

Blood pressure increases as exercise severity increases. It is the systolic pressures that increase most and diastolic pressures demonstrate much smaller increases, therefore pulse pressures widen.

These changes occur rapidly at the beginning of exercise and cease abruptly as exercise stops. This is because of the muscle pump increasing venous return and motor cortical and sympathetic activation. During exercise the increases occur much more slowly and the mechanism controlling the gradual rise in cardiac output is the vasodilatation in muscle and stimulation of the cardiovascular system.

What are the respiratory changes that occur during exercise?

The respiratory changes in exercise mirror the cardiovascular changes somewhat. The tidal volume and respiratory rate rise in proportion to the demand for oxygen and for carbon dioxide elimination. As for cardiac output, these changes occur rapidly at the start of exercise, then more gradually as exercise intensity increases, and they cease abruptly as exercise stops. The ventilation increase is due to stimulation of the respiratory centre from the motor cortex and from proprioceptors from moving limbs. The slower gradual rise during exercise is due to the increased sensitivity of carotid bodies and as lactic acid builds they receive additional stimulation resulting in a disproportionate rise in minute volume and CO_2 removal.

At extremely intense exercise the maximal oxygen consumption is reached and oxygen consumption plateaus. If exercise continues to increase the anabolic threshold will be exceeded and lactic acid will accumulate. In this situation muscle pH can fall from its normal resting value of 7 to as low as pH 6.4, arterial pH can fall to 7.1 and ventilation is stimulated and increases over and above the necessary ventilation to achieve oxygen requirements and CO_2 elimination.

Chapter

1.3

Physiology of the central, peripheral and autonomic nervous systems

1.3.1. Cerebral circulation – Emily K Johnson

Describe the blood supply to the brain

This question could be used as an OSCE station possibly with a diagram where you are required to name vessels and/or discuss with the examiner. It may also come in a structured oral examination question, so a little time spent memorising the arterial supply and venous drainage of the brain will be well worth it! Be able to picture the circle of Willis, and in a structured oral examination scenario it would be helpful to draw it (Figure 1.3.1a).

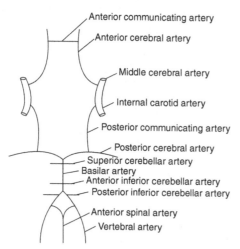

Figure 1.3.1a. The circle of Willis.

The internal carotid arteries and the vertebral arteries ascend to supply the brain. Two-thirds of the brain is supplied by the internal carotids. They ascend through the carotid canal in the petrous temporal bone and enter the skull where they have a tortuous course, ending by dividing into the anterior and middle cerebral arteries. The anterior cerebral arteries supply the superior and medial parts of the cerebral hemisphere and are linked by the anterior communicating artery, making the anterior portion of the circle of Willis. The middle cerebral arteries supply most of the lateral side of the hemisphere, and branches supply the internal

Dr Podcast Scripts for the Primary FRCA, ed. Rebecca A. Leslie, Emily K. Johnson and Alexander P. L. Goodwin. Published by Cambridge University Press. © R. A. Leslie, E. K. Johnson and A. P. L. Goodwin 2011.

capsule. The blood supply to the other one-third of the brain comes from the vertebral arteries. These are branches of the subclavian artery. They ascend in the transverse foramina of the upper six cervical vertebrae and enter the skull by piercing the dura at the foramen magnum. They run on the medulla and join in front of the pons to form the basilar artery, which gives off the cerebellar arteries. The basilar artery then divides into the posterior cerebral arteries, which supply the occipital lobe and medial side of the temporal lobe. The posterior communicating arteries form the anastomoses between the internal carotids and posterior cerebral arteries thus completing the circle of Willis.

Technically you have now answered the question so you could stop and wait for the examiner to lead you down whichever route of questioning they choose. Alternatively you could confidently go ahead and describe the venous drainage to demonstrate your knowledge – they can always stop you if this is not where the question was heading. Try to picture the venous drainage system in order to describe it.

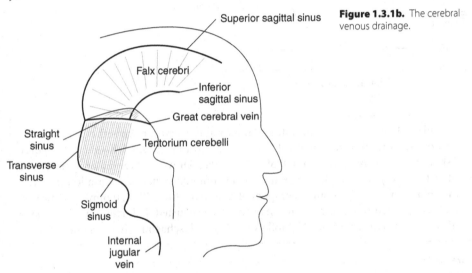

Figure 1.3.1b. The cerebral venous drainage.

The venous drainage is via the dural venous sinuses (Figure 1.3.1b). The superior and inferior sagittal sinuses drain the cerebral and cerebellar cortices. They lie between the dural layers of the falx cerebri. The superior sagittal sinus drains into the right transverse sinus, and the inferior sagittal sinus drains via the straight sinus into the left transverse sinus. The midline great cerebral vein drains deep structures into the inferior sagittal sinus. The transverse sinuses lie in the tentorium cerebelli and become the sigmoid sinuses, pass through the jugular foramen and become the internal jugular veins. The cavernous sinuses lie on either side of the pituitary fossa and drain the eyes and surrounding structures. They also drain into the transverse sinuses.

Define cerebral perfusion pressure

Give a concise definition and don't waffle.

Cerebral perfusion pressure = Mean arterial pressure − Intra-cranial pressure.

Under normal circumstances a mean arterial pressure (MAP) of 90 mmHg and an intra-cranial pressure (ICP) of approximately 10 mmHg would give a cerebral perfusion pressure

(CCP) of 80 mmHg. A CPP of less than 70 mmHg would lead to a rapid decrease in jugular venous bulb saturations representing an increased oxygen extraction by brain tissue. A CPP of 30–40 mmHg is the threshold for critical ischaemia.

What is the Monro–Kellie doctrine?

A diagram of an intra-cranial pressure–volume curve would help illustrate your answer. Draw axis, label axis, add units and draw the curve, see Figure 1.3.1c.

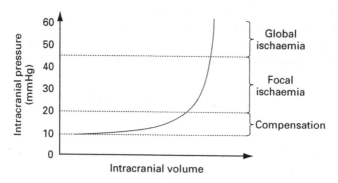

Draw and label the axes as shown. Note that the *x* axis is usually drawn without any numerical markers. Normal intracranial volume is assumed to be at the left side of the curve and should be in keeping with an ICP of 5–10 mmHg. Draw a curve similar in shape to a positive tear-away exponential. Demonstrate on your curve that compensation for a rise in the volume of one intracranial component maintains the ICP <20 mmHg. However, when these limited compensatory mechanisms are exhausted, ICP rises rapidly, causing focal ischaemia (ICP 20–45 mmHg) followed by global ischaemia (ICP >45 mmHg).

Figure 1.3.1c. Intra-cranial volume–pressure relationship. Reproduced with permission from Cross, M. and Plunkett, E. 2008. *Physics, Pharmacology and Physiology for Anaesthetists: Key Concepts for the FRCA.* Cambridge: Cambridge University Press. © M. Cross and E. Plunkett 2008.

The Monro–Kellie doctrine states that the skull has a fixed volume containing brain, blood and CSF. If any one component were to occupy greater volume, unless another component occupied a reduced volume, it would result in a raised ICP.

If the brain volume increases initially CSF is squeezed out into the spinal compartment, its absorption is increased and production decreased. Once these compensatory mechanisms are exhausted a very small increase in volume will result in large increases in ICP.

What is the cerebral blood flow rate and how does it vary between grey and white matter?

The cerebral blood flow is 50 ml/100 g/min. This varies from 20 ml/100 g/min in white matter to 70 ml/100 g/min in grey matter, which is metabolically more active.

The adult brain weighs approximately 1500 g (which is roughly 2% of total body weight) and, therefore, receives 750 ml/min of blood, which is 15% of the total cardiac output.

What is the cerebral metabolic rate for oxygen?

The cerebral metabolic rate for oxygen is the rate of oxygen consumption of the brain. It is approximately 3 ml/100 g/min and is higher in grey matter. It is approximately 20% of the total body oxygen consumption.

The brain requires a large amount of energy and has very limited capacity for anaerobic metabolism so in the absence of a good oxygen supply, energy-dependent processes cease and irreversible cell damage occurs. A good blood supply is therefore essential.

What do you understand by the threshold values for cerebral ischaemia?

The threshold values for cerebral ischaemia are values for cerebral blood flow (CBF) below which known neuronal physiological changes occur. A normal CBF is 50 ml/100 g/min; below this, acidosis occurs. Below 40 ml/100 g/min protein synthesis is impaired, below 30 ml/100 g/min oedema occurs, below 20 ml/100 g/min electrical function begins to fail and cell death occurs below 10 ml/100 g/min.

What factors affect cerebral blood flow?

CBF is affected by a number of factors. Firstly, those factors affecting cerebral perfusion pressure and secondly those factors affecting the radius of cerebral vessels, which can be divided into chemical, metabolic and neurogenic factors.

CPP is the difference between the MAP and the ICP. It will therefore be influenced by changes in MAP or ICP. In a normal brain despite changes in MAP, CBF remains constant with CPP between 60 and 160 mmHg. This is achieved by autoregulation. Metabolic, myogenic and neurogenic factors may contribute to autoregulation.

Your explanation would be aided by a graph showing the relationship between CBF and CPP. You may be asked to draw this graph but it would be favourable to volunteer it as part of your answer. Draw axes, label axes, add units, plot the points between which CBF remains stable and draw the graph, Figure 1.3.1d.

This autoregulation curve would be shifted to the right in people with chronic hypertension and to the left in neonates. Autoregulation may be impaired in disease processes or by drugs. For example the volatile anaesthetic agents abolish autoregulation and cause dose-dependent vasodilatation so increasing CBF. Thiopentone, propofol and benzodiazepines reduce CBF.

The radius of cerebral blood vessels is very important as the increased radius that occurs in vasodilatation leads to an increase cerebral blood volume and so an increased ICP thereby reducing CPP.

Chemical factors include the change in hydrogen ion concentration due to metabolic activity and changes in $PaCO_2$ and PaO_2.

Draw the graph that illustrates these relationships between CBF, PaO_2 and $PaCO_2$. Draw axes, label axes, add units and add scales and talk through the graphs as you are drawing them, see Figures 1.3.1e and 1.3.1f.

Changes in $PaCO_2$ cause almost linear changes in CBF between $PaCO_2$ of 2.7 kPa and 10.6 kPa. For each one kilopascal change in $PaCO_2$ there is a corresponding change in CBF of approximately 15 ml/100 g tissue. At $PaCO_2$ 10.6 kPa the arterioles are maximally dilated and no further increase in flow is possible. Below a $PaCO_2$ of 2.7 kPa no further reduction in

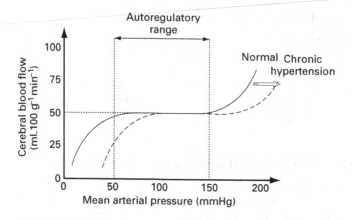

Draw and label the axes as shown. Mark the two key points on the x axis (50 and 150 mmHg). Between these points, mark a horizontal line at a y value of 50 ml.100 g^{-1}.min^{-1}. Label this segment the 'autoregulatory range'. Above this range, cerebral blood flow (CBF) will increase as mean arterial pressure (MAP) increases. There will, however, be a maximum flow at some MAP where no further increase is possible. Below 50 mmHg, CBF falls with MAP; however, the line does not pass through the origin as neither MAP nor flow can be zero in live patients. Demonstrate the response to chronic hypertension by drawing an identical curve displaced to the right to show how the autoregulatory range 'resets' itself under these conditions.

Figure 1.3.1d. Autoregulation. Reproduced with permission from Cross, M. and Plunkett, E. 2008. *Physics, Pharmacology and Physiology for Anaesthetists: Key Concepts for the FRCA.* Cambridge: Cambridge University Press. © M. Cross and E. Plunkett 2008.

CBF occurs, see Figure 1.3.1e. At such a low PaCO$_2$ vasoconstriction results in tissue hypoxia and the build up of local metabolites causes vasodilatation. It is thought that nitric oxide mediates these changes.

Changes in PaO$_2$ have no influence in CBF until PaO$_2$ falls below a threshold of 7.5 kPa, at which point there is a dramatic increase in CBF, see Figure 1.3.1f.

Cerebral metabolic rate influences CBF but under normal circumstances, although local flow may alter, the global CBF remains constant. Thus, blood flow is diverted around the brain to supply the metabolically active parts at any one time.

Any factor such as convulsions or pyrexia which increases the overall cerebral metabolic rate will result in a global increase in CBF. Conversely, factors such as hypothermia and anaesthesia will decrease cerebral metabolic rate and thus CBF. Neurogenic factors have an influence on CBF. Sympathetic fibres cause vasoconstriction and have a role in protecting the brain by shifting the autoregulation curve to the right in hypertension. Parasympathetic fibres cause vasodilatation and may play a role in hypotension and reperfusion injury.

Blood viscosity, which is directly related to haematocrit, affects CBF. The lower the viscosity the higher the flow as stated by the Hagen–Poiseuille's law. There is a balance between flow and oxygen carrying capacity, which is a haematocrit of approximately 30%.

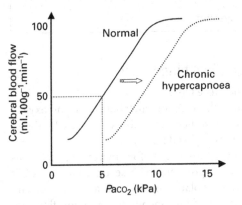

Draw and label the axes.

Normal Mark a point at the intersection of a normal $PaCO_2$ and cerebral blood flow as shown. As CBF will approximately double with a doubling of the $PaCO_2$ extend a line from this point up to a $PaCO_2$ of around 10 kPa. At the extremes of $PaCO_2$ there arise minimum and maximum flows that depend on maximal and minimal vasodilatation, respectively. The line should, therefore, become horizontal as shown at these extremes.

Chronic hypercapnoea The curve is identical but shifted to the right of the normal curve as buffering acts to reset the autoregulatory range.

Figure 1.3.1e. Effects of $PaCO_2$ on cerebral blood flow. Reproduced with permission from Cross, M. and Plunkett, E. 2008. *Physics, Pharmacology and Physiology for Anaesthetists: Key Concepts for the FRCA.* Cambridge: Cambridge University Press. © M. Cross and E. Plunkett 2008.

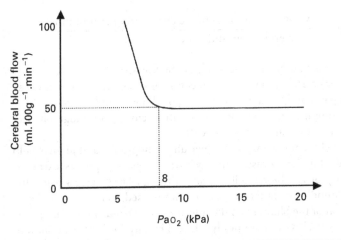

Draw and label the axes. Plot a point at a normal PaO_2 and CBF as shown. Draw a horizontal line extending to the right of this point. This demonstrates that for values >8 kPa on the x axis, CBF remains constant. Below this point, hypoxia causes cerebral vasodilatation and CBF rises rapidly. At flow rates >100 ml.$100g^{-1}$.min^{-1}, maximal blood flow will be attained and the curve will tail off. Remember that the vasodilatory effect of hypoxia will override any other reflexes to ensure maximal oxygenation of the brain tissue.

Figure 1.3.1f. Effects of PaO_2 on cerebral blood flow. Reproduced with permission from Cross, M. and Plunkett, E. 2008. *Physics, Pharmacology and Physiology for Anaesthetists: Key Concepts for the FRCA.* Cambridge: Cambridge University Press. © M. Cross and E. Plunkett 2008.

Give examples of drugs that influence cerebral blood flow

Drugs can influence cerebral metabolism and therefore CBF.

Thiopentone, etomidate and propofol reduce the cerebral metabolic rate for oxygen thereby reducing the CBF. Thiopentone can be infused therapeutically to reduce CBF therefore reducing cerebral blood volume and ICP following head injuries.

Volatile agents cause vasodilatation of cerebral vessels, therefore increasing CBF. This effect can be reduced by hyperventilation and is less profound with sevoflurane. At MACs greater than 1.5 they abolish autoregulation. Newer volatile agents such as isoflurane and sevoflurane also decrease neuronal function and so lead to uncoupling of blood flow and metabolism. This effect is concentration dependent. Nitrous oxide is a potent vasodilator and increases CBF. It also increases $CMRO_2$. Opioids appear to have no direct effects but may have secondary effects if they cause respiratory depression and increase $PaCO_2$. Rapid boluses of strong opioids are thought to be associated with a rise in ICP which could be secondary to autoregulation resulting in vasodilatation due to a rapid fall in MAP.

How is cerebral blood flow measured?

Cerebral blood flow can be measured in a number of ways.

Methods used in research are described below:

The Fick principle can be employed using nitrous oxide. This is referred to as the Kety–Schmidt technique. The equation used is:

$$CBF = \frac{\text{quantity of } N_2O \text{ removed by the brain from the circulation per unit time}}{\text{arteriovenous difference}}.$$

This method gives only an averaged value and measures global flows.

Radioactive techniques can be used. Inhalation or injection of xenon-133 allows its decay to be detected over different parts of the brain therefore regional flows can be measured.

Single photon emission computed tomography and positron emission tomography can be used with radiodense contrast to quantify regional CBF.

Methods used clinically include transcranial Doppler ultrasonography and jugular bulb catheterisation. Transcranial Doppler ultrasonography involves placing probes extracranially to measure the velocity of red blood cells passing through large vessels using the Doppler shift principle. The middle cerebral artery is commonly used, as it is easy to detect and receives a large proportion of the blood from the internal carotid and allows easy probe fixation. The diameter of the vessel is not commonly affected by physiological variables, so provided this and the angle of insonation remains constant, changes in the velocity correlate closely with changes in CBF. These changes in velocity or waveforms can be used to detect ischaemia and vasospasm and to estimate the CPP.

What do you understand by the Doppler effect?

The Doppler effect is when a signal frequency is increased as the signal source approaches and is decreased as the signal source moves away. It is used clinically to detect velocities and flow rates of moving substances. An ultrasound beam is directed along the path of flow of the blood cells and the sound waves reflect from the surfaces of the cells with different frequencies as they move towards and away from the probe. Analysis of the frequencies allows calculation of the velocity of flow.

What is jugular bulb catheterisation?

Jugular bulb catheterisation involves inserting a central venous catheter into one of the jugular veins. The jugular bulb is a dilatation of the internal jugular vein just below the base of the skull – the tip of the catheter should sit within this bulb. The catheter is inserted with the Seldinger technique using the same landmarks as normal central venous cannulation; however, the catheter is directed caudally towards the external auditory meatus.

Once inserted blood can be sampled for pO_2 and oxygen saturation, lactate and other substances. These measurements can give an indication of the adequacy of CBF. Lower values suggest a greater uptake by the brain and therefore decreased blood flow, providing there is no change in oxygen consumption and that it is uniform throughout the brain tissue.

Indwelling oximetric catheters can be used which give a continuous oxygen saturation measurement reflecting global cerebral perfusion. A drop in saturation may reflect cerebral hypoperfusion.

The drawbacks of jugular bulb saturations include the lack of information on regional differences in cerebral perfusion – it only provides an idea of global cerebral function. Furthermore, if the overall CBF and oxygen consumption were to decrease as a result of brain injury this would result in an overall decrease in oxygen uptake and saturations may remain unchanged.

1.3.2. CSF – Sarah F Bell

What is the function of CSF?

This question lends itself to a short introduction and then a descriptive list of functions.

CSF is a specialist extra-cellular fluid that bathes the central nervous system. It has a number of functions. Firstly, it offers mechanical protection for the brain by providing buoyancy. The low specific gravity of CSF reduces the effective weight of the brain from 1.4 kg to 47 g thus reducing brain inertia and protecting it against deformation due to acceleration or deceleration forces. Secondly, the CSF provides a constant chemical environment for neuronal activity. Thirdly it plays a role in the central chemo-receptor control of respiration and finally it helps to regulate ICP.

What is the volume of CSF?

The volume of CSF is between 100 and 150 ml, of this one-third to half of the fluid is contained within the subarachnoid space whilst the rest is in the ventricles.

How is CSF produced?

CSF is produced by the specialised cells of the choroid plexus. A combination of filtration and active transport through the fenestrated capillary of the epithelial cells controls the substances passing through the blood–CSF barrier. (This is distinct from the blood–brain barrier which consists of endothelial cells linked by tight junctions whose function is to protect the brain from chemicals in the bloodstream.) The choroid plexus is located in the third, fourth and lateral ventricles. CSF is produced at a rate of 3 ml/min or 500 ml/day. Its formation is dependent of the cerebral perfusion pressure. When this falls below 70 mmHg, CSF production also decreases because of the reduction in cerebral and choroid plexus blood flow.

Can you describe the circulation of CSF?

CSF flow is aided by the cilliary movements of the ependymal cells. It flows from the lateral ventricles via the foramen of Munro to the third ventricle. It then passes to the fourth ventricle via the aqueduct of Sylvius. CSF leaves the fourth ventricle via the single foramen Magendie which is located in the posterior midline or the two foramina of Luschka which are positioned laterally. CSF then passes either down the spinal cord or up and around the cerebral hemispheres.

How is the CSF reabsorbed?

The CSF is reabsorbed mostly by the arachnoid villi and then passes into the dural sinuses. The mechanism behind resorption is the difference between the CSF and venous pressure. A small amount of CSF may be absorbed into the spinal veins via the spinal nerve cuffs.

Can you suggest any conditions that may cause hydrocephalus?

An increase in CSF production, obstruction in circulation or inadequate resorption may result in hydrocephalus. This may be due to congenital abnormalities, tumours, haemorrhage, infection, meningeal disease or choroid plexus tumours.

Please can you compare the constitution of CSF and plasma?

This question may be difficult to answer because there are many differences to mention. It may be worth writing down a table to help you remember the salient points.

The CSF concentration of sodium ions is approximately 140 mmol/L, calcium ions is 1.2 mmol/L, potassium ions is 3 mmol/L and glucose is 4 mmol/L. These ionic concentrations are all lower than in plasma. In contrast, the CSF concentration of chloride ions is 120 mmol/L which is higher than that in the plasma. The plasma and CSF concentrations of bicarbonate are approximately equal. The osmolality of both plasma and CSF is 290 mOsmol/kgH$_2$O. The pCO$_2$ of CSF is higher than that of plasma, being approximately 6.6 rather than 5.2 kPa and the pH is lower in CSF by approximately 0.8. CSF contains hardly any protein compared to plasma, the figures being 0.2–0.4 g/L compared to 70 g/L. The white blood cell count is also much lower in normal CSF, ranging from 0 to 5 cells per mm^3 compared with 4000 to 110 000 per mm^3 in the plasma.

What is the role of CSF in the control of respiration?

This question is key knowledge so take the time to learn it well.

The central chemoreceptors are sensitive to changes in hydrogen ion concentration. They are situated in the floor of the fourth ventricle and ventral surface of the medulla and are bathed in CSF.

CO_2 freely diffuses into the CSF and then combines with water to form carbonic acid which dissociates to form hydrogen ions and bicarbonate. The CSF hydrogen ions then diffuse into the chemoreceptor tissue and act as an indirect measure of the partial pressure of carbon dioxide and stimulate the chemoreceptors. Owing to the poor protein content in CSF, minimal buffering occurs. Changes in the arterial partial pressure of carbon dioxide therefore cause more sensitive pH changes in CSF than in the plasma.

An increase in the partial pressure of carbon dioxide stimulates the respiratory centre to produce hyperventilation via the central chemoreceptors. If this is sustained a slow compensatory mechanism comes into play due to secretion of bicarbonate into CSF buffering the pH.

What is the purpose of examining the content of CSF?

The examiners are asking a more clinical question to assess your ability to apply your physiological knowledge in a clinical setting.

The purpose of a CSF analysis is to aid diagnosis of disorders affecting the central nervous system. For example, meningitis and encephalitis, syphilis, subarachnoid haemorrhage, de myelinating diseases including MS and Guillain-Barré and metastatic tumours (e.g., leukaemia) and central nervous system tumours that shed cells into the CSF.

What tests can be performed on CSF?

Routine examination of CSF may include visual observation of colour and clarity and tests for glucose, protein, lactate, red blood cell count, white blood cell count with differential, syphilis serology, Gram stain and bacterial culture.

The concentration of glucose in the CSF is normally two-thirds of the fasting plasma glucose. A glucose level that is below one-third of the plasma level is significant and may occur in bacterial and fungal meningitis and malignancy. A raised CSF glucose concentration may occur in viral meningitis.

CSF protein content is normally extremely low. Elevated levels may be seen in bacterial or tuberculous meningitis, demyelinating diseases, subarachnoid haemorrhage, traumatic tap and tumours.

The CSF lactate is used mainly to help differentiate bacterial and fungal meningitis, which cause increased lactate, from viral meningitis, which does not.

The white cell count in CSF is usually very low. An increase may occur in many conditions including infection, allergy, leukemia, demyelination, haemorrhage and traumatic tap. The differential count will help to distinguish between diagnoses.

While not normally found in CSF, red blood cells will appear whenever bleeding has occurred. They therefore signal subarachnoid haemorrhage, stroke or traumatic tap.

Gram stain, culture, acid-fast stain for *Mycobacterium tuberculosis*, fungal culture and syphilis serology may all be performed on CSF samples.

1.3.3. Blood–brain barrier – Rebecca A Leslie

What is the blood–brain barrier?

The blood–brain barrier is a physiological barrier between the blood and the brain which restricts the transfer of molecules from the plasma to the brain.

How do the endothelial cells of the capillaries in the blood–brain barrier alter from those in the rest of the body?

In the rest of the body the endothelial cells of the capillaries are separated by small gaps called fenestrations which allow the passage of molecules from the blood to the tissues and from the tissues back to the blood. However in the brain the endothelial cells are packed very densely and joined together by tight junctions which prevents the passage of molecules from the blood to the brain. In addition the cerebral capillary endothelial cell possesses a greater number and volume of mitochondria than the capillaries in the rest of the body.

Are any other cells involved in the blood–brain barrier?

Yes. The endothelial cells are surrounded by a basement membrane which is in turn in close contact with the foot processes of astrocytes which essentially separates the capillaries from the neurones.

In summary there are three structures which are involved in the blood–brain barrier:

- The endothelium
- The basement membrane
- The astrocytes from the blood–brain barrier.

In addition to this structural barrier there is a metabolic barrier. This consists of enzymes located on the peripheral processes of the astrocytes, which metabolise specific substances before they reach the brain tissue where they could cause significant damage.

Give me three examples of drugs which are metabolised by the blood–brain barrier

Try to give examples of common drugs which are relevant to anaesthesia.

The astrocytes contain monoamine oxidase which breaks down dopamine and nor-adrenaline before they reach the brain tissue. For this reason L-DOPA, the precursor to dopamine, which is able to pass through the blood–brain barrier, is administered for dopamine deficiencies such as Parkinson's disease rather than dopamine.

Ester local anaesthetics are also metabolised by the cholinesterases present on the astro-cytes in the blood–brain barrier protecting the brain from the effects of the local anaesthetic agent.

Ammonia which is potentially neurotoxic is able to cross the brain capillary endothelium but is metabolised before it reaches the brain tissue.

Which substances are able to freely pass though the blood–brain barrier?

The tight junctions of the capillary endothelium mean that only highly lipid-soluble substances that are able to traverse cell membranes are able to freely cross the blood–brain barrier. Examples include carbon dioxide, oxygen, alcohol, steroids and inhalational anaesthetic agents.

In addition there are specialised transport systems that allow the transport of biologically significant water-soluble substances such as D-glucose, phenylalanine, lactate, arginine and choline. Hormones such as thyroxine and insulin can also cross the blood–brain barrier by carrier transport.

In general small, lipid-soluble, unionised and unbound drugs will pass though the blood–brain barrier. Drugs which are large and polar, such as neuromuscular blocking agents, have only a very limited ability to cross the blood–brain barrier.

What are the functions of the blood–brain barrier?

It is important you know the functions of the blood–brain barrier. Start with the most important functions.

The functions of the blood–brain barrier include:

- Protection of the brain from endogenous and exogenous toxins present in the plasma
- Provides tight control of the ionic concentrations of hydrogen, sodium, potassium, calcium and magnesium to which the brain is extremely sensitive
- Protects the brain from transient changes in plasma glucose levels
- Prevents the release of central neurotransmitters into the systemic circulation.

Can you tell me situations where there are pathological changes in the blood–brain barrier?

The integrity of the blood–brain barrier is disrupted by many pathological processes such as inflammation, oedema, hypertension and epilepsy.

In meningitis when the meninges become inflamed there is disruption of the blood–brain barrier. This allows the passage of substances which would not normally be able to enter in to the brain tissue. However it does also have advantages, as it allows anti-biotics to enter the brain interstitium and help treat the meningitis.

In both acute and chronic hypertension the blood–brain barrier also become disrupted. In acute hypertension this is thought to be as a result of the stretching and weakening of the tight junctions.

After an epileptic seizure there is a rise in blood pressure and blood flow which causes weakening of the tight junctions and transiently allows the movement of normally excluded substances. The blood–brain barrier is normally restored within 1 hour of the seizure.

The auto-immune condition, multiple sclerosis also affects the blood–brain barrier. It is thought that in multiple sclerosis the blood–brain barrier is broken down and allows T lymphocytes to cross into the central nervous system and attack the myelin.

It is also thought that in Alzheimer's disease there is a disruption of the blood–brain barrier which allows plasma amyloid plaques to pass into the brain tissue where they are deposited in astrocytes.

How do we administer drugs we wish to act in the central nervous system?

It is a challenge overcoming the difficulty of delivering therapeutic agents to specific regions of the brain. The neuroprotective role of the blood–brain barrier prevents the delivery of many potentially therapeutic agents and diagnostic interventions to the brain.

In order to give drugs to target the brain the drug must either go through or bypass the blood–brain barrier. In order to deliver drugs to the brain, the blood–brain barrier can be disrupted by osmotic means, for example by giving mannitol. It is also possible to disrupt the blood–brain barrier by the use of vasoactive substances such as bradykinin. Another strategy to allow drugs to pass through the blood–brain barrier is to use one of the endogenous transport systems, such as the carrier-mediated transporters for glucose or amino acids.

To avoid the blood–brain barrier completely an alternative method is to give the drugs via an intra-ventricular catheter.

Which parts of the brain lie outside the blood–brain barrier?

Rather than just learning a list of the regions of the brain that lie outside the blood–brain barrier try and learn the reasons behind it. This will make it much easier to understand and remember.

There are several areas of the brain which lie outside the blood–brain barrier, these include the area postrema, the median eminence, the pineal gland, the neurohypophysis of the posterior pituitary and the choroid plexus.

The area postrema is also called the "vomiting center". It lies outside the blood–brain barrier so that when a toxic substance enters the bloodstream it will be sensed in the area postrema and may cause vomiting. This is a protective mechanism where the toxic substance is eliminated from the stomach before more harm can be done.

The pineal gland secretes melanin into the bloodstream and is responsible for circadian rhythms, if it was within the blood–brain barrier the melanin would not be free to pass into the systemic circulation and it would not be able to exert its affects.

The neurohypophysis of the posterior pituitary is responsible for the release of the neurohormones oxytocin and vasopressin (anti-diuretic hormone) into the blood therefore it is important that it lies outside the blood–brain barrier.

The median eminence also lies outside the blood–brain barrier, this is imperative as it regulates the control of the anterior pituitary through the release of neurohormones.

Do neonates have a fully functioning blood–brain barrier?

No. The blood–brain barrier of neonates is not as effective as that of adults. As a result there is an increased passage of drugs into the central nervous system such as opiate analgesics. There is also an increased passage of substances such as bile salts which have the potential to cause kernicterus.

1.3.4. Action potentials – Rebecca A Leslie

What do you understand by the term resting membrane potential?

Cell membranes have an electrical charge across them, with the inside being negative compared to the outside. This is called the membrane potential. The membrane potential depends on the selective membrane permeability to various ions, and the different ionic concentrations on the inside and the outside of the cell. The membranes can be described as semi-permeable, as they let some ions through but will not let others pass. For example, in a resting cell most membranes are permeable to potassium but impermeable to sodium.

The concentration of potassium inside the cell is 150 mmol which is much higher than outside the cells, 5 mmol. Potassium diffuses down this concentration gradient, but only to the point at which the negative potential attracting them into the cell is balanced by the chemical gradient out of the cell. For example there are negatively charged proteins, phosphates and sulphates that are trying to draw in the positively charged potassium ions. At the resting membrane potential of around –70 mV, the electrical and chemical gradients acting on potassium are balanced. The cell membranes are relatively impermeable to cations, including sodium, so these ions contribute little to the resting potential.

What is the Nernst equation?

The Nernst equation is used to calculate the potential difference that any ion would produce if the membrane was fully permeable to it.

In the resting state the cell membranes are almost fully permeable to potassium, therefore the Nernst potential for potassium is similar to resting membrane potential at –94 mV.

This is not true for sodium because the membranes are relatively impermeable to this ion, and the Nernst potential for sodium is +80 mV.

So if the situation is reversed and sodium channels open and all potassium channels are closed, which is the situation in excitable cells, the membrane potential equals the Nernst potential of sodium, +80 mV. If different numbers of sodium and potassium channels are opened then the membrane potential is between these two extremes.

The Nernst equation states that:

$$E = \frac{RT}{zF} \times \ln \frac{[Co]}{[Ci]}$$

where E is the equilibrium potential, R is the universal gas constant, T is the absolute temperature, z is the valency, F is the Faraday constant, [Co] is the concentration of the ion outside the cell and [Ci] is the concentration of the ion inside the cell.

At the normal resting potential of –70 mV both chemical (the concentration gradient) and electrical (the negative charge inside) gradients are tending to move sodium into the cell. Although the cell membranes are relatively impermeable to sodium, some sodium does manage to pass through the cell membrane into the cell. If this sodium was not removed out of the cell by the Na^+/K^+ ATP pump then the membrane potential would gradually diminish. The Na^+/K^+ ATP pump extrudes three sodium ions in exchange for two potassium ions and utilises ATP. This inequality in sodium for potassium contributes to the negative membrane potential within the cell.

Describe the action potential as it passes along a nerve cell

You should draw a diagram whilst describing nerve action potentials, see Figure 1.3.4a.

Nerve cells have a low threshold for excitation. During the action potential the resting membrane polarity reverses so that it becomes positive inside the cell relative to the outside.

When the nerve is stimulated it initiates the opening of ligand-gated ion channels that increase the permeability of sodium. As a result, sodium ions move into the cell initiating depolarisation (phase 1).

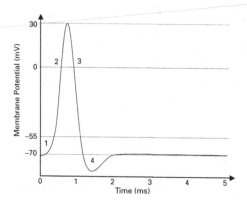

Draw and label the axes as shown.

Phase 1   The curve should cross the y axis at approximately -70 mV and should be shown to rapidly rise towards the threshold potential of -55 mV.

Phase 2   This portion of the curve demonstrates the rapid rise in membrane potential to a peak of $+30$ mV as voltage-gated Na^+ channels allow rapid Na^+ entry into the cell.

Phase 3   This phase shows rapid repolarization as Na^+ channels close and K^+ channels open, allowing K^+ efflux. The slope of the downward curve is almost as steep as that seen in phase 2.

Phase 4   This phase shows that the membrane potential 'overshoots' in a process known as hyperpolarization as the Na^+/K^+ pump lags behind in restoring the normal ion balance.

Figure 1.3.4a. Nerve action potential. Reproduced with permission from Cross, M. and Plunkett, E. 2008. *Physics, Pharmacology and Physiology for Anaesthetists: Key Concepts for the FRCA.* Cambridge: Cambridge University Press. © M. Cross and E. Plunkett 2008.

When the depolarisation reaches a threshold potential of approximately -55 mV the change in membrane potential opens voltage-gated fast sodium channels, allowing sodium to flood into the cell (phase 2). With the movement of sodium the potential of the cell rapidly overshoots the isopotential line to approximately $+30$ mV. This is called the positive spike of the action potential. It could be expected from the Nernst equation that the membrane potential would reach $+80$ mV. This is because it is the Nernst potential for sodium ions, and hence the potential difference which will develop across the cell wall if sodium is freely permeable is $+80$ mV. However the action potential never quite reaches the Nernst potential for sodium because at peak depolarisation the sodium channels inactivate and the permeability to sodium plummets.

As the sodium channels close potassium channels open, causing potassium to move out of the cell in a process called repolarisation (phase 3). This process returns the cell membrane to its resting potential.

During the final stage in the action potential the depolarisation continues past the resting potential, this is due to a continued potassium efflux and this is known as hyperpolarisation (phase 4).

What is the absolute refractory period?

The absolute refractory period starts as the voltage-gated fast sodium channels open when the threshold potential is met and continues until the repolarisation is a third complete. This period is approximately 1 msec long and the nerve cell cannot be excited by any stimulus despite how strong it is.

How does this differ from the relative refractory period?

The absolute refractory period is followed by a period of 2–3 msec which due to high permeability of potassium ions an action potential can be initiated but only with a supra-maximal stimulus. These refractory periods mean that action potentials are only propagated in one direction and also limits the frequency of the conduction of nerve impulses.

1.3.5. Spinal cord – Natasha A Joshi

Describe the anatomy of the spinal cord

If you can draw a basic diagram whilst you are talking, this will enable you to convey informa-tion more quickly and show that you understand what you are talking about (Figure 1.3.5a).

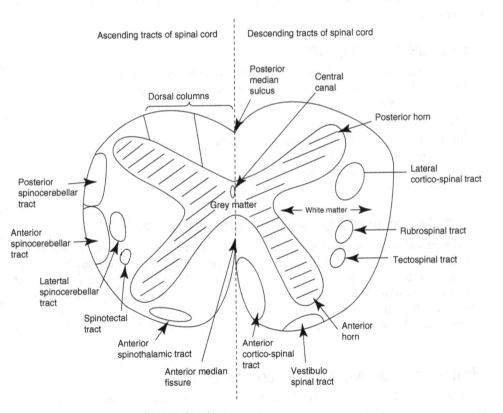

Figure 1.3.5a. The anatomy of the spinal cord.

The spinal cord forms part of the central nervous system. Superiorly, it begins at the foramen magnum, as a continuation of the medulla oblongata. Inferiorly, it terminates at the level of the first or second lumbar vertebrae, where it tapers to form the conus medullaris. From here, the filum terminale (consisting of pia mater) extends inferiorly and attaches to the coccyx. At birth, the spinal cord terminates at the level of the third lumbar vertebra, but it rises to the adult level by the age of 20.

The spinal cord is situated in the vertebral canal and surrounded by the meninges, the pia, arachnoid and dura mater. It is bathed in cerebrospinal fluid, occupying the subarachnoid space, and stabilised within the dura, by the denticulate ligaments.

In cross section, it is roughly a cylindrical structure, with an anterior median fissure (which is a deep longitudinal fissure), and a posterior median sulcus (which is more of a shallow longitudinal furrow). Working from the inside outwards, there is a central canal, which contains CSF. This is surrounded by an H-shaped area of grey matter. The "points of the H" correspond to the anterior and posterior horns. In the thoracic region of the spinal cord, there are also two lateral horns, which convey the sympathetic tracts. White matter surrounds the grey matter, and consists of ascending and descending tracts (most of which are myelinated), hence its white appearance. Grey matter contains the cell bodies of neurones, hence its grey appearance.

Throughout its length, the spinal cord gives off 31 pairs of spinal nerves. It has dorsal and ventral roots. The dorsal roots convey sensory or afferent fibres from peripheral sensors to the spinal cord, whereas the ventral roots convey motor or efferent fibres from the spinal cord to their effector organs.

Describe the ascending tracts

The ascending tracts convey sensory information from peripheral sensors to higher centres in the brain. To describe them logically, in their anatomical arrangement from posterior to anterior, they consist of:

- The posterior/dorsal columns
- The posterior and anterior spinocerebellar tracts
- The lateral spinothalamic tract
- The anterior spinothalamic tract and
- The spinotectal tract.

Can you tell me more about the posterior/dorsal columns?

The posterior/dorsal columns convey sensory information about fine touch, proprioception and vibration sense, from the ipsilateral side of the body, ultimately to the sensory cortex in the brain. The fibres decussate (or cross over) in the medulla. The dorsal columns are divided anatomically into two bundles, or fasciculi. The gracile fasiculus is found medially, and carries information from the lower half of the body, (below the level of T6). The cuneate fasiculus is found laterally, conveying information from the upper half of the body (above the level of T6).

What do you know about the spinocerebellar tracts?

The posterior and anterior spinocerebellar tracts convey sensory information about proprioception, from the ipsilateral side of the body, to the cerebellum.

What is the difference between the spinothalamic tracts and the spino-tectal tract?

The lateral spinothalamic tract conveys sensory information about pain and temperature from the contralateral side of the body, to the thalamus and ultimately the sensory cortex.

The anterior spinothalamic tract conveys sensory information about crude touch and pressure from the contralateral side of the body, to the thalamus and ultimately the sensory cortex.

In contrast, the spinotectal tract conveys sensory information to the brainstem, required for the processing of spino-visual reflexes.

Describe the descending tracts

The descending tracts carry motor information from higher centres in the brain to the effector organs of the body. To describe them in their anatomical arrangement, from posterior to anterior, they consist of:

- The lateral cortico-spinal tract
- The rubrospinal, tectospinal and vestibulospinal tracts
- The anterior spinothalamic tract.

The lateral cortico-spinal tract conveys motor information from the cerebral cortex, to the contralateral side of the body, via the pyramidal tracts.

The rubrospinal, tectospinal and vestibulospinal tracts convey extra-pyramidal fibres from the brainstem nuclei, to lower motor neurones.

The anterior spinothalamic tract conveys motor information from the cerebral cortex, to the ipsilateral side of the body, via the extra-pyramidal tracts.

Describe the arterial blood supply to the spinal cord

The blood supply to the spinal cord is from a single anterior spinal artery, two posterior spinal arteries, and several radicular branches.

The anterior spinal artery is formed at the level of the foramen magnum, by the union of two branches of the vertebral arteries. It lies in the anterior median sulcus, and descends along the length of the spinal cord, supplying the anterior two-thirds of the cord with arterial blood.

The posterior spinal arteries arise from the posterior inferior cerebellar arteries. Each then divides into two branches, which descend along the lateral aspect of the spinal cord, one branch posterior, and one anterior to the dorsal nerve roots. These vessels supply the posterior one-third of the cord with arterial blood.

The radicular branches arise segmentally, from local arteries, such as the cervical, intercostal and lumbar arteries. They supply local areas of the spinal cord. The most important radicular branches are those at T1 and T11–L3, the so called "artery of Adamkiewicz". This is crucial in supplying the lower two-thirds of the spinal cord with arterial blood and occlusion of the artery may result in cord ischaemia and subsequent paralysis.

What are the effects of an acute spinal cord injury?

Always try to classify if you can, be this early and late effects, or systems of the body.

The features of an acute spinal cord injury may be subdivided into the systems of the body that are affected:

Cardiovascular

Initially hypertension and peripheral vasoconstriction are seen. Arrhythmias are also common. With lesions at the level of T6 and above, hypotension may be observed, as a result of vasodilatation and blood pooling. At T1 and above, bradycardia is common, due to sympathetic disruption- so called "spinal shock".

Respiratory

The effects of an acute spinal cord injury on the respiratory system depend upon the level of the lesion. Obviously the higher the lesion, the greater the effects are on ventilation.

- Lesions at C4 and above will result in diaphragmatic paralysis, with gross impairment of ventilation.
- Lesions at C6 and below will leave the diaphragm intact, however intercostal muscle paralysis and a diminished cough will be seen.
- Lesions at T7 and above will cause alterations in oxygenation and ventilation due to a diminished vital capacity, FEV1 and expiratory reserve volume.

Neurological

Following an acute spinal cord injury, flaccid paralysis is seen. This may last for 2–3 weeks and is followed by a spastic paralysis. There is also visceral and somatic sensory loss below the level of the lesion.

With cervical lesions, neurogenic pulmonary oedema is common.

Gastrointestinal

Gastric paralysis and paralytic ileus are commonly seen and lead to abdominal distension, which may further impair ventilation. The risks of gastric aspiration are also increased due to excess gastric secretions, gastric dilatation and an ineffective cough.

Metabolic

Thermoregulation is often impaired. Other common features include a respiratory acidosis (as a result of hypoventilation), metabolic alkalosis and hypokalaemia (due to vomiting and gastric suctioning).

Can you describe Brown–Sequard syndrome?

Brown–Sequard syndrome results from hemisection of the spinal cord. The clinical features include:

- Loss of fine touch on the ipsilateral side of the body
- Loss of proprioception and vibration sense on the ipsilateral side of the body
- Loss of pain and temperature sensation on the contralateral side of the body, a so-called "dissociative sensory loss"
- Motor weakness is observed on the ipsilateral side, below the level of the spinal cord lesion.

These findings occur as a result of the points at which the sensory and motor tracts decussate in the central nervous system.

Can you describe the anatomical structures that the Tuohy needle passes through, when performing an epidural?

From the outside moving inwards, the structures passed through are:

- Skin
- Subcutaneous tissue
- Suspraspinous ligament
- Interspinous ligament
- Ligamentum flavum
- Epidural space.

For a spinal the structures passed through are:

- Dura mater
- Subarachnoid space.

1.3.6. Reflex arc – Emily K Johnson

What is a reflex arc?

A reflex arc is a pathway involving the nervous system resulting in a predictable repetitive response to a particular sensory input and generally not involving voluntary control. The pathway consists of:

- A sense organ
- An afferent neurone
- One or more synapses
- An efferent neurone
- An effector

Can you tell me a little more about different types of reflex arc?

The reflex arc can be classified according to its complexity, which is the number of synapses involved. They can be monosynaptic, such as stretch reflexes, or polysynaptic with two or more synapses such as the withdrawal reflex. Activation of a simple reflex may have widespread effects due to ascending, descending pathways and excitatory and inhibitory interneurone involvement. In addition to involving skeletal muscle, reflex arcs are the basis of the functioning of the autonomic nervous system.

Autonomic reflex arcs can be classified according to the source of the afferent input:

- The autonomic nervous system – for example a tachycardia in response to baroreceptor stimulation in hypotension
- The central nervous system – such as a "vaso-vagal" episode in response to unpleasant visual stimulus.

The autonomic reflex arcs can also be classified according to whether the efferent limb is part of the parasympathetic or the sympathetic nervous system.

Give an example of a monosynaptic reflex arc

You should be able to draw a basic reflex arc and talk through it to help you answer such questions.

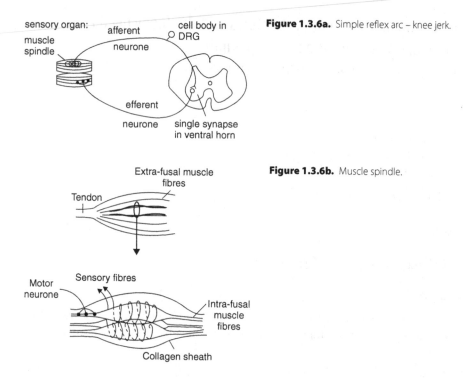

Figure 1.3.6a. Simple reflex arc – knee jerk.

Figure 1.3.6b. Muscle spindle.

An example of the simplest type of reflex arc, a monosynaptic reflex arc, is the knee jerk (Figure 1.3.6a). The sense organ is a muscle spindle which is stimulated by passive stretching of the muscle. Then a group 1a afferent neurone transmits an impulse straight to the ventral horn of the spinal cord. Here there is a synapse directly onto an α motor neurone which results in activation of extra-fusal muscle fibres and contraction of the quadriceps muscle. The excitatory transmitter released is glutamate which produces an excitatory postsynaptic potential (EPSP). The EPSPs summate to generate a motor neurone action potential. The afferent neurone also synapses on an inhibitory interneuron which relaxes the opposing muscle group allowing the unopposed contraction of the quadriceps. The neurotransmitter released at the inhibitory interneurone is glycine which hyperpolarises the motor neurone membrane by opening chloride channels. This produces an inhibitory post-synaptic potential, an IPSP.

Tell me more about muscle spindles and how they work

A quick sketch of a muscle spindle would be helpful to illustrate this answer, see Figure 1.3.6b.

Muscle spindles are capsules of fibres present in skeletal muscle that detect muscle length and movement. Their fibres are called intra-fusal fibres and are parallel and attached to the skeletal muscle fibres, also called extra-fusal fibres. The intra-fusal fibres are modified muscle fibres with contractile ends but a central non-contractile portion, and each spindle contains 3 to 10 such fibres enclosed in a collagen sheath. There are three types of intra-fusal fibres:

- The dynamic nuclear bag or bag 1 fibres
- The static nuclear bag or bag 2 fibres
- The nuclear chain fibres.

The muscle spindles have sensory and motor innervation. There are two sensory supplies to each spindle, primary and secondary afferents. They terminate on the central non-contractile element of the intra-fusal fibres. Primary afferents are also known as 1a or dynamic fibres and are more sensitive to rate of change of fibre length. They connect to nuclear bag and nuclear chain fibres at junctions called annulospiral endings. They are the larger and faster fibres and fire when the muscle is stretching but adapt and stop firing when the muscle stops changing length, therefore conveying proprioceptive information about the rate of change of the muscle concerned. Secondary afferents are also known as 2 or static fibres and are more sensitive to absolute fibre length.

The motor innervation is by γ-motor neurones which cause a slight contraction in the ends of the fibres when activated. The γ-motor neurones are classified according to the intra-fusal fibres they innervate. Static motor neurones innervate the nuclear chain or bag 2 fibres and dynamic motor neurones innervate the bag 1 fibres and increase the sensitivity of the 1a afferent fibres. The γ-motor neurones do not supplement overall muscle contraction; they modify the sensitivity of the muscle spindle to stretch. At the γ-motor neurone neuromuscular junction when acetylcholine is released, the contractile end portions of the intra-fusal fibres contract. This stretches the non-contractile central portion of the fibre and opens stretch sensitive ion channels on the afferent axons positioned on the central part of the intra-fusal fibre. These channels allow entry of sodium therefore increasing the resting potential and making an action potential more likely, so increasing fibre sensitivity.

What are the different types of motor neurone?

Define and classify.

A motor neurone is a neurone that originates in the central nervous system and extends its axon into the periphery to innervate skeletal muscle directly or indirectly. Motor neurones can be classified as upper motor neurones or lower motor neurone.

Upper motor neurones are neurones of the motor pathways in the CNS. Lower motor neurones are neurones that directly innervate muscle. A lower motor neurone is often referred to as an efferent neurone and there are two types: α and γ. The α-motor neurones are large with axons of 10 to 20 μm in diameter and innervate the extra-fusal fibres of skeletal muscle. The γ-motor neurones are smaller with axon diameters of approximately 3 to 6 μm in diameter and innervate the intra-fusal fibres of muscle spindles. The cell bodies of α- and γ-motor neurones lie in the ventral horn of the spinal cord. They can be excited or inhibited by descending pathways or as part of a reflex arc by afferent neurones synapsing directly onto the cell bodies.

Tell me about the different sensory receptors

Sensory receptors are the receptors initiating the reflex arc. They can be classified according to the stimulus that they react to. They include mechanoreceptors, chemoreceptors, thermoreceptors, photoreceptors and nociceptors.

Mechanoreceptors detect changes both inside and outside the body. They include muscle spindles that detect stretching of muscle fibres, tendon organs that respond to muscle tension, baroreceptors responding to change in blood pressure and pressure receptors responding to external pressure.

Chemoreceptors detect changes in hydrogen ion concentration in body fluids and are also involved in taste and smell.

Thermoreceptors include hypothalamic temperature receptors and cutaneous temperature receptors.

Photoreceptors on the retina are involved in sight.

Nociceptors are a broad name for the classification of pain receptors. These react to any potentially harmful stimulus such as mechanical or chemical stimulus, and include the receptor classes already mentioned.

What are the mechanisms that cause activation of the sensory receptors?

Sensory receptors are usually activated as the afferent nerve endings are depolarised by certain stimuli such as sodium influx due to increased membrane permeability to sodium. This localised depolarisation of the nerve terminal is known as the generator potential. Generator potentials vary according to the stimulus intensity and can fire off action potentials in the afferent nerve axon. The nerve terminals can take the form of free or unmyelinated nerve endings, Pacinian corpuscles where lamellae cover the free nerve ending and sense changes in pressure, or be connected to specialised receptor cells such as in muscle spindles, vision and hearing.

What are Golgi tendon organs?

Golgi tendon organs are mechanoreceptors located at the site where skeletal muscle fibres insert into tendons. They exist in series with muscle fibres and sense tension in the muscle contraction. They are innervated by 1b afferent fibres which are large myelinated fibres. The 1b afferents either ascend to the cerebellum or synapse on interneurones in the spinal cord and are involved in reflexes. The overall function of Golgi tendon organs is to provide sensory feedback to help the regulation of muscle contraction via reflex pathways and central control.

1.3.7. The autonomic nervous system and adrenoceptors – Rebecca A Leslie

What is the role of the autonomic nervous system?

The autonomic nervous system provides the efferent pathways for the involuntary control of most organs, with the exception of the motor innervation of skeletal muscle. The autonomic nervous system consists of the parasympathetic and the sympathetic nervous systems.

Both the parasympathetic and the sympathetic nervous systems contain pre-ganglionic neurones which originate in the central nervous system and synapse with post-ganglionic neurons in the autonomic ganglia and innervate target organs. The pre-ganglionic fibres are slow-conducting B fibres that release acetylcholine which acts on the cholinergic nicotinic receptors of the post-ganglionic fibres. The post-ganglionic fibres are unmyelinated slow-conducting C fibres and the neurotransmitter varies depending on whether they are sympathetic or parasympathetic fibres.

Tell me more about the parasympathetic nervous system

The pre-ganglionic fibres of the parasympathetic nervous system have a cranial and a sacral outflow. The cranial efferents originate in the brainstem and travel in the third, seventh, ninth and tenth cranial nerves. The parasympathetic outflow in the third, seventh and ninth cranial nerves supplies the parasympathetic function of the head, whilst the parasympathetic fibres in the tenth cranial nerve supply the thoracic and abdominal viscera.

The sacral outflow originates in the second, third and fourth sacral nerves and supplies the pelvic viscera.

The parasympathetic nervous system tends to have long pre-ganglionic fibres and short post-ganglionic fibres. The post-ganglionic nerve fibres release acetylcholine and act on cholinergic muscarinic receptors.

The parasympathetic nervous system can be described as coordinating "rest or digest" responses. For example the parasympathetic nervous system controls secretion from many glands, such as tear glands, salivary glands and mucus glands in the gut. It is also responsible for increased motility of the gut, relaxation of the pyloric and ileocolic sphincters.

What are the similarities and differences between the sympathetic and the parasympathetic nervous systems?

In contrast to the parasympathetic nervous system, the outflow of the sympathetic nervous system originates from the lateral horns of the spinal cord at the thoracic and upper lumbar levels, typically T1 to L2. These efferents leave the spinal cord through the ventral roots with the spinal nerves. They then leave the spinal nerves as white rami communicantes and synapse with post-ganglionic fibres in the sympathetic ganglion. The post-ganglionic fibres leave the sympathetic ganglion as grey rami communicantes and supply the target viscera or they re-join the spinal nerves.

The pre-ganglionic fibres of the sympathetic nervous system are short due to the presence of the sympathetic ganglion, and the post-ganglionic fibres are much longer. This is the opposite situation to the parasympathetic nervous system, which has long pre-ganglionic and short post-ganglionic fibres. In both the parasympathetic and the sympathetic nervous system the pre-ganglionic fibres are myelinated B fibres, whilst the post-ganglionic fibres are unmyelinated C fibres. The pre-ganglionic fibres of both the parasympathetic and the sympathetic nervous system release acetylcholine and act on cholinergic nicotinic receptors on the post ganglionic fibre. However the majority of post-ganglionic fibres in the sympathetic nervous system release noradrenaline at target sites which acts on adrenoceptors, whilst the post-ganglionic fibres of the parasympathetic system release acetylcholine and act on cholinergic muscarinic receptors.

Which post-ganglionic sympathetic nerve fibres do not release noradrenaline?

The exception to the rule that post-ganglionic sympathetic nerve fibres release noradrenaline is the sympathetic innervation to sweat glands and the adrenal gland.

Post-ganglionic innervation to the sweat glands uses the neurotransmitter acetylcholine.

The pre-ganglionic fibres of the adrenal medulla release acetylcholine which acts directly on chromaffin cells, causing the release of adrenaline into the circulation. Therefore there are no post-ganglionic fibres in the adrenal medulla.

What different types of adrenoceptor have you heard of?

There are two main classes of adrenergic receptors: α and β. The α-adrenergic receptors are further classified into $\alpha 1$ and $\alpha 2$, and the β-adrenergic receptors into $\beta 1$, $\beta 2$ and $\beta 3$.

Describe the structure of an adrenergic receptor

All adrenergic receptors are G-protein coupled receptors. This means they are membrane-bound proteins with a serpentine structure that traverse the cell membrane seven times. Noradrenaline or other adrenergic agonists bind to the extra-cellular side of the receptor and as a result activates a G-protein on the cytosolic side of the receptor. This in turn activates intermediate messengers at the expense of GTP which gets broken down to GDP. These intermediate messengers then activate or inhibit effector proteins to bring about the intra-cellular change.

Which different G proteins do you know about, and why is this relevant to adrenoceptors?

The G-proteins consist of three subunits: α, β and γ. There are three different classes of G-protein as a result of different α-subunits.

G_s (stimulatory) proteins have α-subunits which stimulate adenylyl cyclase therefore increasing the amount of cyclic AMP. The cAMP is then responsible for the biochemical effect. In contrast G_I (inhibitory)-proteins have α-subunits which inhibit adenylyl cyclase so reduce levels of intra-cellular cAMP. G_q have α-subunits which activate phospholipase C. Phospholipase C controls the breakdown of phosphoinositides to form inositol triphosphate (IP_3) and diacylglycerol (DAG). IP_3 causes calcium release from the endoplasmic reticulum, which then causes membrane hyperpolarisation or enzyme release. DAG causes activation of protein kinase C, which results in biochemical effects specific to the nature of the cell.

The different types of G-proteins are of relevance when discussing adrenoceptors because the different adrenoceptors are linked with different G-proteins. For example, $\alpha 1$ adrenoceptors are linked to G_q-proteins and therefore mediate their effects by activating phospholipase C causing the release of IP_3. In contrast $\alpha 2$ adrenoceptors are linked to G_i proteins and are inhibitory in nature, inhibiting adenylyl cyclase, and reducing the intra-cellular levels of cAMP.

All the β-adrenoceptors are linked to G_s proteins and stimulate adenylyl cyclase to produce cAMP.

Where would you find adrenoreceptors?

All adrenoreceptors except $\alpha 2$-receptors are found on the post-synaptic membrane of the end organs. For example, they are found in vascular smooth muscle, the heart, bronchial smooth muscle, the liver and the uterus. The $\alpha 2$-receptors are pre-synaptic receptors.

What effect does stimulation of adrenergic receptors have?

When trying to remember the effects of each of the different receptors, think about drugs you use on a regular basis and what effects they have. For example you know that salbutamol is a $\beta 2$-agonist and causes bronchodilation.

Each of the adrenoreceptors have different effects when they are stimulated.

Activation of the $\alpha 1$-receptors causes vasoconstriction, relaxation of gut smooth muscle, hepatic glycogenolysis and saliva secretion.

In contrast activation of the $\alpha 2$-receptors inhibits the release of the neurotransmitter noradrenaline from autonomic nerves, as well as stimulating platelet aggregation.

β1-receptor activation causes positive inotropy and chronotropy, thus increases heart rate and myocardial contractility. β1-receptor stimulation also relaxes smooth muscle of the gut and can cause lipolysis.

Activation of β2-receptors causes bronchiolar dilatation, vasodilatation to skeletal muscle, relaxation of smooth muscle including uterus, bladder and urinary sphincter, hepatic glycogenolysis and gluconeogenesis, muscle tremors, increased renin release and inhibition of histamine release from mast cells.

β3-receptor activation mediates lipolysis, especially in brown fat and in addition mediates thermogenesis.

Classify sympathomimetic drugs

When describing classes of drugs it is always a good idea to have a classification system. Sympathomimetics lend themselves very nicely to being classified, and there are a number of different methods available. For example they can be classified by direct or non-direct acting, catecholamine or non-catecholamine and naturally occurring or synthetic. Choose one classification system and stick to it. For your information we describe all three methods here.

Mechanism of action

Sympathomimetic drugs can be classified according to their mechanism of action; direct acting or indirect acting drugs. Direct acting sympathomimetic drugs attach directly to the receptors whilst indirect sympathomimetics cause the release of noradrenaline to then produce their effects via these receptors. Examples of direct acting sympathomimetics include adrenaline, noradrenaline, phenylephrine, isoprenaline, dobutamine and dopexamine. Ephedrine and metaraminol have both indirect and direct mechanism of action.

Structure

The basic structure of a sympathomimetic is a benzene ring with an amine side chain at C1. If a hydroxyl group is also present at C3 and C4 it is known as a catecholamine. Adrenaline, noradrenaline, dopamine, dopexamine, isoprenaline and dobutamine are all catecholamines, whilst ephedrine, metaraminol and phenylephrine are non-catecholamines.

Naturally occurring or synthetic

A further classification for sympathomimetic agents would be to divide them into naturally occurring and synthetic agents. Adrenaline, noradrenaline and dopamine are all naturally occurring catecholamines, whilst isoprenaline, dobutamine, dopexamine, ephedrine and metaraminol are synthetic agents.

Can you tell me on which receptors the commonly used sympathomimetics exert their effects?

Adrenaline has both α-and β-agonist actions. Its effects vary according to the dose. At low doses the β-adrenergic effects predominate increasing the cardiac output, but at high doses, such as the 1 mg given after a cardiac arrest, α1 effects predominate causing a rise in systemic vascular resistance.

The actions of noradrenaline are mediated predominantly through α1-adrenoceptors, but it also acts on β-receptors.

Metaraminol has both α- and β-agonist effects, but like noradrenaline the α effects are most pronounced.

Ephedrine also has both α- and β-agonist effects but in contrast to metaraminol the β effects predominate.

Dopamine is an agonist at α1-, β-receptors and dopamine receptors. The receptors that dopamine works on is dependent on the dose. When given at a low dose, initially only dopamine receptors are activated, but as the dose is increased β-receptors and then α-receptors are activated.

Phenylephrine is a potent α1-agonist whilst clonidine only activates α2 receptors. Neither drug has any effect on β-receptors.

Isoprenaline is a non-specific β-adrenoceptor agonist.

Dobutamine also acts on both β1- and β2-receptors, but its β1 effects predominate.

Dopexamine acts as a β2-agonist and at dopamine receptors.

Salbutamol is a potent β2-agonist

For more information about inotropes please see our Inotrope section, section 2.8.3

Physiology of the neuromuscular junction

1.4.1. Neuromuscular junction – Emily K Johnson

What is the neuromuscular junction?

The neuromuscular junction consists of a motor neurone and a muscle cell separated by a synaptic cleft. Action potentials are transmitted across the junction, from the nerve to the muscle by the release of acetylcholine.

Describe the neuromuscular junction in more detail

A diagram of the neuromuscular junction may help to illustrate your answer (Figure 1.4.1a).

The motor neurones originate in the ventral horn of the spinal cord and end in a pre-synaptic nerve terminal. The axons are myelinated, and the myelin sheath is separated by nodes of Ranvier to speed conduction. Before the nerve reaches the neuromuscular junction it branches into several terminals to innervate several muscle cells. In the nerve terminal acetylcholine is synthesised and stored in vesicles. These vesicles release acetylcholine into the synaptic cleft either spontaneously or in response to a nerve impulse.

The synaptic cleft is a gap approximately 20 nm wide, and it separates the nerve terminal and the motor end-plate which is a specialised area of muscle, rich in acetylcholine receptors. It is an oval area with deeply folded clefts all with a high concentration of acetylcholine receptors on their surfaces. There are between 1 and 10 million acetylcholine receptors at each end-plate. Acetylcholine travels across the synaptic cleft and binds with post-synaptic receptors on the motor end-plate of the muscle cell. This causes an action potential to travel through the muscle cell.

What is a motor unit?

A motor unit is a motor neurone and the muscle cell which it innervates.

Tell me about the acetylcholine receptors

Again, a diagram may help you to illustrate you answer, but you should practice drawing this many times so it looks correct and can be drawn quickly without wasting time (Figure 1.4.1b).

Dr Podcast Scripts for the Primary FRCA, ed. Rebecca A. Leslie, Emily K. Johnson and Alexander P. L. Goodwin.   Published by Cambridge University Press. © R. A. Leslie, E. K. Johnson and A. P. L. Goodwin 2011.

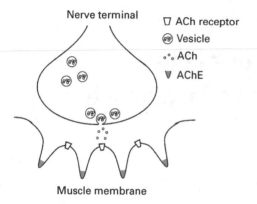

Nerve terminal

▽ ACh receptor
◉ Vesicle
∘°∘ ACh
▼ AChE

Muscle membrane

The diagram shows the synaptic cleft, which is found at the junction of the nerve terminal and the muscle membrane.

Vesicle You should demonstrate that there are two stores of acetylcholine (ACh), one deep in the nerve terminal and one clustered beneath the surface opposite the ACh receptors in the so-called 'active zones'. The deep stores serve as a reserve of ACh while those in the active zones are required for immediate release of ACh into the synaptic cleft.

ACh receptor These are located on the peaks of the junctional folds of the muscle membrane as shown. They are also found presynaptically on the nerve terminal, where, once activated, they promote migration of ACh vesicles from deep to superficial stores.

Acetylcholinesterase (AChE) This enzyme is found in the troughs of the junctional folds of the muscle membrane and is responsible for metabolizing ACh within the synaptic cleft.

Figure 1.4.1a. Neuromuscular junction. Reproduced with permission from Cross, M. and Plunkett, E. 2008. *Physics, Pharmacology and Physiology for Anaesthetists: Key Concepts for the FRCA.* Cambridge: Cambridge University Press. © M. Cross and E. Plunkett 2008.

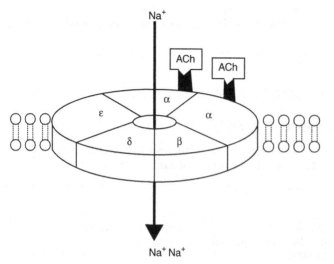

Figure 1.4.1b. The structure of the acetylcholine receptor.

Acetylcholine receptors can be nicotinic or muscarinic. The pre-ganglionic acetylcholine receptors throughout the autonomic nervous system are nicotinic, and the post-ganglionic receptors in the parasympathetic nervous system are muscarinic. Acetylcholine receptors at the motor end-plate of the neuromuscular junction are nicotinic.

The acetylcholine receptor has been studied in electric eels. It is a transmembrane protein with a molecular weight of 250 000 Da composed of five subunits. Each subunit is a glycosylated protein that projects into the synaptic cleft. The subunits are named α, β, γ and δ. There are two α-subunits, and the γ-subunit is thought to be replaced by an ε-subunit in mammals. The subunits are arranged in a cylinder with a central ion channel. The two α-subunits on each receptor carry the acetylcholine binding site. When acetylcholine binds to the two α-subunits a conformational change is induced in the receptor, opening the ion channel. Sodium, potassium and calcium then flow through the channel in a direction dictated by their concentration gradients. This movement of ions causes depolarisation of the cell membrane and initiation of an action potential in the muscle.

Other than this post-junctional acetylcholine receptor, what other nicotinic receptors are present around the neuromuscular junction?

There are three types of acetylcholine receptor that have been identified at the neuromuscular junction. As well as the post-junctional receptors involved in traditional neuromuscular transmission there are also pre-junctional receptors and extra-junctional receptors.

Pre-junctional acetylcholine receptors are situated in the cell membrane of the nerve terminal. When activated by two acetylcholine molecules binding to their sites on the α-subunits they open their ion channel and permit the flow of sodium ions through it. This results in the mobilisation of further acetylcholine storage vesicles in the nerve terminal into the active zone, the area closest to the synaptic cleft, where the vesicles are imminently ready to release their contents into the synaptic cleft.

Extra-junctional receptors are generally only present in small numbers at sites in the muscle membrane distant to the motor end-plate. They are significant in denervation when they proliferate over the muscle membrane. This occurs in conditions such as severe burns and some muscle diseases.

What is denervation hypersensitivity?

Denervation hypersensitivity is a condition that may occur 4 to 5 days following denervation of skeletal muscle. It is when skeletal muscle has increased sensitivity to acetylcholine and is due to the proliferation of extra-junctional acetylcholine receptors. It is this mechanism that is thought to cause the amplified response to suxamethonium following peripheral nerve injuries and hyperkalaemia.

Tell me about acetylcholine, including its synthesis, storage and breakdown

You should be able to draw the structure of acetylcholine. It is worth learning this because then you can also draw the structure of suxamethonium, which is two acetylcholine molecules linked together (Figure 1.4.1c).

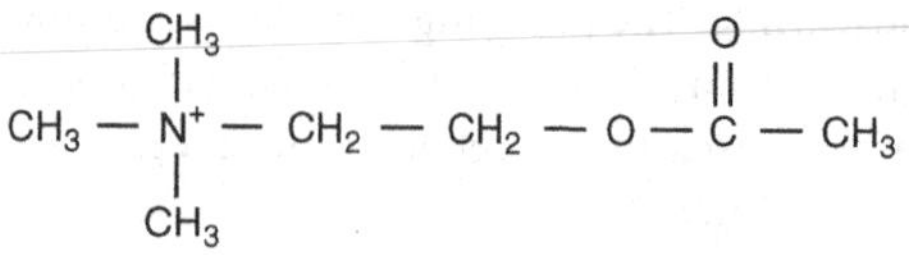

$$CH_3 - \overset{\overset{\displaystyle CH_3}{|}}{\underset{\underset{\displaystyle CH_3}{|}}{N^+}} - CH_2 - CH_2 - O - \overset{\overset{\displaystyle O}{||}}{C} - CH_3$$

Figure 1.4.1c. Acetylcholine structure.

Acetylcholine is an acetyl ester of the base choline. It is a neurotransmitter at autonomic ganglia, parasympathetic post-ganglionic nerve endings, sympathetic post-ganglionic nerve endings at sweat glands and some blood vessels, the neuromuscular junction and extensively within the CNS.

Acetylcholine is synthesised from acetylcoenzyme A and choline. Acetylcoenzyme A is made in the mitochondria and choline is actively transported into the nerve terminals. The reaction occurs in the cytoplasm of the nerve terminal and is catalysed by the enzyme choline acetyltransferase.

Acetylcholine is then stored in the nerve terminals in vesicles which are moved into position near the synaptic cleft when pre-junctional acetylcholine receptors are stimulated. The vesicles fuse with the pre-junctional membrane to release acetylcholine. The fusion of vesicles is a calcium-dependent process.

Acetylcholine is broken down by hydrolysis to acetate and choline. The enzyme responsible for this breakdown is acetylcholinesterase, and it is situated mostly on the post-synaptic membrane but also exists in red blood cells and the placenta. There are other esterases that are also able to break down acetylcholine, such as plasma cholinesterase, which is also known as pseudocholinesterase and is largely responsible for the hydrolysis and breakdown of suxamethonium.

Discuss in more detail the breakdown of acetylcholine

A diagram with acetylcholine drawn out would definitely help explain how it is broken down. Make sure you are able to draw it quickly and you understand which parts of the molecule are the choline and the acetate.

Acetylcholine is broken down by the enzyme acetylcholinesterase. The enzyme has six enzyme sites, each with an anionic site and an esteratic site. The $N(CH_3)^{3+}$ part of acetylcholine binds to the anionic site of the enzyme, and the acetate end of acetylcholine forms an intermediate bond with the esteratic site. Choline is then released, and the complex of the acetate end and enzyme is subsequently hydrolysed to release acetate.

What is an end-plate potential?

An end-plate potential is the depolarising potential produced at the post-synaptic motor end-plate by acetylcholine binding to nicotinic acetylcholine receptors.

What is a miniature end-plate potential?

End-plate potentials can vary in magnitude depending on the amount of acetylcholine released in the synaptic cleft, the amount of acetylcholinesterase available to breakdown the acetylcholine and the number of receptors available to bind acetylcholine. Miniature end-plate potentials occur when the potential is less than 1 mV and are produced due to spontaneous release of acetylcholine from single vesicles. These potentials occur with a frequency of around 2 Hz. One vesicle contains between 4 and 10 000 molecules of acetylcholine. The reason for their random release in the absence of motor nerve stimulus is not known. When neuronal depolarisation occurs roughly 200 of the vesicles are released and end-plate depolarisation ensues, initiating muscle contraction.

1.4.2. Muscle physiology – Dana L Kelly

What different types of muscle are you aware of?

Muscle tissue is divided into three types: skeletal, cardiac and smooth muscle.

What are the functions of skeletal muscle?

The primary function of skeletal muscle is movement. This includes both voluntary movements and involuntary movements. In addition, muscle contraction also fulfils some other important functions including the maintenance of posture, joint stability, and heat production. Maintenance of muscle tone and posture is achieved by summation. The tendons of many muscles extend over joints and in this way contribute to joint stability. Heat production is an important by-product of muscle metabolism. Skeletal muscle contraction is the body's predominant means of maintaining normothermia.

What are the differences between cardiac and skeletal muscle?

In terms of their structure, skeletal muscle is uniquely striated whereas cardiac muscle forms a functional syncitium. Skeletal muscle has motor end-plates present and a more extensively developed sarcoplasmic reticulum, and contains muscle spindles to regulate the contraction. Cardiac muscle has many more mitochondria and has more capillaries to avoid hypoxia.

In terms of functional differences, skeletal and cardiac differ in terms of the mechanism of their depolarisation. In skeletal muscle there is a nerve action potential depolarising each muscle cell which then spreads to the motor end-plate, whereas in cardiac muscle depolarisation is spread by specialised muscle cells within the conducting system, then from cell to cell.

The duration of the muscle depolarisation also varies. Skeletal muscle has short durations of depolarisation, approximately 5–10 msec, compared to long durations for cardiac muscle e.g. 150–250 msec.

The duration of muscle contraction is different: 7.5–100 msec for skeletal muscle (depending on fibre type) and approximately 300 msec for the ventricle with a normal heart rate.

In addition, the control of skeletal muscle contraction is voluntary compared to the involuntary control (via pacemaker cells) of cardiac muscle.

What is a sarcomere?

A sarcomere is the basic unit of a muscle's cross-striated myofibril (Figure 1.4.2a). Sarcomeres are multi-protein complexes composed of different filaments, known as thick and thin.

The thick filaments are composed of myosin. They also contain myosin-binding protein C, which binds at one end to the thick filament and the other to actin. The thick filaments produce the dark **A band**.

The thin filaments are composed of actin. They also involve tropomyosin, a dimer which coils itself around the core of the thin filaments. The thin filaments extend in each direction from the **Z line**. Where they do not overlap the thick filaments, they create the light **I band**.

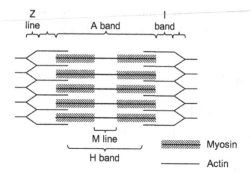

The diagram should be drawn carefully so that the actin and myosin filaments are shown to overlap while ensuring that enough space is left between them to identify the various lines and bands.

Z line The junction between neighbouring actin filaments that forms the border between sarcomeres. It has a Z-shaped appearance on the diagram.

M line The 'middle' zone of the sarcomere, formed from the junction between neighbouring myosin filaments. There are no cross-bridges in this region.

A band This band spans the length of the myosin filament although it is confusingly given the letter A.

I band This band represents the portion of actin filaments that are not overlapped by myosin. It comes 'in between' the Z line and the A band.

H band This band represents the portion of the myosin filaments that are not overlapped by actin.

Figure 1.4.2a. Sarcomere. Reproduced with permission from Cross, M. and Plunkett, E. 2008. *Physics, Pharmacology and Physiology for Anaesthetists: Key Concepts for the FRCA.* Cambridge: Cambridge University Press. © M. Cross and E. Plunkett 2008.

The **H zone** is that portion of the A band where the thick and thin filaments do not overlap.
The **I bands** are bisected by the **Z line**.
The sarcomere is the area between the **Z lines**.

Can you explain the mechanism of muscle contraction in skeletal muscle?

The sliding filament theory is used to explain the mechanism of skeletal muscle contraction. Contraction occurs because of the sliding of the thin filaments between the thick filaments. This involves the formation of cross-linkages between actin and myosin to provide the "pull". These cross-linkages break after some shortening. The actin then forms a new cross link with the next myosin and further shortening occurs. This cycle continues repeatedly to cause shortening of the muscle. Each cycle shortens the muscle by approximately 1% of its original length.

Therefore in each sarcomere, when a muscle contracts, the Z lines come closer together, and the width of the H zones and the I bands decreases, but there is no change in the width of the A band.

Conversely, as a muscle is stretched, the width of the H zones and I bands increases, but there is still no change in the width of the A band.

Describe the sequence of events between motor neurone excitation and muscle contraction

Skeletal muscle contraction occurs via excitation–contraction coupling.

This is a term used to refer to the physiological process of converting an electrical stimulus to mechanical response. In muscle physiology, the electrical stimulus is an action potential and the mechanical response is contraction.

Initially, acetylcholine released by the axon of the motor neurone crosses the cleft and binds to receptors/channels on the motor end-plate. An action potential is generated in response to binding of acetylcholine. This depolarises the adjacent muscle, and subsequent end-plate potentials are propagated across the surface membrane and down the T tubules of muscle cell. The action potential in the T-tubule activates the voltage-gated L-type calcium channels (also known as the dihydropyridine receptors). This has two effects: some calcium ions enter the cytoplasm via the calcium channel, and there is also a "charge movement" across the membrane.

This "charge movement" leads to the opening of the sarcoplasmic calcium ion release channels (also known as the ryanodine receptors). Calcium ions are released from the sarcoplasmic reticulum and diffuse to the thick and thin filaments. Calcium ions bind to troponin C on the thin actin filaments. This interacts with troponin I and leads to tropomyosin being physically moved aside to uncover cross-bridge binding sites on actin, where the myosin heads bind. Myosin attaches to actin and forms a cross link. The sliding of the filaments is powered by the hydrolysis of ATP by the ATPase activity of the myosin heads.

How is contraction terminated?

Contraction persists until the cytoplasmic calcium ion concentration falls. Calcium ions are then released from troponin C, tropomyosin slips back to its blocking position over binding sites on actin and actin is no longer able to interact with the myosin heads. This occurs due to active rapid pumping of calcium ions (via the calcium/magnesium ATPase pump) back into the sarcoplasmic reticulum. The calcium ions then diffuse to the terminal cisternae adjacent to the T tubules ready to be released in the event of a further contraction.

What is the source of energy for muscle metabolism?

Most muscle cells only store enough ATP for a small number of muscle contractions. Muscle cells also store glycogen; however, most of the energy required for contraction is derived from phosphagens such as creatine phosphate.

What various types of skeletal muscle are you aware off?

Type I or *slow oxidative fibres* have a slow contraction speed and a low myosin ATPase activity. These cells are specialised for steady, continuous activity and are highly resistant to fatigue. Their motor neurones are often active, with a low firing frequency. These cells have a high surface to volume ratio with a good capillary supply for efficient gas exchange. They are rich in mitochondria and myoglobin, and thus have a red appearance. They require aerobic metabolism and use fat as a preferential source of energy.

Type IIA or *fast oxidative-glycolytic fibres* have a fast contraction speed and a high myosin ATPase activity. They are progressively recruited when additional effort is required, but are still very resistant to fatigue. Their motor neurones show bursts of intermittent activity. These cells again have a high surface to volume ratio with a good capillary supply for efficient gas exchange. Like type I fibres, they are rich in mitochondria and myoglobin. Their metabolism is aerobic, using either glucose or fats as a source of energy.

Type IIB or *fast glycolytic fibres* have a fast contraction speed and a high myosin ATPase activity. They are only recruited for brief maximal efforts and are easily fatigued. Their motor neurones transmit occasional bursts of very high-frequency impulses. These are large cells with a poor surface to volume ratio and their limited capillary supply slows the delivery of oxygen and removal of waste products. They have few mitochondria and little myoglobin, resulting in a white colour. They generate ATP by the anaerobic metabolism of glucose to lactic acid.

Describe the neuronal pathways which are involved in the initiation of voluntary movement

The thought that triggers voluntary movement starts from the pre-motor area. Voluntary movement starts in the motor cortex (pre-central gyrus). The impulse then descends through the internal capsule before decussating into the cortico-spinal tract to the anterior horn cell and then to the α-motor neurone. Within the cortico-spinal tract, there is input from the intermediate cerebellum which compares motor cortex requirements to the actual movement made, and thereby modulates cortical activity to produce a controlled movement.

What is the mechanism of the knee jerk?

The stretch reflex is a clinical and classic example of the monosynaptic reflex arc (Figure 1.4.2b). Striking the patellar tendon stretches the quadriceps tendon. This stimulates the muscle spindle afferent neurone from the spindle passes into the spinal cord through the dorsal root. The afferent neurone then synapses in the anterior horn with the motor neurone to that muscle fibre. The transmitter at the synapse is glutamate. The efferent motor neurone stimulates the muscle to contract.

The muscle spindle is a complex sensory organ, consisting of intra-fusal fibres. Nerves leaving the spindle are of two types: Ia fibres (which are fast, primary fibres to the cord) and also type II fibres (slower fibres to the cerebral cortex). The motor innervation of the muscle spindle is via Aγ fibres, which cause a tightening of the intra-fusal fibres. The purpose of the motor innervation of the muscle spindle is to increase both the dynamic and static response of the muscle. Fast motor fibres, known as Aα fibres, are the efferent neurones responsible for muscle contraction. In addition to muscle spindles, an important component of the reflex system is the Golgi tendon organ. There are nerve endings amongst the fascicles of a tendon. They are activated by passive stretch and active contraction of a muscle. They make intra-neurone connections which are both excitatory and inhibitory.

How do smooth muscles contract?

Smooth muscle cells do not have ordered sarcomeres. T tubules and sarcoplasmic reticulum are largely absent from smooth muscle and, here, calcium influxes mainly from the cell surface. In smooth muscle, the effect of calcium is mediated by calmodulin, a widely distributed

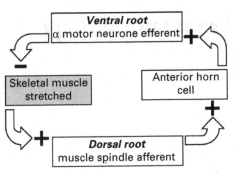

Stretching of the muscle is sensed in the muscle spindle and leads to firing in muscle spindle afferent. These nerves travel via the dorsal root and synapse in the anterior horn of the spinal cord directly with the motor neurone to that muscle. They stimulate firing of the motor neurones, which causes contraction of the muscle that has just been stretched. The muscle spindle afferent also synapses with inhibitory interneurons, which inhibit the antagonistic muscles. This is called reciprocal innervation.

Figure 1.4.2b. Stretch reflex. Reproduced with permission from Cross, M. and Plunkett, E. 2008. *Physics, Pharmacology and Physiology for Anaesthetists: Key Concepts for the FRCA.* Cambridge: Cambridge University Press. © M. Cross and E. Plunkett 2008.

intra-cellular calcium binding protein. Calmodulin activates myosin light chain kinase and myosin phosphorylation before myosin can bind to actin, making contraction a much slower process.

What is the role of nitric oxide in vascular smooth muscle?

Nitric oxide is an important chemical messenger. It is a major determinant of the basal resting tone of vascular smooth muscles in arterioles. It has very localised effects as it is a highly reactive free radical with a short half-life. Nitric oxide is produced in vascular endothelium from L-arginine by nitric oxide synthase. It diffuses to vascular smooth muscle cells and stimulates guanylate cyclase, leading to the formation of cGMP, and ultimately to relaxation of vascular smooth muscle. It also contributes to the thrombo-resistance of the vessel wall because of its inhibition of platelet aggregation and adhesion.

Fluids and renal physiology

1.5.1. Fluid balance – Rebecca A Leslie

What is your total body water?

A large proportion of body weight is water. In young male adults water composes approximately 60% of total body weight. This percentage varies with build, sex and age. Adipose tissue contains very little water, therefore total body water will vary with individual differences in adipose tissue. Total body water in females is lower than in males, and is approximately 50–55%. Neonates have a relatively high total body water, which can be as high as 80%.

A rough formula to determine total body water is 600 ml of water per kg of body weight. Therefore a 70-kg man will contain approximately 42 litres of water.

What are body fluid compartments?

The total body water is considered to exist in physiologic collections which are known as compartments. The main two fluid compartments are called the intra-cellular fluid compartment and extra-cellular fluid compartment.

What are the sizes of the body's fluid compartments?

Intra-cellular fluid is approximately two thirds of total body water, whilst extra-cellular fluid makes up the remaining third. Therefore a 70-kg man will contain approximately 28 litres of intra-cellular water and 14 litres of extra-cellular fluid.

Extra-cellular fluid can be further divided into:

- Interstitial fluid
- Intra-vascular fluid
- Transcellular fluid.

The intra-vascular compartment equates to plasma volume and makes up 5% of body weight.

Transcellular fluid is a term used to refer to a compartment consisting of a diverse group of fluid collections. All these fluid collections are formed from the transport activities of cells

Dr Podcast Scripts for the Primary FRCA, ed. Rebecca A. Leslie, Emily K. Johnson and Alexander P. L. Goodwin. Published by Cambridge University Press. © R. A. Leslie, E. K. Johnson and A. P. L. Goodwin 2011.

and are found in epithelial lined spaces. The composition of transcellular fluid differs from both plasma and interstitial fluid because it is controlled by the secretory cells.

Give me some examples of transcellular fluids

Examples of transcellular fluid include:

- Cerebrospinal fluid
- Joint fluid
- Intra-ocular fluid
- Gastrointestinal fluid
- Bile
- Pleural fluid
- Peritoneal fluid
- Pericardial fluid
- Sweat.

What controls the distribution of fluid between the intra-cellular and extra-cellular fluid compartments?

A bi-phospholipid cell membrane separates the intra-cellular fluid compartment from the extra-cellular fluid compartment. Water is free to cross the cell membrane but solutes cannot. Water will move across the cell membrane until the osmolality is the same on both sides of the membrane. This process is described as osmosis. As a result of this process the osmolality of the intra-cellular fluid compartment is the same as the osmolality of the extra-cellular fluid compartment. If the osmolality of the extra-cellular fluid is increased then this will draw fluid from the cells into the extra-cellular fluid until the osmolality within the intra-cellular and the extra-cellular fluid compartments are the same. This means that factors that change the extra-cellular fluid osmolality will determine the distribution of total body water between the intra-cellular and extra-cellular fluid compartments.

What is the definition of osmolality, and what is the normal osmolality of extra-cellular fluid?

Osmolality is the number of osmoles of solute per kilogram of solvent. The normal osmolality of extra-cellular fluid, and therefore plasma, is 285–290 mOsmol/kg.

How is the osmolarity different from the osmolality?

The osmolarity is the number of osmoles of solute per litre of solution, whilst the osmolality is the number of osmoles of solute per kilogram of solvent.

What is the osmotic pressure?

The osmotic activity of solute particles in an aqueous solution can be thought of as exerting an "osmotic pressure", which is the potential to draw water into the solution.

Imagine two aqueous solutions separated by a semi-permeable membrane through which only water can pass. One of the solutions is pure water, whilst the other solution contains dissolved particles. Water will move across the membrane from the pure water into the solution. The osmotic pressure is a measure of the osmotic tendency for water to cross the membrane.

How is total body water controlled?

Total body water is kept fairly constant from day-to-day. It is easy to think of water control as a simple model with three components:

- Sensors
- A central integrator
- Effectors.

Osmoreceptors, volume receptors and high-pressure baroreceptors sense changes in fluid osmolality and total body fluid volume. These messages are sent to the hypothalamus which then stimulates or decreases the sensation of thirst and causes a release or inhibits the release of anti-diuretic hormone (ADH).

Thirst regulates fluid intake and ADH regulates fluid output.

How does anti-diuretic hormone increase water reabsorption?

ADH is a nonapeptide which is produced in the hypothalamus and secreted from the posterior pituitary in response to hypovolaemia, hypotension, increased plasma tonicity, angiotensin II and stress.

ADH acts in the kidney; more specifically on the basolateral membrane of cells in the collecting duct. Through a second messenger system aquaporins or water channels are then integrated into the luminal surface of the cell membrane. This allows water to be reabsorbed down its osmotic gradient. If ADH is not present then the luminal membrane is impermeable to water.

Which other cell membranes are impermeable to water?

Most cell membranes allow water to pass through easily. However, there are a few which are relatively impermeable to water because of their functional requirements. Examples include:

- The bladder epithelium to prevent the urine becoming isosmotic
- The ascending loop of Henle so that urine that enters the distal convoluted tubule is hypotonic
- The cortical and medullary collecting ducts in the absence of ADH.

How is fluid lost from the body compartments?

When a patient becomes dehydrated fluid is lost from all body compartments. Pure dehydration implies loss of water alone, with no lack of electrolytes. However, in reality there is always some electrolyte loss. Dehydration occurs as a result of prolonged lack of fluid intake, protracted pre-operative fasting or in conditions where the patients become unable to swallow.

Other causes of fluid depletion include conditions where electrolytes and water are lost together such as vomiting, diarrhoea, inappropriate diuretic therapy, intestinal obstruction and pre-operative bowel preparation.

The intra-vascular compartment will be depleted by blood loss as a result of trauma or during surgery.

What is the definition of a crystalloid and a colloid?

A crystalloid is a solution which contains small molecules that dissociate into ions to form a true solution which is able to easily pass through semi-permeable membranes. Examples of crystalloid solutions include 0.9% saline, Hartmann's and 5% dextrose.

Colloids are larger molecules that are dispersed throughout a solvent rather than forming true solutions. The particles tend to arrange as groups of molecules, and they do not readily pass through semi-permeable membranes. Examples of colloids are gelatins such as Gelofusin and Haemaccel and starches such as Hetastarch.

What are the advantages and disadvantages of crystalloids?

Crystalloids are cheap, readily available and can be rapidly infused in large volumes.

The main disadvantage of crystalloids is that they only remain in the intra-vascular compartment for a very short period of time after infusion. This results in an increased potential for over-infusion, with possible circulatory over-load and pulmonary oedema.

What happens when you rapidly infuse 1000 ml of 0.9% saline?

When you rapidly infuse 1000 ml of 0.9% saline the intra-vascular compartment will initially be expanded. This causes an increase in the venous return to the heart, which in turn will increase the cardiac output and the mean arterial pressure.

The body has several mechanisms which sense the increased blood volume and act to help return it back to normal. These mechanisms include an immediate neural response, and slower humoral responses by ADH, aldosterone and atrial natriuretic peptide (ANP).

The neural response is initiated by baroreceptors in the carotid sinus. They detect the increase in blood pressure from the 0.9% saline infusion and cause a reflex systemic vasodilation to return the mean arterial blood pressure back to normal. This reflex occurs quickly.

Later, stimulation of low pressure–volume receptors by the increase in blood volume causes an inhibition in the release of ADH from the posterior pituitary. This will prevent water from being reabsorbed in the collecting ducts of the kidney and a diuresis will ensue.

The increased blood volume will also lead to a reduction in the production of renin in the kidney. This reduces the amount of circulating aldosterone and leads to a reduction in the amount of sodium and water which are reabsorbed. Over time this reflex will help to return blood volume back to normal.

ANP is released in response to stretching of the atrium by fluid over-load. If 1 litre of fluid is infused rapidly, the atria are stretched and ANP is released. ANP increases glomerular filtration rate (GFR) and the urinary sodium and water excretion, again helping to try and return circulating blood volume back to normal.

How much of 1000 ml of 0.9% saline will eventually remain in the vascular compartment?

The 0.9% saline is isotonic. Therefore, it will tend to distribute within the extra-cellular compartment. The intra-vascular compartment makes up approximately 25% of the extra-vascular fluid compartment. Therefore roughly 250 ml of 0.9% saline will remain in the intra-vascular compartment. The remaining 750 ml will distribute between the interstitial compartment and the transcellular compartments.

How will this differ if 1000 ml of 5% dextrose was administered?

When 5% dextrose is administered the glucose is metabolised, leaving 1000 ml of water.

As we have already mentioned water will distribute equally into the total body water. The intra-cellular fluid compartment contains two thirds of total body water, whilst the extra-cellular fluid compartment contains only one third of total body water. This means that only 333 ml of 5% dextrose when administered will enter the extra-cellular fluid compartment. The intra-vascular compartment is only 25% of the extra-cellular fluid compartment; therefore, only approximately 84 ml of 1000 ml of 5% dextrose will remain in the intra-vascular compartment after infusion.

Tell me about the different types of colloids you know about

There are several different types of colloids; gelatins, starches, dextrans and human albumin solutions.

Gelatins, such as Gelofusin and Haemaccel, contain chemically modified polypeptides predominantly derived from bovine collagen. They have an average molecular mass of 35 kDa with an effective plasma expansion time of approximately 2 hours. Gelatins carry a risk of allergic reactions with the incidence of severe anaphylactic reactions approximately 1:13 000.

Starches, such as hydroxyethyl starch (HES), consist of amylopeptin which is a polymer of glucose with branches every 24–30 glucose units. Hydroxyethyl groups are substituted on the glucose molecules throughout the polymer. The more hydroxyethyl groups within the polymer, the longer the starch takes to be metabolised. HES solutions can be categorised according to their molecular weight:

- Low molecular weight HES has an average molecular mass of 70–130 kDa
- Medium molecular weight HES has an average molecular mass of 200–260 kDa
- High molecular weight HES has an average molecular mass of >450 kDa.

Solutions containing large molecular weight molecules are not readily metabolised by the body and therefore remain in the plasma for longer. Medium and high molecular weight HES solutions have been found to cause a reduction in the levels of Factor VIII and von Willebrand factor and can cause coagulopathies. Low molecular weight HES solutions do not have this drawback.

Dextrans contain branched polysaccharides which are produced from lactic-acid producing bacteria. They are classified according to their molecular weight: Dextran 40 has an average molecular mass of 40 kDa, whilst Dextran 70 has an average molecular mass of 70 kDa. They are presented either in 0.9% saline or 7.5% saline. Their use has been associated with renal failure, coagulopathies and anaphylactic reactions, and for these reasons they are not commonly used in clinical practice.

Human albumin solution (HAS) contains 96% human albumin. It is derived from pooled human plasma, serum or normal placentas. It is subsequently sterilised by heat and ultrafiltration to prevent disease transmission. In the UK, because of concerns about prion protein transmission, all HAS is sourced from the USA. It can be supplied as 4.5% solution to reflect

Table 1.5.2.a. Equivalent values for pH and H^+ concentration

pH	$[H^+]$(nmol/L)
6.8	158
6.9	126
7.0	100
7.1	79
7.2	63
7.3	50
7.4	40
7.5	32
7.6	25
7.7	20
7.8	16
7.9	13
8.0	10

normal plasma or as a 20% solution. HAS has good plasma expanding properties, and has an intra-vascular half-life of approximately 24 hours. Side effects of HAS are rare.

1.5.2. Acid–base physiology – Emily K Johnson

Why is it important to control pH in body tissues?

pH is the negative logarithm to the base 10 of the hydrogen ion concentration.

Write down the formula for pH:

$$pH = -\log_{10}[H^+].$$

It is a measure of the acidity of a solution and a normal arterial pH is 7.35 to 7.45, which corresponds to an H^+ concentration of 34–46 nmol/L. The maintenance of a stable body pH is important for a number of essential functions. Enzymes require a specific pH to perform their reactions and may become deranged outside a narrow range. Likewise membrane excitability and energy production are affected. pH influences the state of ionisation of molecules in the body and therefore whether they are intra- or extra-cellular. Nervous and endocrine systems can suffer indirect effects of abnormal pH.

Explain the pH scale a little more and give some examples of the relationship between pH and hydrogen ion concentration

The relationship between H^+ concentration and pH is inverse, so as pH decreases H^+ concentration increases. The negative logarithmic scale of pH is non-linear which means that for every reduction by 1 in the pH there is a 10 times increase in activity. For example if the pH falls from 7.4 to 7.3, the concentration increases from 40 to 50 nmol/L. At a pH of 6.8 the concentration is 158 nmol/L, compared to at a pH of 8.0 when the concentration is 10 nmol/L (Table 1.5.2a).

What is a hydrogen ion?

A hydrogen ion is a hydrogen molecule without its electron, which makes it a proton.

Define acid and base

An acid is a substance that donates a proton, for example HA.

A base is a substance that accepts a proton, for example A^-.

What is the Henderson–Hasselbalch equation?

You should write down the equation and explain it using the necessary equations described. You will need to practice writing the equations and explaining them several times. It is worthwhile trying to explain this to as many different people as possible, whether they are medical or non-medical. If they are generous enough to listen, take advantage of the opportunity and teach them these useful pieces of information!

The Henderson–Hasselbalch equation describes the relationship between the pH, the dissociation constant and the concentrations of a weak acid and its base salt.

It is:

$$pH = pKa + \log[A^-]/[HA].$$

In solution an acid dissociates into a H^+ ion and a base A^- as shown in the equation:

$$HA \underset{k^2}{\overset{k^1}{\rightleftharpoons}} H^+ + A^-.$$

The proportions of the acid and base are dependent on the dissociation constants, k^1 for the forward reaction and k^2 for the backward reaction. If k^1 is greater than k^2 there is more H^+ and A^- in solution and vice versa. The law of mass action dictates that:

$$K = k^1/k^2 \text{ (where K is the dissociation constant)}$$

Therefore,

$$[H^+] = K[HA]/[A^-].$$

Thus the hydrogen ion concentration depends on the dissociation constant and the ratio of the buffers A^- and HA.

By applying a logarithmic conversion of this equation the Henderson–Hasselbalch equation is produced:

$$pH = pKa + \log[A^-]/[HA].$$

pKa is the negative log of the dissociation constant and is equal to the pH at which the substance is 50% dissociated.

The lower the pKa, the stronger acid. Therefore, whether a substance is an acid or base, that is, its ability to donate or accept a proton depends on its pH and its degree of dissociation, pKa.

How does the body maintain the pH within its normal range?

The body maintains the pH between 7.35 and 7.45, therefore maintaining the H^+ concentration between 34 and 46 nmol/L by three mechanisms:

- Buffering
- Compensation
- Correction

Buffering by various systems works instantly to maintain pH, compensation occurs more slowly and correction of the disorder causing the disturbance is the ultimate goal, but may take longer to achieve.

What is a buffer?

A buffer is a substance which resists a change in pH by absorbing or releasing hydrogen ions. It normally consists of a weak acid and its conjugate base resisting pH change when a stronger acid or base is added.

If asked this question it would be a good idea to follow up your definition with examples.

What buffer systems in the body are you aware of?

Buffer systems in the body can be extra-cellular or intra-cellular. There are several buffer systems in the blood:

- Carbonic acid–bicarbonate buffer system
- Haemoglobin
- Plasma proteins
- Phosphate buffer system

The carbonic acid–bicarbonate buffer system is the most important in extra-cellular fluid. It works as carbonic acid (H_2CO_3) is formed from the reaction of CO_2 and water. This reaction is catalysed by carbonic anhydrase. H_2CO_3 dissociates into H^+ and HCO_3^-. When a strong acid is added the H^+ ions are buffered by the bicarbonate ions and more H_2CO_3 is formed. This subsequently dissociates into H_2O and CO_2.

$$CO_2 + H_2O \leftrightarrow H_2CO_3 \leftrightarrow H^+ + HCO_{3-}.$$

Increased arterial CO_2 stimulates ventilation and respiratory compensation occurs. This system has a pKa of 6.1. This means at a pH of 6.1 there is an equal amount of carbonic acid, H^+ and HCO_3^- ions, so it can be said the system is in equilibrium. At physiological pH of 7.4, the low pKa means the carbonic acid buffer system is good at buffering acids but not so useful for buffering alkalis. However, due to the abundance of carbonic acid, the ability of the lungs to excrete CO_2 and the kidneys to regulate bicarbonate this is the main buffer system.

How can you use the Henderson–Hasselbalch equation to determine the hydrogen ion or bicarbonate ion concentration?

Again, it is essential you can write and explain the equations described in answer to this or similar questions.

The Henderson–Hasselbalch equation is:

$$pH = pKa + \log[A^-]/[HA].$$

Bicarbonate ion concentration is substituted for $[A^-]$ and carbonic acid, H_2CO_3 is substituted for $[HA]$. As H_2CO_3 concentration is related to CO_2 concentration, and CO_2 concentration is related to partial pressure of CO_2 and a solubility factor (0.03 mmol/L/mmHg or 0.23 mmol/L/kPa) the $[HA]$ can also be substituted by pCO_2 multiplied by the appropriate solubility factor. The pKa of the carbonic acid–bicarbonate buffer system is 6.1 so this is also substituted so the final equation is:

$$pH = 6.1 + \log[HCO_3^-]/pCO_2 \times 0.03 \text{ (if } pCO_2 \text{ is measured in mmHg)}.$$

The bicarbonate ion concentration and pCO_2 can be measured and substituted in to calculate pH and therefore H^+ concentration. Under normal conditions:

$$pH = 6.1 + \log 24/(40 \times 0.03) = 7.4.$$

You mentioned the enzyme carbonic anhydrase, can you tell me a little more about it?

Carbonic anhydrase is the enzyme that catalyses the reaction of carbon dioxide and water to form carbonic acid. Carbonic acid then dissociates into hydrogen and bicarbonate ions.

Carbonic anhydrase is present in large amounts in red blood cells, renal tubules and lung alveolar cells and plays an important role in buffering as well as in CO_2 and O_2 transport. It is also present in gastric mucosa where it is involved in hydrochloric acid production and in the ciliary body for aqueous humour production.

Tell me a little more about the other buffer systems

The other buffer systems are haemoglobin, plasma proteins and the phosphate buffer system.

Haemoglobin is the other main buffer system for acids in the body. It is present in red blood cells as a weak acid HHb, and its potassium salt KHb. Its pKa is 6.8. It buffers H^+ ions, and HCO_3 increases in proportion. Red cell bicarbonate increases and diffuses out of the cell and may be detected in the plasma. The buffering action is due to the dissociation of the histidine residues located in the globin chain. Each haemoglobin has 38 histidine residues so there is a lot of buffering capacity. Deoxygenated haemoglobin is a better buffer than oxygenated haemoglobin as it dissociates to a greater extent, this is the Haldane effect.

Plasma proteins containing amino and carboxyl groups can buffer H^+ ions. The pKa of these groups is 9 and 2, respectively, which means that at a physiological pH of 7.4 they do little buffering. However, within cells the pH is lower and the concentration of proteins is higher, so they do contribute to intra-cellular buffering.

Phosphate is an effective buffer, with a pKa of 6.8. Extra-cellular phosphate levels are low so it is of negligible importance; however, intra-cellular levels are higher and the intra-cellular pH is closer to the pKa allowing more effective buffering to occur. Phosphate is also an important buffer in the urine.

Can you tell me about the compensatory mechanisms the body uses to maintain pH in the normal range?

The body compensates for disturbances in the acid–base balance using respiratory or renal compensation. Respiratory compensation occurs within minutes. It operates by control of plasma partial pressure of CO_2, which causes increased ventilation, subsequent excretion of excess CO_2 and the plasma pH is returned towards normal. Acid–base status cannot be completely corrected via this mechanism.

Renal compensation occurs more slowly over hours to days. It operates to control plasma bicarbonate by altering the renal secretion of H^+ and the production and the reabsorption of bicarbonate. These mechanisms can correct the acid–base balance.

What is an anion gap and how do you calculate it?

An anion gap is the difference between the measured cation and anion concentrations in the plasma. It is therefore calculated by the concentration of sodium plus potassium minus the concentrations of chloride plus bicarbonate.

$$\text{Anion gap} = [K^+] + [Na^+] - [Cl^-] - [HCO_3^-].$$

It is useful in the differential diagnosis of a metabolic acidosis. The normal anion gap is 8 to 16 mmol/L and it represents the unmeasured anions present in plasma such as phosphate, sulphate, acetate and ketones.

In what conditions may the anion gap be deranged?

A high anion gap acidosis indicates the presence of unmeasured anions which could be lactate, ketoacids, exogenous acids or ethanol. Therefore, inadequate tissue perfusion causing lactic acidosis, diabetic ketoacidosis and poisoning will increase the anion gap. Renal failure will increase the anion gap as organic acids accumulate.

A normal anion gap acidosis may be due to hyperchloraemia and bicarbonate loss or retention of hydrogen ions. The causes of this include GI losses, inappropriate 0.9% saline infusion in large volumes and renal tubular acidosis.

What is the base excess?

The base excess or deficit is the amount of acid or base required to restore a litre of blood back to a normal pH at PCO_2 5.3 kPa and temperature of 37°C. It has a negative value in acidosis and positive value in alkalosis. It is useful clinically to give an idea of the severity of the metabolic component of an acid–base derangement.

What is a Siggaard–Andersen nomogram?

Familiarise yourself with the Siggaard–Andersen nomogram as it could be shown to you in an OSCE or structured oral examination to start off a question on acid–base balance or pH or pCO_2 measurement.

The Siggaard–Andersen nomogram is a graph showing the log of the arterial pCO_2 on the y axis and the plasma pH on the x axis. Base excess, bicarbonate and buffer base are added as separate lines. It is derived from the analysis of many blood samples. It is used to measure the arterial pCO_2. Modern blood gas machines calculate the pCO_2 automatically.

1.5.3. Renal physiology – Rebecca A Leslie

What is the normal renal blood flow?

You must know the regional blood flows to the main organs. Take a few minutes to learn them.

The kidneys receive 20–25% of the cardiac output, which equates to 1000–1250 ml/min. The kidneys only weigh 1% of the body weight.

Although the kidneys have a high metabolic rate the renal blood flow is still 10 times more than is needed. The very high renal blood flow is required for the production of large amounts of renal filtrate, which is necessary for urinary excretion of waste products.

The renal cortex receives 500 ml/min/100 g, the outer medulla 100 ml/min/100 g and the inner medulla only 20 ml/min/100 g.

What is autoregulation?

Give short precise definitions to demonstrate your understanding.

Autoregulation is the protective mechanism of the body organs to maintain blood flow over a wide range of blood pressures. In the kidneys the blood flow remains constant over a mean arterial pressure of 75–170 mmHg.

What mechanisms are responsible for autoregulation of renal blood flow?

The autoregulation of the renal blood flow is by two mechanisms: myogenic control and tubuloglomerular feedback.

Myogenic control is where the afferent arterioles dilate or constrict as a response to transmural pressure. For example if the renal perfusion pressure increases, the transmural pressure will increase which causes a reflex action on the smooth muscle of the arterioles to constrict. The constriction of the arterioles causes an increase in the resistance and returns blood flow back to normal.

The macula densa is situated in the wall of the ascending loop of Henle, and is the sensing unit for the tubuloglomerular feedback mechanism. If the renal perfusion pressure increases, then the glomerular capillary pressure increases and therefore the glomerular filtration increases. This results in a larger concentration of sodium in the loop of Henle. This is sensed by the macula densa cells which then release adenosine in response. The adenosine acts as a vasoconstrictor at the afferent arterioles, reducing glomerular capillary pressure, and therefore GFR.

What is the normal glomerular filtration rate and what determines the rate of filtration?

Remember to classify your answer in order to help give a good structure to your answer. To prevent getting confused you may find it beneficial to draw a diagram whilst describing Starling's forces, see Figure 1.5.3a.

The glomerular filtration rate is normally 125 ml/min which is equivalent to 180 L/day.

There are two main factors which determine the filtration at the glomerulus: the balance of filtration forces such as hydrostatic and oncotic pressures and the type of molecules involved.

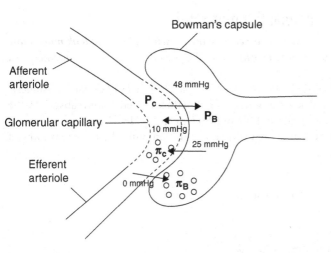

Bowman's capsule

Afferent arteriole

Glomerular capillary

48 mmHg

P_c

P_B

10 mmHg

25 mmHg

π_c

Efferent arteriole

0 mmHg

π_B

Figure 1.5.3a. The hydrostatic and oncotic forces acting on the glomerulus. Where, P_c = hydrostatic pressure of glomerular capillary, P_B = hydrostatic pressure of Bowman's capsule, Π_c = oncotic pressure of glomerular capillary and Π_B = oncotic pressure of Bowman's capsule.

The GFR is dependent on the difference between the hydrostatic and colloid oncotic pressures within the glomerular capillaries and Bowman's capsule. The relationship is explained by Starling's equation:

Glomerular filtration pressure $= [Pc - P_B] + [\pi_B - \pi_C]$

where Pc = glomerular capillary hydrostatic pressure, P_B = hydrostatic pressure in Bowman's capsule, π_C = oncotic pressure of the glomerular capillary and π_B = oncotic pressure in Bowman's capsule.

The glomerular capillary hydrostatic pressure is greater than elsewhere in the body because of the unique arrangement of afferent and efferent arterioles and is approximately 48 mmHg. The hydrostatic pressure in Bowman's capsule which is responsible for moving fluid from Bowman's capsule back into the glomerular capillaries is roughly 10 mmHg. So the net hydrostatic force driving filtration is approximately 38 mmHg.

This is opposed by the oncotic pressure of the capillary plasma trying to hold fluid in the capillaries. This is approximately 25 mmHg. The filtrate oncotic pressure in Bowman's capsule is essentially zero and can be disregarded in the calculation.

Therefore:

Glomerular filtration pressure $= [Pc - P_B] + [\pi_B - \pi_C]$
$$= [48 \text{ mmHg} - 10 \text{ mmHg}] + [0 - 25 \text{ mmHg}]$$
$$= 13 \text{ mmHg}.$$

The molecule size and charge is also another important determinate of the glomerular filtration rate. Molecules which are smaller than 7000 Da are freely filtered by the glomerulus, molecules which are less than 70 000 Da are partially filtered, and particles larger than 70,000 Da are not filtered.

The charge of molecules is also an important determinant of glomerular filtration. The basement membrane contains heparin sulphate proteoglycan molecules and the foot processes contain sialoglycoproteins. These are both negatively charged so repel negatively charged molecules, thus preventing their filtration.

How can you measure glomerular filtration rate?

Try to write down the equations as you are describing the principles. You will look much more knowledgeable if you are able to explain the principles behind GFR measurement instead of just reproducing the formula.

The GFR is measured indirectly by measuring the renal clearances of certain substances.

If substance x is freely filtered at the glomerulus but neither excreted nor reabsorbed, the amount in the urine must equal the amount filtered. So we can say, the plasma concentration multiplied by the GFR must be equal to the urine concentration multiplied by the volume of urine.

Therefore,

$$[Plasma] \times GFR = [Urine] \times Urine\ volume.$$

If this is rearranged,

$$GFR = [Urine] \times Urine\ volume \div [Plasma].$$

Inulin is most commonly used for the measurement of the glomerular filtration rate. This is because it has a small molecular mass at 5500 Da so is freely filtered. In addition it is not reabsorbed, secreted, metabolised or synthesised in the kidney. Therefore its clearance represents the GFR.

Creatinine is often used to approximate the GFR. Creatinine is released at a steady state from skeletal muscle cells. It is freely filtered and not reabsorbed. A small amount is secreted into the tubules; however, this only introduces a small error and the error is constant.

Would it be sensible to use urea or glucose to measure GFR?

Do not panic, you may not have thought about this before but using basic principles it is easy to work out the answer.

No, neither urea nor glucose would give accurate results for measuring the glomerular filtration rate.

Urea would not be suitable because it is not only reabsorbed in the proximal tubule, but variable amounts are also reabsorbed in the medullary collecting ducts. This will underestimate the GFR.

Glucose is freely filtered but in health is totally reabsorbed in the proximal convoluted tubule. This means it would be impossible to measure the glomerular filtration rate using glucose, and in health would give a value of zero.

What is meant by the term filtration fraction?

The filtration fraction is the fraction of plasma (not blood) which is filtered by the glomerulus. Renal plasma flow is 600 ml/min and GFR approximately 125 ml/min, therefore the filtration fraction is 125/600 which is approximately 20%.

How do you measure renal blood flow?

To measure renal blood flow para-aminohippuric acid (PAH) is used. At low concentrations PAH is completely filtered at the glomerulus and is also secreted in to the proximal convoluted tubules. As a result no PAH remains in the venous outflow. The amount appearing in the urine must therefore equal the amount entering the kidney, and thus the clearance of PAH is equal to renal plasma flow.

It is important to remember that this will give you renal plasma flow and not blood flow. Renal blood flow (RBF) is a function of renal plasma flow (RPF) and the haematocrit (how dense the red blood cells are). Blood is composed of approximately 45% blood cells and 55% plasma.

Therefore,

$$RBF = RPF/(1 - Haematocrit)$$

What happens to the concentration of sodium, glucose and inulin as the filtrate passes down the proximal convoluted tubule?

As sodium passes down the proximal convoluted tubule the concentration remains unchanged. This is because when sodium is reabsorbed, water is also reabsorbed.

In health glucose is completely reabsorbed by the proximal convoluted tubule, therefore by the end of the proximal convoluted tubule the concentration of glucose is zero.

Inulin is filtered at the glomerulus and neither reabsorbed or secreted, as a result its concentration increases as it progresses along the proximal convoluted tubule.

Can you describe the counter-current mechanism of the kidney?

This is a tough question, but the examiners know this. Start by drawing a simple diagram of the loop of Henle. As you are describing the different permeabilities add these on to the diagram so the principles are very clear. If possible add on the key osmolarities as you describe the mechanism.

Fluid entering the loop of Henle is isotonic with the plasma, with an osmolarity of approximately 290 mOsmol/kg.

The thin descending loop is permeable to water but impermeable to urea, whereas the ascending limb is permeable to urea but impermeable to water. In addition, the thick ascending limb is also incredibly permeable to sodium and chloride.

Sodium and chloride are actively reabsorbed from the thick ascending loop of Henle into the tubular cells by means of an apical sodium–potassium–chloride co-transporter. The sodium is then transported out of the tubular cell into the interstitial fluid by three mechanisms, the Na-K ATPase pump, the Na-HCO$_3$ co-transporter and by diffusion with chloride ions. Because the thick ascending loop of Henle is impermeable to water the osmolality in the tubule drops, whilst the osmolality in the interstitium rises, creating an osmotic difference of approximately 200 mOsmol/kg.

The increased interstitial osmolality causes fluid to move out of the water-permeable descending loop of Henle, and sodium and chloride ions to diffuse into the descending loop, concentrating the tubular fluid. As this concentrated fluid descends, more tubular water is reabsorbed into the still higher osmotic areas deep in the medulla.

This counter-current arrangement creates an osmotic gradient causing sodium and chloride to diffuse out of the ascending loop and water to diffuse out of the descending loop. This effect is potentiated by the recycling of urea from the medullary collecting ducts.

The osmolarity at the tip of the loop of Henle can reach as high as 1400 mOsmol/kg. This is due in equal parts to sodium chloride and urea.

As this fluid then passes through the ascending loop of Henle which is impermeable to water but permeable to sodium chloride so the osmolarity starts to drop. By the time the fluid leaves the loop of Henle the osmolarity is approximately 90 mOsmol.

What do we mean by the recycling of urea in the kidneys?

The medullary collecting tubules are permeable to urea. As a result it diffuses down its concentration gradient into the medulla, it then continues to move down its concentration gradient into the ascending limb of the loop of Henle. Urea is therefore partially recycled, and provides 50% of the osmolality of the medulla.

What role does the vasa recta play in the counter-current mechanism?

The vasa recta, which are the blood vessels supplying the loops of Henle and collecting ducts, are also arranged with hairpin loops. Like in the loop of Henle, as they descend into the medulla, water is lost and salt is absorbed into the vessels. However, in the ascending vasa recta fluid is absorbed and solutes lost, so the plasma osmolality as it leaves is back to the normal 320 mOsmol/kg.

This counter-current exchange between the descending and ascending vessels ensures that blood flow to the medulla does not wash away the interstitial medullary gradient, and it removes the water reabsorbed from the loop of Henle and the medullary collecting ducts.

How is a dilute urine produced?

The distal convoluted tubule is impermeable to water but permeable to sodium and chloride ions. In states of excess water the urine is diluted by the reabsorption of more sodium and chloride ions in the distal convoluted tubule without reabsorption of water.

Similarly, the collecting ducts are relatively impermeable to water, as they need anti-diuretic hormone to open the aqua pores or water channels. However sodium and chloride are still reabsorbed and leave the urine. In this way large quantities of dilute urine are produced.

How is a concentrated urine produced?

During fluid deprivation, the distal convoluted tubule initially acts in the normal way by reabsorbing sodium chloride and remaining impermeable to water. Therefore the fluid leaving the distal convoluted tubule is dilute with an osmolarity of less than 100 mOsmol/kg.

However, anti-diuretic hormone is released from the hypothalamus when baroreceptors and osmoreceptors detect reduced plasma volume, or increased osmolality. Anti-diuretic hormone acts on the collecting tubules in both the cortex and the medulla to allow reabsorption of water.

In the medulla, a lot of water can be reabsorbed because of the high interstitial fluid osmolality produced by the loop of Henle. This allows the production of a small quantity of very concentrated urine to be excreted. The maximum urine osmolarity the kidneys can produce is 1400 mOsmol/kg. Urea accounts for half of the osmolality of this concentrated urine, and sodium, chloride, potassium and creatinine the remainder.

Chapter

1.6

Liver and endocrine physiology

1.6.1. Glucose and metabolism – Rebecca A Leslie

What do you understand by the term metabolism?

Metabolism is the physical and chemical changes that occur within an organism. It involves anabolism or building up of substances for structural maintenance and growth, and catabolism or breaking down of molecules to extract energy.

The main macronutrients involved in these processes are carbohydrates, fats and proteins. Once ingested the macronutrients are broken down by digestive enzymes to smaller molecules, which are metabolised by many different pathways.

Carbohydrates are the energy source for immediate use, fats are the longer-term energy store and proteins are the building blocks for the tissues which make up the structure of the body.

Define the basal metabolic rate

The basal metabolic rate is the amount of energy used per unit time in a subject under standardised conditions at mental and physical rest, in an environmental temperature and fasted for 12 hours. In a healthy adult it is approximately 70–100 kcal/hr.

Where does the circulating glucose come from?

Glucose comes from three main sources:

- Dietary intake of carbohydrates
- Breakdown of glycogen in a process called glycogenolysis
- Generation of glucose from smaller precursor molecules in the process gluconeogenesis.

Tell me more about glycogen

Gycogen is a branched polymer of glucose and is the major storage form of carbohydrate in the body. It is produced in a process called glycogenesis. First glucose molecules are phosphorylated under the action of hexokinase in tissue cells and glucokinase in liver cells to produce glucose-6-phosphate. Glucose-6-phosphate is then converted into glucose-1-phosphate

Dr Podcast Scripts for the Primary FRCA, ed. Rebecca A. Leslie, Emily K. Johnson and Alexander P. L. Goodwin. Published by Cambridge University Press. © R. A. Leslie, E. K. Johnson and A. P. L. Goodwin 2011.

by phosphoglucomutase. These molecules are subsequently joined together under the action of glycogen synthase to produce glycogen.

There are roughly 325 g of glycogen in the body and this is stored in skeletal muscle and the liver, in the ratio 3:1.

When glucose is required enzymes cleave the terminal glucose molecule from the glycogen chain. This is called glycogenolysis. The storage and retrieval of glucose to and from glycogen is very energy efficient.

What is gluconeogenesis?

Gluconeogenesis is an important process where glucose is synthesised from non-carbohydrate precursors such as lactate, pyruvate, glycerol and amino acids.

The importance of gluconeogenesis is that it is one of two ways that the body has to maintain plasma glucose levels. The second way the body maintains the blood glucose level is through the breakdown of glycogen in a process called glycogenolysis. Gluconeogenesis predominantly occurs in the liver but it can also occur to a smaller extent in the kidneys. Gluconeogenesis occurs during periods of fasting, starvation, extreme exercise and in low-carbohydrate diets.

The pathway starts with the generation of lactate from muscle and other tissues. It is then transported to the liver where it is converted into pyruvate under the influence of lactate dehydrogenase. Pyruvate, the first designated substrate in the gluconeogenesis pathway, is then converted into glucose through a number of steps. In addition to pyruvate other substances such as glycerol from fat cells, alanine from skeletal muscle and all intermediates in the tricarboxylic acid cycle (TCA) can enter the glucogeneogenesis pathway at different points.

Glucagon and glucocorticoids promote gluconeogenesis, whilst insulin inhibits it.

What are the main pathways of carbohydrate metabolism?

In this question they are trying to ascertain if you have a clear understanding about the three pathways of carbohydrate metabolism:

- *Glycolysis*
- *TCA or Krebs cycle*
- *Hexose monophosphate shunt.*

Glucose is the basic unit of carbohydrates. However the active form of glucose is glucose-6-phosphate which is produced in a reaction catalysed by two different enzymes depending on the site. Hexokinase catalyses the reaction in tissue cells, and glucokinase catalyses the reaction in the liver cells.

Glucose-6-phosphate can be metabolised by three pathways, most importantly, glycolysis and the TCA cycle and less importantly the hexose mono-phosphate shunt.

What is glycolysis?

You will not be expected to know all the intermediate steps in glycolysis, just remember the key facts that glucose-6-phosphate is converted into two molecules of pyruvate and that two molecules of ATP are generated.

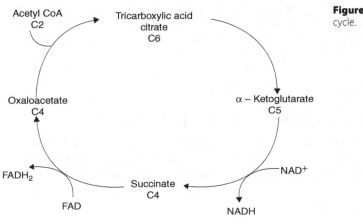

Figure 1.6.1. Tricarboxylic acid cycle.

Glycolysis can also be called the Embden–Meyerhof pathway. It is the first stage of glucose breakdown and occurs in the cytoplasm of the cell. Glycolysis is a six-stage metabolic process whereby one molecule of glucose is metabolised into two molecules of pyruvate which can then enter the TCA cycle.

Pyruvate is a triose sugar, therefore has three carbon molecules, and under aerobic conditions will enter the TCA cycle. Under anaerobic conditions, on the other hand, pyruvate goes on to form lactate which is less energy efficient.

Glycolysis produces four molecules of ATP for one glucose molecule, but two molecules of ATP are required in the process, so the net gain is only two molecules of ATP.

Tell me about the tricarboxylic acid cycle

The TCA cycle is very complicated, and the examiners are not expecting you to be able to name all the different molecules in the cycle. There are four main molecules that you should remember; citrate C6, α-ketoglutarate C5, succinate C4 and oxaloacetate C4. It will be much easier to explain if you draw a diagram. Citrate should be in the 12 o'clock position of the cycle, α-ketoglutarate in the 3 o'clock position, succinate at 6 o'clock and oxaloacetate in the 9 o'clock position, see Figure 1.6.1. Remember that acetyl CoA enters the cycle by joining with oxaloacetate to produce citrate.

The TCA cycle occurs in the mitochondria. It is a sequence of reactions that leads to the majority of ATP production from fat and carbohydrate oxidation.

Pyruvate is transported across the inner mitochondrial membrane and oxidatively decarboxylated to acetyl CoA. Acetyl CoA is essentially an activated acetyl group, and therefore has two carbon molecules. Acetyl CoA reacts with the 4-carbon acid oxaloacetate to produce the 6-carbon tricarboxylic acid citrate. Three subsequent reactions take place which produces α-ketoglutarate, which has five carbon atoms. After two further reactions, another carbon molecule is cleaved off and succinate is produced. Oxaloacetate is then regenerated from succinate in three further reactions.

During these reactions a number of intermediate compounds are produced, including oxoglutarate, malate and fumarate. Most importantly the oxidation of the acetyl groups produces carbon dioxide and this reaction is coupled with the reduction of NAD^+ to NADH and FAD to $FADH_2$. These act as intermediate energy storage compounds and carry electrons to the electron transfer chain in the inner membrane of the mitochondria.

In the electron transfer chain the electrons are transferred through a series of carriers from high to lower potentials. NADH is oxidised to NAD^+ and ATP is formed by the phosphorylation of ADP. This process is called oxidative phosphorylation. In the final reaction in the electron transfer chain oxygen is required.

Thirty-six molecules of ATP are eventually synthesised by the oxidation of each glucose molecule via the glycolytic pathway and the TCA cycle.

Tell me briefly what the hexose monophosphate shunt is?

The hexose monophosphate shunt is an alternative pathway for glucose metabolism. It produces pentose sugars which are essential for nucleotide and nucleic acid synthesis. It does not use ATP or oxygen. It is also sometimes called the pentose phosphate pathway.

How are fats metabolised?

Fats are digested and broken down by lipases into fatty acids and glycerol. Fatty acids undergo β-oxidation to form acetyl CoA which can then enter the TCA cycle within the mitochondrion. Short and medium chain fatty acids directly enter the mitochondrion but long chain fatty acids have to be bound to carnitine before crossing the inner mitochondrial membrane.

When large amounts of acetyl CoA are formed by β-oxidation ketone bodies (acetoacetate and β-hydroxybutyric acid) are produced in the liver. This occurs during starvation and pathologically in diabetes. The liver is the only organ which is able to produce ketone bodies; however, it cannot utilise them as it lacks the essential enzymes. Therefore acetoacetate and β-hydroxybutyric acid are released by the liver and utilised in preference to glucose by cardiac muscle, skeletal muscle and the kidney.

Fatty acids can be synthesised from acetyl CoA in response to a high glucose load. This process, known as lipogenesis, is stimulated by insulin and occurs mostly in the liver and adipose tissue.

1.6.2. Pituitary and endocrine function – Emily K Johnson

What is the function of the endocrine system?

Questions about the endocrine system are often feared and frequently get asked. If you learn some basic principles and definitions it will help you get a good handle on the topic and give structured answers.

The endocrine system is a system of communication within the body. In combination with the nervous system it allows signalling between different parts of the body. The endocrine system mediates slow communication between a large number of cells at different sites, compared to the nervous system which acts more rapidly and at more specific sites. The endocrine system is concerned with basal processes such as metabolism, growth and reproduction. It consists of secretory cells forming ductless glands, which release hormones into the bloodstream. The hormones are transmitter substances which exert their effects on specific target tissues.

What is a hormone?

A hormone is a substance which is secreted into the bloodstream and exerts its effects on a target tissue distant to its site of release.

What are neuroendocrine cells and can you give examples?

A neuroendocrine cell is a cell that, when stimulated by a nervous stimulus, releases transmitter substances into the circulation. Examples include the release of hormones into the portal circulation of the hypothalamus and the release of hormones from the adrenal medulla into the general circulation.

What are the structures of hormones?

Hormones can be broadly divided into three different types based on their structures. There are derivatives of single amino acids such as thyroxine and catecholamines, polypeptide chains containing amino acids with carbohydrate chains attached such as growth hormone and insulin, and steroid hormones which are based on the steroid nucleus, such as aldosterone and cortisol.

How do hormones exert their effects?

Different hormones act in different ways. Each hormone has specific receptors on its target cells. There are broadly two types of receptor: intra-cellular receptors and membrane bound receptors.

Intra-cellular receptors are the targets for fat-soluble hormones such as steroid hormones. Fat-soluble hormones can diffuse easily across the cell membrane into the cytoplasm. The receptor may be present in the cytoplasm or in the nucleus. Once bound the hormone–receptor complex alters gene expression thereby exerting its effect, which may be coding for a different protein or changing synthesis of an existing protein.

Membrane bound receptors could be tyrosine kinase-linked receptors or G-protein coupled receptors. These types of receptors usually respond to water-soluble hormones such as the polypeptide hormones. When the hormones bind to the receptor they release intra-cellular second messengers to stimulate cellular processes, thereby exerting their effects.

Describe and give an example of a negative feedback system

A negative feedback system in its simplest form is when the product from the target cells inhibits the hormone secretion from the endocrine cells. It can be more complex than this, for example if the product inhibits release of more than one hormone. An example of a negative feedback system is the release of thyroid stimulating hormone (TSH) from the anterior pituitary. This stimulates the release of thyroxine, and high levels of thyroxine feedback and inhibit the release of TSH.

What are the anatomical relations of the pituitary?

The pituitary is approximately 1 cm in diameter and sits at the base of the brain in the pituitary fossa, or sella turcica. The fossa is covered superiorly by the diaphragma sellae which is a fold of dura mater. It is connected superiorly to the hypothalamus by the pituitary stalk or infundibulum which passes through a central aperture in this fold. Below is the body of the sphenoid and laterally lies the cavernous sinus and its contents, with the intercavernous sinuses communicating in front, behind and below. The optic chiasm lies above and in front of the infundibulum.

What is the structure of the pituitary gland?

If you can remember the embryological origins of the pituitary you can work out the structure of the lobes.

The pituitary consists of three lobes, anterior, posterior and a very small intermediate lobe, or pars intermedia. These reflect its embryological origin. The posterior lobe originates from a down-growth of the hypothalamus and the anterior and intermediate lobes originate from up-growth of the primitive mouth cavity. These lobes fuse together and develop direct vascular connections. The anterior lobe consists of many cells which are classified according to the hormones they secrete. The pars intermedia contains numerous colloid vesicles resembling thyroid tissue. The posterior lobe is made up of nerve fibres with their cell bodies lying in the hypothalamus. The long portal veins connect the hypothalamus and the anterior pituitary and the anterior and posterior lobes of the pituitary are connected via the short portal veins.

What are the functions of the hypothalamus?

The hypothalamus acts as a control centre for a variety of functions of the body. It controls autonomic nervous system activity, temperature regulation, thirst, hunger, sexual activity and in fact exerts control over most of the endocrine system. It receives input from higher centres and releases factors that stimulate or inhibit release of other hormones, such as pituitary hormones.

How is body temperature maintained?

Maintenance of body temperature is a complex mechanism coordinated by the temperature regulation centre in the hypothalamus. There are central and peripheral thermoreceptors. These detect changes in the temperature of regional blood supply and such changes affect the neuronal firing rates. The central thermoreceptors are mostly situated within the hypothalamus where much, but not all, of the integration occurs. Other structures within the CNS are likely to play a part but such structures have yet to be identified. The central control system compares the afferent signals to a base value and evokes a proportional response.

Under normal conditions body temperature fluctuates by less than $0.5°C$. This is achieved by the integration of different responses. The body is divided into two compartments, the core consisting of deep tissues including brain, thoracic and abdominal organs and the periphery including subcutaneous tissues and skin. The periphery may be altered by vasomotor control, and this contributes to core temperature control.

The responses can be thought of as those to conserve heat and those to lose heat. In each category we can consider behavioural and physiological temperature regulation. Behavioural temperature regulation is conscious and voluntary and includes dressing and undressing appropriately, body positioning to conserve or lose heat and exercising to increase heat production.

Physiological heat conservation is achieved by autonomic activation, resulting in peripheral vasoconstriction resulting in reduced convection and the activation of effector signals for shivering. Shivering is controlled by motor innervation and is an involuntary response of skeletal muscles. It is an energy consuming process and can lead to more heat loss due to movement of limbs and reduced tissue insulation as blood is diverted to the vessel rich muscle groups. Sympathetic activation of sweat glands results in sweat production and the evaporation of sweat cools the skin.

Physiological heat loss is achieved by peripheral vasodilatation, resulting in an increase in heat loss by convection. Sweat glands undergo sympathetic stimulation, resulting in sweating, and evaporation of sweat from the skin cools the skin.

Discuss the functions of the posterior pituitary

The posterior pituitary secretes two hormones, anti-diuretic hormone (ADH), also called vasopressin, and oxytocin. These hormones are synthesised in the supra-optic and paraventricular nuclei and travel down nerve axons into the posterior pituitary where they are released into the bloodstream in response to nervous stimuli.

ADH is a nine amino acid polypeptide synthesised in the supra-optic nucleus. Its primary function is to conserve body water. It achieves this by acting on the renal distal tubules and collecting ducts to increase their permeability to water, allowing it to pass back into the interstitium. This results in a decreased urine output, an increased urine concentration and increased extra-cellular fluid volume. In high concentrations ADH also causes vasoconstriction and therefore raises the blood pressure. ADH is released in response to an increased blood osmolality, which is sensed by the hypothalamic osmoreceptors. It is also released in response to hypovolaemia.

Oxytocin is also a nine amino acid peptide synthesised in the paraventricular nuclei. It stimulates smooth muscle in the breast and uterus. It is released in response to nipple stimulation.

Which hormones are released by the anterior pituitary?

As a general rule when answering any question never say there are a definite number of answers, for example it would be best to avoid saying there are six anterior pituitary hormones. This is because then if you can only remember four or five it is obvious you have forgotten some. It would be better to say "there are several hormones released by the anterior pituitary", and then if you forget one the examiner may not notice and you can continue with your answer without getting stuck trying to remember one hormone. In the following answers I have not followed this rule to help you learn and to add clarity.

The anterior pituitary contains cells that secrete a number of hormones. Five cell types have been identified and six hormones are released by the anterior pituitary. Somatotrophs secrete growth hormone, lactotrophs secrete prolactin, corticotrophs secrete adrenocorticotrophic hormone (ACTH), thyrotrophs secrete thyrotrophin or TSH and gonadotrophs secrete luteinising hormone (LH) and follicle stimulating hormone (FSH).

The anterior pituitary hormones can be thought of in two groups: the stimulating hormones ACTH, TSH, LH and FSH; and the directly acting hormones growth hormone and prolactin.

Describe the regulation of the anterior pituitary by the hypothalamus

The hypothalamus controls anterior pituitary secretions. Nuclei in the hypothalamus synthesise releasing or inhibiting factors which are released into the portal veins in response to higher signals. These then circulate to the anterior pituitary in the long portal veins where they regulate release of anterior pituitary hormones.

There are seven hypothalamic hormones involved in regulating anterior pituitary secretion:

- Adrenocorticotrophic releasing hormone
- Thyroid releasing hormone
- Growth hormone releasing hormone
- Prolactin releasing hormone
- Prolactin inhibiting hormone or dopamine
- Gonadotrophin releasing hormone
- Somatostatin
- Somatostatin inhibits the release of growth hormone, prolactin and thyroid stimulating hormone.

What are the functions of growth hormone?

Growth hormone is a polypeptide hormone released from the anterior pituitary. It is composed of 191 amino acids. It is controlled by hypothalamic hormones; growth hormone releasing hormone which stimulates its release and somatostatin which inhibits its release. Growth hormone itself has a negative feedback effect and inhibits its own release.

Growth hormone has the overall effect of promoting growth, mostly skeletal growth and cell division. It is an anabolic hormone but it antagonises the effects of insulin. It stimulates amino acid uptake into muscle and liver protein synthesis. As part of the stress response it reduces glucose uptake into muscle and stimulates lipolysis and gluconeogenesis. Its release is stimulated by hypoglycaemia, exercise, stress such as the stress response to surgery, trauma, infection or psychological stress, a protein meal, glucagons and dopamine receptor agonists.

Growth hormone's actions are mediated by other peptide hormones called somatomedins. These are produced by the liver in response to growth hormone. The main somatomedins are called insulin-like growth factor (IGF) 1 and 2. They are so named because of their structure. IGF 1 is mostly responsible for skeletal growth and IGF 2 for anabolic response and tissue repair.

What are the functions of prolactin?

Prolactin is a polypeptide hormone with 199 amino acids. It acts on female milk-producing alveolar cells. The release of prolactin is controlled by the hypothalamic hormones prolactin releasing and prolactin inhibiting hormone (also known as dopamine). Its release is also stimulated by nipple stimulation. Circulating prolactin levels also rise with sexual intercourse and as part of the stress response. Its role in these circumstances is not clear.

Tell me about the anterior pituitary stimulating hormones

The anterior pituitary stimulating hormones are thyroid stimulating hormone (TSH), adrenocorticotrophic hormone (ACTH), and the gonadotrophins, FSH and LH.

TSH stimulates the synthesis and secretion of thyroid hormones. Its secretion is controlled by the hypothalamic hormones thyroid releasing hormone which stimulates its release and somatostatin which inhibits its release. Its release is also subject to negative feedback from thyroid hormones. If there is a deficiency of thyroid hormones due, for example, to a lack of iodine then the levels of TSH would rise and result in a goitre.

ACTH is a 39 amino acid polypeptide hormone which stimulates the release of corticosteroid from the adrenal glands. This effect is on glucocorticoids and aldosterone. ACTH release is controlled by adrenocorticotrophic releasing hormone from the hypothalamus transmitted to the anterior pituitary in the long portal vessels. It is also subject to negative feedback of cortisol on the hypothalamus and anterior pituitary.

The gonadotrophins, LH and FSH, promote the development of the egg in females and the sperm in males and the production of the sex hormones oestradiol in females and testosterone in males.

1.6.3. Thyroid – Emily K Johnson

What can you tell me about the anatomy of the thyroid gland?

The thyroid gland is situated in the pre-tracheal fascia in the anterior part of the neck. It is one of the largest endocrine glands weighing approximately 20 g. It consists of two lobes lying either side of the trachea with a small bridge of tissue connecting the lobes called the isthmus. This lies across the trachea at the level of C6. The lateral lobes extend from the sides of the thyroid cartilage down to the sixth tracheal ring. There is often a pyramidal lobe projecting up from the isthmus on the left which represents the embryological descent of the thyroid. It develops from a bud from the floor of the pharynx and descends into its final position in the neck.

Anterior to the thyroid are the strap muscles, overlapped by the sternocleidomastoids. The anterior jugular vein runs anteriorly over the thyroid isthmus. Deep to the thyroid lies the larynx and trachea, and further posteriorly lie the pharynx and oesophagus with the carotid sheath on either side. Between the trachea and the oesophagus lies the recurrent laryngeal nerve and deep to the upper pole of the thyroid lies the external branch of the superior laryngeal nerve on route to supply the cricothyroid muscle.

The blood supply to the thyroid is one of the richest of any organ and consists of three arteries and three veins. The superior thyroid artery from the internal carotid and inferior thyroid artery from the thyrocervical trunk of the first part of the subclavian supply the upper pole and inferior and posterior part of the gland respectively. The thyroid ima artery is absent in many people. When present it arises from the arch of the aorta or the brachiocephalic artery. The superior and middle thyroid veins drain into the internal jugular vein and the inferior thyroid vein drains into the brachiocephalic veins.

What do you know about the histological composition of the thyroid?

It would be a good idea to sketch a picture to illustrate your answer (Figure 1.6.3a).

The thyroid tissue is composed of follicles. These consist of cuboidal cells forming a sphere, in which there is a protein-rich material called colloid. The colloid is made up of thyroglobulin. Thyroglobulin is a large glycoprotein. The protein component is synthesised in the rough endoplasmic reticulum of the cells and a carbohydrate moiety is added in the Golgi apparatus.

How is thyroid hormone formed?

There are two main thyroid hormones, thyroxine or T4 and triiodothyronine or T3. These are formed from iodination of the amino acid tyrosine. Iodine is obtained from the diet in

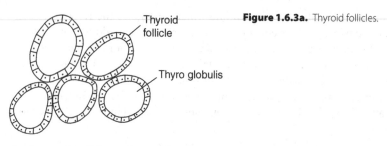

Thyroid
follicle

Thyro globulis

Figure 1.6.3a. Thyroid follicles.

the form of iodide, and actively taken up into the thyroid follicular cells. Here it diffuses to the apical surface of the cell where it is oxidised to iodine and diffuses into the adjacent colloid where it is stored as thyroglobulin. Cell surface enzymes catalyze the iodination of tyrosine residues in thyroglobulin to form two compounds, monoiodotyrosine or MIT and diiodotyrosine or DIT. Two DIT molecules form the precursor of T4 and one DIT, and one MIT forms the precursor of T3.

When the thyroid cells are stimulated to produce thyroid hormone, villi extend from the follicular cells and engulf some of the colloid. The thyroglobulin containing colloid droplets are combined in the cell with lysosomes, which break down the thyroglobulin to produce T3 and T4. The hormones are then released into the general circulation.

There are two forms of thyroid hormone T3 and T4. T4 is the principle secretion with much smaller secretions of T3. However T3 is much more potent and tissues convert T4 to T3.

What factors stimulate the synthesis and secretion of thyroid hormone?

Thyroid hormone synthesis is stimulated by thyroid stimulating hormone (TSH) which is released from the anterior pituitary. This in turn is controlled by thyrotropin releasing hormone (TRH), from the hypothalamus.

The hypothalamus releases TRH in response to signals from higher centres in the brain, for example, the thermoregulatory centre in response to reduced temperature. The subsequent release of TSH results in increased synthesis and release of T3 and T4. These thyroid hormones exert a negative feedback effect on the anterior pituitary and the hypothalamus.

How is thyroid hormone transported?

Thyroid hormone is fairly insoluble. Therefore, it is transported bound to plasma proteins. These proteins are mostly thyroid binding globulin and to a lesser extent albumin. T4 is more closely associated with plasma proteins than T3 and therefore more free T3 is available. Consequently T3 is removed from the circulation more rapidly.

What are the functions of thyroid hormone?

Thyroid hormone has many actions. Primarily it controls the basic metabolic rate and the production of heat. It works slowly and has a long duration of action. High levels of thyroid hormone cause an increase in the basic metabolic rate and oxygen consumption of most tissues. Therefore high levels increase myocardial contractility and heart rate to aid increased oxygen delivery. For the same reason ventilation increases and red cell concentration rises.

Thyroid hormone enhances the glycogenic effect of insulin and the effects of catecholamines by increasing number and sensitivity of β-adrenoceptors. Normal levels of thyroid hormone enhances fat storage; however, high levels results in increased breakdown of fats and proteins resulting in loss of fat stores and lean body mass.

Thyroid hormones also increase growth hormone levels. They are vital in growth and development of the nervous system, and they influence mental alertness and speed of nerve conduction.

What are the causes of hyperthyroidism?

Excess thyroid hormone results in hyperthyroidism or thyrotoxicosis. There are many causes of hyperthyroidism. A total of 99% of cases are due to autoimmune disease, usually Graves' disease. In Graves' disease anti-bodies bind to and activate TSH receptors causing increased unregulated production of thyroid hormone. This abnormality can be triggered in pregnancy, iodine excess, lithium therapy, viral or bacterial infection and withdrawal of glucocorticoids. It is 7 to 10 times more common in women. Other causes of hyperthyroidism are carcinoma, increased TSH secretion or administration of exogenous thyroid hormones.

What are the features of hyperthyroidism?

The features of hyperthyroidism can be divided into general features and specific eye and cardiac features.

General features include weight loss, malaise, tremor, heat intolerance, proximal myopathy, gynacomastia and presence of a goitre.

Eye features include lid retraction, proptosis and occasionally visual disturbances.

Cardiac features include palpitations, atrial fibrillation, tachycardia and sometimes cardiac failure.

What are the possible anaesthetic implications of hyperthyroidism?

The anaesthetic considerations can be broken down into pre-, intra-, and post-op considerations.

Pre-operatively the thyroid function should be checked and the possibility of other autoimmune disease explored. Airway obstruction should be excluded clinically and if necessary with imaging such as a CXR with thoracic inlet views. Damage to laryngeal nerves should be considered and assessed if necessary. Tracheal intubation may be difficult and reinforced tubes may be necessary.

Intra-operatively patients undergoing thyroid surgery have a risk of bleeding which can be profuse and adrenaline solutions can be injected as well as hypotensive and head up anaesthesia. Patients are at higher risk of arrhythmias due to poor thyroid control and possible inadvertent carotid sinus massage.

Post-operatively airway obstruction is a risk if the patient has undergone thyroid surgery. This may be due to haemorrhage, tracheomalacia, laryngeal nerve damage or hypocalcaemia causing tetany due to hypoparathyroidism.

What are the causes of hypothyroidism?

An underactive thyroid can be congenital or acquired. Congenital hypothyroidism is rare; acquired is more common and affects 2–4% of women of all ages. It is 10 times less common in men. It is mostly caused by iodine deficiency in the developing world. Other causes include autoimmune disease called Hashimoto's thyroiditis, surgery, radioiodine therapy or excessive iodine intake. It can also follow treatment with other drugs such as amiodarone and lithium. More rarely it can be due to pituitary disease.

What are the features of hypothyroidism?

The features of hypothyroidism can be divided into general and cardiac features.

The general features are lethargy, delayed tendon reflexes, coarse skin and hair, increased weight, reduced appetite, constipation, hoarse voice, a lower temperature, menorrhagia, myopathy, confusion, a myxoedema coma and cretinism in children.

Cardiac features are bradycardia, cardiomegaly and sometimes a pericardial effusion. High cholesterol and ischaemic heart disease can occur.

What are the anaesthetic considerations in hypothyroidism?

Anaesthetic considerations include the possibility of other autoimmune diseases being present. Carbon dioxide and heat production are reduced because of the slower metabolic rate. Also drug metabolism and excretion is reduced, leading to higher sensitivity to depressant drugs, particularly opioids. Hypoventilation and coma can occur.

What are the functions of calcium in the body?

Calcium has several functions and is vital to a number of physiological processes. Plasma calcium is essential to the permeability of nerve tissues to sodium ions. If calcium levels fall nerves spontaneously depolarise causing tetany. If respiratory muscles are affected the subject is unable to breathe. Calcium functions as an intra-cellular messenger, mostly mediating the actions of hormones. It is also crucial to excitation–contraction coupling in muscle and to acetylcholine release at the neuromuscular junction. Calcium is involved in blood clotting and in the function of many enzyme systems and protein secretion. It also helps in the control of the body's acid–base status.

How is calcium present in the body?

Of the calcium in the body 99% is in bone, 0.3% is in muscle and 0.7% is contained in other tissues. The plasma calcium is normally approximately 10 mg/100 ml. Forty per cent of this is protein bound mostly to albumin, 10% is forms complexes with other molecules such as phosphate and bicarbonate, and 50% is ionised. It is the ionised fraction that is active and is therefore under tight homeostatic control.

How is phosphate present in the body and what are its major functions?

Of phosphate in the body 80% is in the bone, 15% is in soft tissue and only 0.1% is in extra-cellular fluid. It has several essential physiological functions. It is involved in cell membranes, enzyme regulation, energy storage as ATP, oxygen transport in 2,3-diphosphoglycerate and in acid–base buffering.

How is calcium homeostasis achieved?

Calcium homeostasis is achieved by a balance among three hormones:
- Parathyroid hormone
- Calcitonin
- Vitamin D metabolites

These hormones act on bone, the GI tract and the kidney to regulate the extra-cellular calcium concentration.

Parathyroid hormone is a polypeptide produced in the chief cells of the parathyroid glands. A decrease in plasma calcium stimulates parathyroid hormone secretion. Parathyroid hormone then mobilises calcium from bone stores by stimulating osteoclasts. It also increases the gastrointestinal absorption of calcium and phosphate indirectly by the production of a vitamin D metabolite, 1,25-hydroxy-cholecalciferol.

Calcitonin is a 32 amino acid polypeptide produced by the thyroid's parafollicular C cells. It has a minor role in calcium homeostasis as without it other mechanisms adequately maintain plasma calcium within normal limits. It is secreted in response to an increase in plasma calcium and an increase in some gastrointestinal hormones such as gastrin. Its actions are to increase deposition of calcium in bone by inhibition of osteoclasts. It also has a weak action on the kidney decreasing tubular readsorption of calcium and phosphate.

Vitamin D3 or cholecalciferol comes from the diet or the action of ultraviolet light on the skin. It is modified by the liver then by the kidney to form 1,25-hydroxy-cholecalciferol which is hormonally active. The conversion to the active form is controlled by parathyroid hormone acting on the kidney. If calcium levels fall PTH levels increase and the kidney converts more vitamin D3 to its active metabolite. This works to increase calcium levels by promoting calcium and phosphate readsorption in the kidney and gastrointestinal tract. It works mostly in the GI tract by up-regulating the number and activity of the calcium transport proteins in intestinal mucosal cells. The 1,25-hydroxy-cholecalciferol levels also increase in response to a low phosphate as its effects are to increase plasma calcium and phosphate levels.

1.6.4. Adrenals – Caroline V Sampson

Can you describe the anatomy of the adrenal glands?

This is not a hard question and the examiners will expect a well-organised answer. For those of you who like mnemonics, I remember the layers of the cortex (outside to inside) as GFR – for zona glomerulosa, zona fasciculata and zona reticularis and the hormone production from these different cortex layers (again outside to in) as ACTH – for aldosterone, cortisol, testosterone (and the H is for hormones!)

The adrenals are a pair of triangular glands that are situated at the superior pole of each kidney. Similar to the kidneys they are retroperitoneal and encased in a protective fat pad. In adults they measure approximately 5 cm × 2.5 cm × 1 cm and are found at the level of the 12th thoracic vertebra. They are each formed of two distinct parts with different embryological origins, an outer cortex and an inner medulla. The cortex forms 70% of the gland by volume and is sub-divided into three distinct sections, which from outermost to innermost are the zona glomerulosa, zona fasciculata and zona reticularis. The medulla makes up the remaining 30% of the gland and is essentially a modified sympathetic ganglion formed of hormone producing chromaffin cells.

Which hormones are synthesised by the adrenal cortex?

The zona glomerulosa makes up 15% of the adrenal gland by volume and secretes aldosterone. The zona fasciculata makes up 50% of the adrenal gland and secretes mainly cortisol with some sex steroid production. Finally the innermost zona reticularis makes up 7% of the gland and mainly secretes sex steroids and a small amount of cortisol.

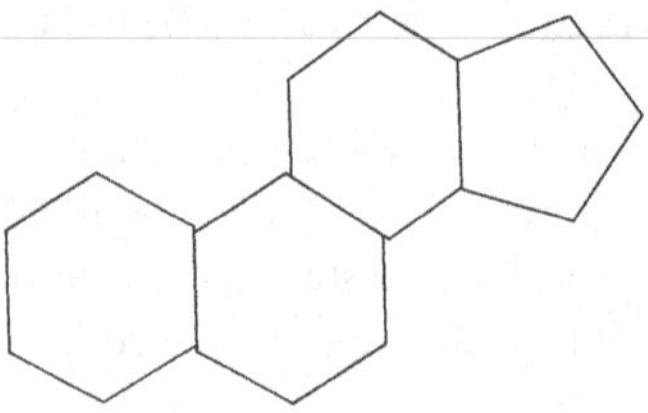

Figure 1.6.4a. Steroid nucleus.

What can you tell me about steroid hormone synthesis?

Although you will not be expected to know every step in the synthesis of corticosteroids, it is worth knowing a brief outline as this has come up in the past. It would be easier to present this as a flow diagram in the exam. It is possible this may appear in a pharmacology structured oral examination as etomidate suppresses steroid synthesis by inhibiting 21β- and 11β-hydroxylase. You should also be able to draw a steroid nucleus – not difficult if you remember it is basically two hexagon carbon rings then a step up to another hexagon carbon ring and a pentagon carbon ring – think block busters! See Figure 1.6.4a.

All corticosteroids are synthesised in the adrenal cortex from cholesterol. Cholesterol is a 27-carbon molecule which is broken down in a series of enzymatic reactions to form firstly pregnenolone via the action of cholesterol desmolase. Within the zona fasciculata pregnenolone is converted by the enzymes 17α-hydroxylase, followed by 21β-hydroxylase and 11β-hydroxylase to form cortisol. Pregnenolone is also converted into progesterone. Progesterone is also acted on by 17α-hydroxylase in the zona reticularis, to form the sex steroids. In the zona glomerulosa progesterone is further converted via deoxycorticosterone to corticosterone again under the actions of 21β- and 11β-hydroxylase and then onto aldosterone by aldosterone synthase.

Can you describe the actions of glucocorticoids?

The actions of cortisol are quite wide ranging so it is really important to classify them so you don't forget anything – personally I break them down into catabolic effects, cardiovascular, anti-inflammatory and "others". This is a physiology structured oral examination so the examiners shouldn't be looking for adrenal pathophysiology (for example what happens in Cushing's or Addison's – even though you probably know that very well!)

Cortisol makes up 95% of total glucocorticoid activity and is known as the stress hormone. Its actions can be divided into several main groups.

- Firstly catabolic effects – protein catabolism, gluconeogenesis, glycogen storage and mobilisation of adipose stores are all promoted, so cortisol has an anti-insulin effect, increasing the supply of glucose to the body tissues.
- Secondly, the cardiovascular effects – cortisol is essential for the normal cardiovascular responses to stress and is therefore said to have a permissive effect on the peripheral vascular response to vasoconstrictors.
- Next comes cortisol's anti-inflammatory effects – it is a potent anti-inflammatory agent by various mechanisms including reducing neutrophil and macrophage migration and cytokine production and stabilising lysosomal membranes. This is obviously its main use therapeutically.

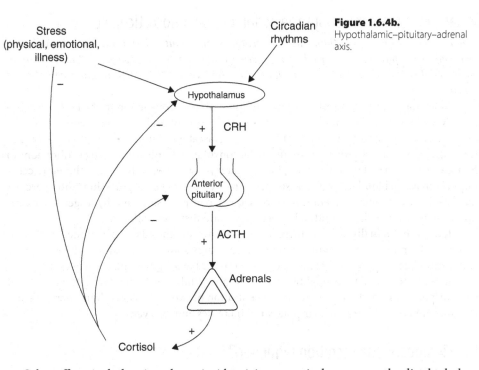

Figure 1.6.4b.
Hypothalamic–pituitary–adrenal axis.

- Other effects include mineralocorticoid activity so cortisol can act on the distal tubule in the kidney causing an increase in sodium and therefore water reabsorption and increased potassium excretion.
- Finally cortisol also acts on the thyroid axis, inhibiting the conversion of T4 to the active form T3.

How is cortisol secretion regulated?

You must be able to draw a simple diagram demonstrating negative feedback in the endocrine system – this is very likely to form part of a structured oral examination question on adrenal, thyroid or parathyroid physiology. In this case it is of course the hypothalamic, pituitary, adrenal (or HPA) axis, see Figure 1.6.4b. However remember also that cortisol is the stress hormone – so you must mention the factors that cause CRH secretion – namely stress as well as the normal diurnal variation.

Cortisol output is 15–30 mg a day, and the most important stimulus for its secretion from the adrenal cortex is the release of adrenocorticotrophic hormone (or ACTH) from the anterior pituitary. ACTH release is itself stimulated by corticotrophic hormone (CRH), which is released by the hypothalamus. Cortisol then exerts a negative feedback onto both ACTH and CRH release. CRH release depends on various factors, including stress, time of day and as I've just mentioned, the levels of cortisol in the blood. Time of day is important as CRH release is modulated by a normal circadian pattern so that cortisol levels peak early in the morning and reach a trough in the middle of the night. Stress refers to physiological stressors on the body which can take many forms including pain, infection, inflammation, anxiety and extremes of temperature.

What can you tell me about the action of mineralocorticoids?

Don't be put off by the question, this is basically asking about aldosterone. Likewise you may be asked to compare corticosteroid and mineralocorticoid actions – again don't let your mind go blank this is just "tell me about aldosterone and cortisol" in slightly more complicated language!

Aldosterone accounts for the majority of mineralocorticoid action in the body (approximately 95%) with the remainder being made up by cortisol. Aldosterone's main action is to increase sodium reabsorption in the kidneys, gut, sweat and saliva. This is most obvious in the kidney where aldosterone acts on the distal convoluted tubule stimulating sodium ions to be actively reabsorbed into the blood, taking water passively with them and, therefore causing an increase in blood volume. The sodium ions are exchanged for potassium and hydrogen ions, so that the sodium excretion is decreased whereas potassium and hydrogen ion excretion is increased which can lead to hypokalaemia and metabolic alkalosis.

Aldosterone actually acts in three different ways on the distal convoluted tubule, it increases the number of sodium channels, it increases sodium/potassium ATPase activity and it stimulates activity in the mitochondria responsible for powering the reactions.

Aldosterone also acts throughout the body at a cellular level, increasing the activity of sodium/potassium ATPase so that the concentration of extra-cellular sodium increases and the concentration of intra-cellular potassium increases and vice versa.

How is aldosterone secretion regulated?

You must be able to explain the renin–angiotensin–aldosterone system succinctly as it comes up in so many physiology and pharmacology structured oral examination questions.

There are three ways in which aldosterone secretion is regulated. The most important is the renin–angiotensin–aldosterone system. A decrease in extra-cellular sodium content or extra-cellular fluid volume is detected by the juxta-glomerular apparatus in the distal convoluted tubule in the kidney and causes the release of the hormone renin. Renin acts on angiotensinogen produced in the liver to convert it to angiotensin I. This then converted to angiotensin II in the lungs by angiotensin-converting enzyme. Angiotensin II has many actions including promoting the release of aldosterone from the zona glomerulosa. It also stimulates the production of more aldosterone as little is stored in the adrenal glands.

The second aldosterone regulator is plasma potassium concentration. Hyperkalaemia acts to increase aldosterone secretion directly from the adrenal cortex and hypokalaemia decreases its secretion.

Finally ACTH production by the anterior pituitary as part of the hypothalamic–pituitary–adrenal axis is not thought to be very important in the normal regulation of aldosterone secretion but may play a minor role.

What can you tell me about the adrenal medulla?

The adrenal medulla is the innermost part of the adrenal gland comprising of 30% of its volume. Its embryological origin is from the neural crest and it is formed from hormone-producing chromaffin cells. It is essentially a modified sympathetic ganglion. It is responsible for producing catecholamines, namely dopamine, noradrenaline and adrenaline. Catecholamine secretion is stimulated by the activation of the sympathetic nervous system.

List the various amino acid precursors and describe the steps in catecholamine synthesis

You do need to know these and be able to present them as a flow diagram to talk through in the structured oral examination. It is very important to point out that the rate-limiting step is the conversion of tyrosine to DOPA (so the examiners know that you know!). You might score extra brownie points if you can draw tyrosine or indeed all the precursors and catecholamines, but I have to admit I never learnt this!

The precursor for all catecholamines is tyrosine which undergoes a series of enzyme-catalysed steps involving hydroxylation and decarboxylation to form the catecholamines. Tyrosine is first converted to dihydroxyphenylalanine (DOPA) by tyrosine decarboxylase. This is the rate-limiting step in catecholamine synthesis. DOPA is then converted by DOPA decarboxylase to dopamine which is further converted to noradrenaline by dopamine β hydroxylase. Finally noradrenaline is converted to adrenaline (or epinephrine) by phenylethanolamine-N-methyl transferase (or PNMT). This final reaction can only take place in the adrenal medulla.

In adults which is produced in greater quantity, adrenaline or noradrenaline?

This is a gift question and you must know it!

Adrenaline is produced in greater quantities, forming approximately 80% of output whilst noradrenaline forms 20% of adrenal medulla output.

Does the adrenal medulla secrete any other substances apart from adrenaline and noradrenaline?

This is small print and probably a 2+ question – so don't worry if you don't know.

Yes, the adrenal medulla also secretes small quantities of dopamine, chromogranin A, acetylcholine and metenkephalin.

1.6.5. Starvation and the stress response – Emily K Johnson

What happens during starvation?

Define and classify

Starvation is when nutrition is either totally absent or present but inadequate, resulting in the body having to use its endogenous stores.

The body's response to starvation can be divided into behavioural and metabolic responses.

Behavioural responses involve reduction of the body's energy expenditure. This is achieved by a reduction in spontaneous activity and unnecessary movement being eliminated. In severe starvation all but critical life-saving movements will cease.

Metabolic responses can be subdivided into three phases: glycogenolysis, gluconeogenesis and ketogenesis, which occur as major pathways at different durations of starvation.

What happens in the first 24 to 48 hours of starvation?

Initially during starvation when food intake ceases, blood glucose levels fall, resulting in a decrease in insulin and an increase in glucagon. This hormonal change is not only triggered by the blood glucose levels but by the autonomic nervous system. The α-adrenoceptor stimulation results in inhibition of insulin and glucagon, whereas β-adrenoceptor stimulation results in stimulation of the two hormones.

These changes result in mobilisation of glycogen stores, i.e., glycogenolysis. The body stores glycogen in the liver and muscle. Liver glycogen, between 50 and 120 g in total, is broken down to glucose-6-phosphate and then to glucose which enters the blood. Muscle stores of glycogen, totalling 350 to 400 g, undergo glycolysis and pyruvate is produced, which is converted to lactate and released into the circulation. Lactate is a substrate for gluconeogenesis and is converted to glucose in the liver.

The liver and muscle stores of glycogen are exhausted after 24–48 hours of starvation and other pathways take over if starvation continues.

What happens after several days of starvation?

During the first 48 hours of starvation when the major source of energy is from glycogenolysis, gluconeogenesis is increasing providing another source of glucose for the body. After this initial increase in gluconeogenesis over the following 1 to 2 weeks it slowly declines as tissues adapt to metabolise ketone bodies and the basic metabolic rate decreases.

Gluconeogenesis is the synthesis of glucose from amino acids, glycerol and lactate. It is stimulated by the drop in insulin levels and increase in glucagon. These hormonal changes stimulate peripheral tissues to release amino acids. The amino acids are converted to glucose in the liver and to a lesser degree in the kidney. This process is inefficient, as it requires twice the amount of protein to make half the amount of glucose.

Skeletal muscle is the largest protein store and therefore the main source of the precursors for gluconeogenesis, which are lactate and amino acids. This causes muscle wasting and weakness.

Glycerol also undergoes gluconeogenesis, and this comes from fat stores. It is mobilised by lipolysis which is when triglycerides are converted to free fatty acids and glycerol. The glycerol is released into the blood and then converted to glucose in the liver.

Ketogenesis is the final process in starvation. Normally free fatty acids undergo esterification in the liver to triglygerides, under the influence of insulin. When there are low insulin levels free fatty acids are converted to ketone bodies, acetoacetate and β-hydroxybutyrate. Most tissues in the body, including the brain, are able to metabolise these ketones instead of glucose. Normal levels of ketones are approximately 0.2 mmol/L, and in starvation these go up to 6–7 mmol/L.

Summarise the hormonal changes in starvation

In response to decreased blood glucose levels and autonomic activation insulin levels decrease and glucagon levels increase. The net result is glycogenolytic and lipolytic pathways are activated and free fatty acids produced. Glucagon also promotes gluconeogenesis.

T3 levels fall and reverse T3 levels rise, which decreases the basal metabolic rate and has a protein sparing effect.

Sympathetic activity is reduced over a long period of starvation resulting in problems with blood pressure and temperature control.

What are the total body reserves of carbohydrate, fat and protein?

Carbohydrate is stored as liver and muscle glycogen with a total quantity of approximately 0.5 kg which is exhausted by 24 hours.

Fat is stored as adipose tissue at approximately 12–15 kg. This will last up to approximately 25 days.

Protein is mostly in muscle and there is 4–6 kg which lasts up to 12 days.

What is meant by the protein sparing effect of glucose?

Small amounts of glucose reduce protein breakdown. This is thought to be due to the effects of insulin preventing protein catabolism.

How long can someone survive complete starvation?

Death would normally occur between 60 and 70 days. When fat stores run out body protein is oxidised for fuel. Once half the muscle mass is lost there is such weakness respiratory secretions cannot be adequately cleared and pneumonia would normally cause death.

What markers of nutritional state do you know?

The nutritional state of patients can be assessed in a number of ways. The assessments can be a clinical history, an examination or biochemical testing. A clinical history may yield information about diet, bowel habit, previous surgery or other factors that may influence the patient's nutritional state. Examination and assessment of BMI and general appearance can also give useful information. Skin fold thickness (known as anthropometric measurements) can be used to assess malnutrition and also monitor progress following intervention. Biochemical markers can be used and albumin, transferrin and pre-albumin can be useful. However, albumin can fall as part of the acute phase response so is not a reliable marker.

Describe the stress response

Define and classify

The stress response is the term used to describe the widespread metabolic and hormonal changes which occur in response to trauma, including surgical trauma. It is a complex neuroendocrine response with the net effect of substrate mobilisation, muscle protein loss and sodium and water retention. The magnitude of this response is proportional to the severity of the trauma.

The stress response can be considered in three phases:

- The ebb phase
- The catabolic flow phase
- The anabolic flow phase.

The ebb phase defines the initial period of shock following trauma and lasts up to 24 hours. It is the time period when substrate is mobilised but the body remains in shock and does not make use of the substrate that has become available. It is therefore a period of hypometabolism with a reduced basal metabolic rate and reduced body temperature. Cardiac output is reduced and a lactic acidosis accumulates. The catabolic flow phase defines the period after this associated with fat and protein metabolism, increased nitrogen excretion and weight loss. The anabolic flow phase is restoration of fat and protein stores and weight gain. In the flow phase the body makes use of the substrate available and goes into a period of regeneration and repair with an increased basal metabolic rate and an increased body temperature. Cardiac output is high, and the lactic acidosis resolves.

The hormones mediating these responses are those involved in the "fight or flight" response associated with activation of the sympathetic nervous system. Adrenal secretion of catecholamines increases, resulting in tachycardia and hypertension. The α-adrenoceptor stimulation predominates and, therefore, decreased insulin release and increased glucagon results. Glycogen is broken down, and glucose is mobilised from the liver. Lipolysis is stimulated, and free fatty acids are released from adipose tissue. Renin is released from the kidney due to sympathetic stimulation and promotes angiotensin I conversion to angiotensin II. This stimulates aldosterone release from the adrenal cortex and results in water and sodium retention.

Cortisol increases as part of the stress response, but this is a more gradual rise. Cortisol stimulates protein metabolism, gluconeogenesis and lipolysis, it also has an anti-insulin effect by inhibiting peripheral glucose utilisation and anti-inflammatory effects. Hypothalamic releasing factors increase in response to trauma which stimulates the anterior pituitary. ACTH is released and this stimulates the glucocorticoid release from the adrenals, also GH increases. GH has protein anabolic effects. It also promotes lipolysis and has an anti-insulin effect. Prolactin rises, but there is no clear reason for this. Other anterior pituitary hormones change little. The posterior pituitary secretes increased ADH which has an anti-diuretic effect and acts as a vasopressor.

The body also mounts an inflammatory response as part of the stress response. This involves release of cytokines including interleukins, interferons and tumour necrosis factor. Il-6 is the main cytokine released in response to surgery. It induces acute phase protein synthesis, including CRP, fibrinogen, complement proteins and many others. The function of these proteins is to limit tissue damage and promote haemostasis and recovery of tissues.

Can you summarise the metabolic component to the stress response?

The metabolic component of the stress response can be considered with respect to carbohydrate, protein and fat metabolism.

Carbohydrate metabolism is affected by reduced insulin levels, decreased tissue sensitivity to insulin and increased glucagon. The blood glucose rises in proportion to the severity of injury.

Protein metabolism is increased with the overall effect being loss of protein and muscle mass. Released amino acids are used for gluconeogenesis and acute phase protein synthesis.

Lipid metabolism following trauma undergoes few changes. Lipolysis is promoted and ketone production increases.

What is the relevance of the stress response to the anaesthetist?

It is suggested that attenuation of the stress response may improve patient outcomes. Clear evidence on this subject is lacking, but the stress response can have obvious harmful effects in susceptible patients. For example the sympathetic activation causing hypertension and tachycardia should be prevented in patients with ischaemic heart disease. Abolishing the stress response could have logical benefits for all patients. Reducing the hyperglycaemic response may be beneficial as hyperglycaemia is associated with poor wound healing, increased infection risk, water and electrolyte loss and damage to the nervous system and myocardium. Other benefits include reducing the water retention and electrolyte imbalance, reducing the protein catabolism and nitrogen loss and reducing the hypercoaguable state and thrombogenesis.

What factors do you know that influence the stress response?
Classify your answer.
The stress response can be modified by regional anaesthetics and analgesics.

Abolition of the stress response can be achieved by epidural anaesthesia. Lumbar epidurals when used for lower abdominal, pelvic or lower limb surgery have been shown to be most effective at attenuating the stress response. Thoracic epidurals are less effective as they achieve a less complete block of the lumbar autonomic nerves. Although regional techniques prevent afferent input and inhibit the neuroendocrine responses they do not affect the cytokine-mediated responses. Morphine does inhibit the hypothalamic–pituitary–adrenal axis, but no evidence has demonstrated any difference in outcomes from surgery despite good analgesia and patient satisfaction.

General anaesthesia does not alter the stress response. However the induction agent etomidate is a potent inhibitor of steroidogenesis and is therefore not licensed for use in critically ill patients.

1.6.6. The liver and clotting – Matthew C Thomas
This podcast accompanies the podcast called "anti-coagulants".

What are the functions of the liver?
Remember to classify your answer; this will make answering the question significantly easier. We only briefly mention drug metabolism in this podcast, as it is covered more comprehensively under Pharmacokinetics, in Section 2.1.1.

The functions of the liver can be divided into three broad categories: metabolic, immune and exocrine.

The metabolic functions are probably the best known and most extensive. The liver has key anabolic and catabolic roles in carbohydrate, protein and fat metabolism. For example, it is responsible for the conversion of the end products of digestion into macromolecules such as glycogen, proteins and phospholipids, and for breakdown of amino acids into urea via ammonia.

Proteins synthesised by the liver have many different functions, including transport for example, albumin, acute phase reactants such as CRP and pro- and anti-coagulant factors such as fibrinogen and protein C. Levels of these proteins are better markers of liver synthetic ability than traditional liver function tests (LFTs).

The liver is also important for drug and toxin metabolism, with both redox and conjugation reactions within hepatocytes.

The liver's immune role is less well recognised but it contains many lymphocytes and macrophages that are exposed to high levels of immune activating cells and antigens as the liver has a high blood flow and filters much of the gut venous drainage. It also secretes IgA into bile.

Production of bile is the major exocrine function of the liver. Bile salts and other alkaline fluids are used for the digestion and absorption of fats and for the neutralisation of gastric acid in the intestines. Another function of bile is the excretion of bilirubin, cholesterol and other waste products.

Can you describe the blood supply to the liver?

The blood supply to the liver is unique, as it is derived from the hepatic artery and the hepatic portal vein.

The liver receives 25% of the cardiac output, which equates to approximately 1.5 L/min. Around a quarter of the weight of a healthy liver is blood. One third of the liver's blood supply is supplied by the hepatic artery, and two thirds by the hepatic portal vein. Blood in the hepatic artery is approximately 98% saturated, as you would expect in most arteries, but as the hepatic portal vein drains blood from the large and small bowel, spleen, stomach, pancreas and gallbladder the oxygen saturation of blood in the portal vein is significantly lower. In the fasting state it is approximately 85%, but this decreases further with gut activity and can be as low as 70%.

Branches of the hepatic artery and the hepatic portal vein travel together with a bile canaliculus, forming what are called hepatic triads. Eventually the portal venule and the arteriole join together to produce sinusoids, which are a specialised capillary system designed to optimise exchange with hepatocytes.

Venous blood from the liver returns to the inferior vena cava through the right and left hepatic veins. A separate set of veins drain the caudate lobe of the liver.

How is liver blood flow regulated?

Try to classify the different mechanisms which regulate liver blood flow before describing each individually.

Arterial supply is regulated by intrinsic and extrinsic mechanisms, and portal venous flow regulated by extrinsic factors only.

The first intrinsic mechanism is myogenic autoregulation. If the hepatic arterial pressure drops, then the flow is maintained by a decrease in hepatic arterial resistance. The portal vein has no autoregulation, and as a result flow is proportional to the pressure gradient and resistance, which increases in cirrhotics.

A second intrinsic mechanism is known as the hepatic arterial buffer response. Essentially, if there is a reduction in flow in the portal vein there is a compensatory decrease in resistance in the hepatic artery so that arterial blood flow increases. Adenosine is thought to be responsible for this: if portal flow reduces then adenosine concentrations around the hepatic triads increase, leading to arterial vasodilatation. If there is a reduction in blood flow in the hepatic artery the portal vein does not dilate with increasing adenosine, so there is little compensatory change in portal flow.

Liver blood vessels are innervated by the sympathetic nervous system. The hepatic artery contains α- and β-adrenoceptors, whilst the portal vein has only α-adrenoceptors. The role of the sympathetic nervous system is important in the stress response when vasoconstriction and venoconstriction reduces hepatic blood flow and produces an autotransfusion of blood from the hepatic venous reservoir.

Finally, many circulating factors like angiotensin, endothelin, vasopressin, glucagon and histamine have effects on the hepatic vasculature. For example, glucagon causes vasodilation of the hepatic artery and portal vein, and therefore increases hepatic blood flow whereas vasopressin constricts the hepatic vasculature and thus decreases hepatic blood flow. It is not clear if these are important physiological regulators of flow.

Is there anything else that affects liver blood flow?

Right heart function has effects on liver blood flow. As the central venous pressure rises there may be hepatic congestion as the transhepatic gradient falls. To some extent this may be mitigated by sphincters around hepatic venules, at least in animals. If CVP falls then there is an autotransfusion effect similar to that produced with venoconstriction.

Yes, and how does hepatic blood flow alter during respiration?

This is important to an anaesthetist so make sure you know how hepatic blood flow alters during the respiratory cycle.

During normal spontaneous breathing, hepatic venous outflow is increased during inspiration as venous return increases with negative intra-thoracic pressure. So, during positive-pressure ventilation there is a decrease in hepatic blood flow during inspiration as the reverse is true, and there is also reduced cardiac output. Liver blood flow may even by cyclical at extremes of positive intra-thoracic pressure or PEEP.

Partial pressure of carbon dioxide also influences hepatic blood flow. Hypocapnia causes a reduction in hepatic blood flow due to a reduction in portal vein blood flow rather than hepatic arterial blood flow, as a result of increasing resistance in the portal system. The reverse occurs in hypercapnia.

Are there any other anaesthetic factors that might be relevant?

Liver blood flow may be altered by the anaesthetic agent used, and its haemodynamic consequences, but surgical factors such as packing or retraction may have much greater effects than any anaesthetic drugs.

What is the functional unit of the liver?

It is a good idea to draw a simple diagram of a lobule as you describe it to the examiner.

The traditional anatomical unit is the hepatic lobule. Each of the lobes of the liver is made up of tens of thousands of hexagonal lobules which are only 1–2 mm in diameter, arranged around a central vein which will eventually become part of the hepatic vein. Radiating out from this central vein are many single columns of hepatocytes. Between the hepatocytes are small canaliculi which eventually drain in bile ducts. At each corner of the lobule lies a portal triad, consisting of branches from the hepatic artery, hepatic portal vein and the bile duct.

More recent thinking emphasises three functional zones differentiated by their distance from the portal triads and therefore the prevailing oxygen saturation. Periportal hepatocytes receive most oxygen and are believed to be most metabolically active; a lot of protein synthesis occurs here. Centrilobular hepatocytes work at lower saturations and contain a lot of cytochrome P450.

Tell me about bile

The hepatocytes secrete a fluid known as bile. It is an isotonic aqueous solution containing bile salts, bile pigments, cholesterol, lecithin, amino acids, proteins, mucus and metabolites for excretion. As this fluid passes along the bile duct it is modified and bicarbonate and water are added to it. The liver can produce between 500 and 1000 ml of bile per day.

The bile will pass through the bile duct into either the right or left hepatic duct, then into the common bile duct, where it is stored in the gallbladder or passes into the duodenum.

Let's move on to clotting. If you cut yourself how does your body act to stop it bleeding?

It is important that you describe the process in a simple and logical manner. It is a complicated topic, and discussing it in a logical format will help you structure your answer.

Haemostasis is an extremely complex event involving many factors, but can initially be considered as a combination of two processes: primary and secondary. Primary haemostasis begins within seconds and involves muscular contraction of the vessel wall, if possible, and formation of a platelet plug at the site of damage. Secondary haemostasis is the strengthening of this plug by fibrin produced by the clotting cascade.

How does the platelet plug form?

There is a process of adhesion, mediator release and aggregation. Endothelial damage exposes collagen which binds platelet glycoproteins in the presence of von Willebrand factor. This is one stimulus to platelet activation, a term for many events including shape and surface membrane changes, increased synthesis of mediators like thromboxane and ADP, and mediator release. These enhance vasoconstriction and platelet adhesion and aggregation. The plug is held together initially by platelet surface glycoproteins, like glycoprotein IIb/IIIa, linked via fibrinogen and von Willebrand factor.

Tell me more about the clotting cascade

The examiners are unlikely to ask you to write down the whole clotting cascade, but you will need to sound knowledgeable about the basic factors involved. Remembering key points, such as targets for drug actions, will give you an air of authority.

Classically the clotting cascade is considered to consist of two distinct pathways, the intrinsic pathway and the extrinsic pathway, converging on the final common pathway of fibrin production from fibrinogen by thrombin. The contemporary approach focuses more on the interaction of tissue factor, factor VIIa, platelets and thrombin, but the basic idea of activation of inactive precursors of clotting factors with positive feedback at each subsequent step remains.

There are four steps in the new cell based model of coagulation: initiation, amplification, propagation and stabilisation. Tissue factor binds the tiny fraction of circulating factor VII that is activated and, with factor V as a co-factor, the complex activates factors IX and X. Activated factor X generates a small amount of thrombin from prothrombin that then feeds in to the amplification step occurring mainly on the surface of the activated platelet. In essence, there are a number of positive feedback loops involving thrombin and other clotting factors that result in sustained production of activated factor X. This produces clot propagation by catalysing the "thrombin burst" that will then result in conversion of fibrinogen to fibrin. Finally, thrombin monomers stimulate factor XIII to cross-link and stabilise the fibrin clot.

So how is coagulation controlled?

In order to prevent uncontrolled coagulation, there are powerful inhibitors of coagulation in the plasma. These factors ensure that the haemostatic response is confined to the vicinity of the vascular injury and platelet plug. These inhibitors can be classified as serine protease inhibitors, such as anti-thrombin III, and the coagulation co-factor inhibitors such as protein C and S.

Anti-thrombin III forms complexes with the serine protease factors, IXa, Xa, XIa and XIIa, and inactivates them. Protein C is a vitamin K-dependent factor, which is activated by thrombin and cleaves the co-factors Va and VIIIa. Protein S enhances the action of protein C. There is also tissue factor pathway inhibitor (TFPI) that binds and inactivates the tissue factor-VIIa and Xa factors.

How do we test clotting?

Think of the tests we use regularly to test a patient's clotting.

The standard laboratory tests are the activated partial thromboplastin time (APTT), the international normalised ratio (INR) and the platelet count. Many other tests can be done, for example fibrinogen and factor levels, ACT, thrombin and bleeding times and inhibitor tests. Clotting can also be assessed dynamically using thromboelastography.

What are the APTT and INR measuring?

The APTT and INR use different reagents to measure the time taken to form a clot in vitro after platelet-poor plasma from blood collected in a calcium chelating tube is re-calcified.

The APTT is prolonged with deficiency of all factors except VII and XIII. Heparin therapy, disseminated intra-vascular coagulation and liver disease can prolong the APTT.

The INR is prolonged with factor VII deficiency in particular, but is also affected with factor I, II, V and X depletion. Clinically, this is usually warfarin administration, vitamin K deficiency, disseminated intra-vascular coagulation or liver disease.

What is fibrinolysis?

Fibrinolysis is the process by which clots are broken down.

Plasminogen is bound up in the clot as it forms. Several factors like tissue plasminogen activator, or t-PA, from damaged endothelium, and circulating urokinase and activated factors IX and XII convert it to active plasmin. As a serine protease, plasmin breaks covalent bonds within the fibrin mesh. The resulting degradation products enhance plasmin generation.

The fibrin degradation products (FDPs) can be measured to assess fibrinolysis but because FDPs are also produced from the breakdown products of fibrinogen, their presence does not definitively indicate that fibrin has been degraded. A more accurate measure of fibrinolysis is the presence of D-dimers which are produced only be the digestion of cross-linked fibrin.

What factors inhibit and enhance fibrinolysis?

This may initially seem like a daunting question, but think carefully about the drugs we use clinically to prevent someone clotting, or to break down a clot and you'll probably surprise yourself by managing to produce an answer.

There are significant effects of cold and acidosis on fibrinolysis, as well as disease processes such as trauma or sepsis that all may lead to DIC.

Streptokinase and urokinase activate tissue-type plasminogen and, therefore, enhance fibrinolysis.

Aprotonin and tranexamic acid are serine protease inhibitors that inhibit the action of plasmin and as a result inhibit fibrinolysis.

1.6.7. Proteins and haemoglobin – Rebecca A Leslie

What is the basic structure of a protein?

The basic building block of a protein is the amino acid. Amino acids are characterised by having a carboxyl group (COOH) and an amine group (NH_2). Amino acids join together into polypeptide chains by forming peptide bonds between the amine group of one amino acid and the carboxyl group of another amino acid. Proteins consist of long, complex polypeptide chains. The proteins can twist and wind together to form a secondary structure. When the twisted chains assume complex structures such as sheets or fibres a tertiary structure is produced. In a quarternary protein, several tertiary proteins join together to form an extremely complex protein molecule.

Can you give an example of a quarternary protein?

An example of a quarternary protein is haemoglobin. Haemoglobin consists of four globin subunits, each of which is a complex polypeptide chain.

Each globin chain is covalently bound to its own haem group, which is a porphyrin ring with a central iron atom in the ferrous (Fe^{2+}) state. Each haem group is able to bind a single atom of oxygen; therefore, a haemoglobin molecule can carry four oxygen molecules.

The four polypeptide chains are joined together by electrostatic interactions rather than covalent bonds, which not only hold the haemoglobin molecule together in a stable form but are also responsible for the conformational change that takes place in the haemoglobin molecule with oxygenation.

Tell me more about the conformational changes that occur in the haemoglobin molecule when oxygen binds

The haemoglobin molecule can be thought of as opening and closing as oxygen is taken up and released. When deoxygenated the haemoglobin is in a taut or closed configuration, however when oxygen binds the configuration becomes more relaxed and some of the electrostatic bonds between the globin chains are broken. The first oxygen to be taken up by the haemoglobin molecule is relatively weakly bound because energy is required to break the electrostatic bonds holding the tight conformation of the haemoglobin molecule. Less energy is required for the binding of the subsequent oxygen molecules because less electrostatic links must be broken. This sequential increase in the affinity of oxygen explains the shape of the oxygen-haemoglobin dissociation curve.

Why are proteins required in a healthy diet?

Proteins are required to replace the proteins which are lost continuously by catabolism. Body proteins are continuously broken down into amino acids. These amino acids are subsequently re-utilised; however, additional dietary proteins are required to maintain the protein balance.

The amino acids which are formed from protein breakdown not only go on to produce proteins but also contribute to the production of purines and pyrimidines, hormones and neurotransmitters.

Other amino acids will:

- Enter the tricarboxylic acid cycle (TCA cycle, also known as the Krebs cycle) to produce energy
- Take part in gluconeogenesis to help maintain plasma glucose levels
- Contribute to fatty acid synthesis.

What do you understand by the term *essential amino acids*?

Essential amino acids are amino acids which the body cannot synthesise and are therefore dependent on dietary intake alone. They are also essential for human life. Examples include; methionine, arginine, threonine, tryptophan, valine, leucine, phenylalanine and lysine.

Other amino acids can be synthesised from the breakdown products of carbohydrates or fats.

You mentioned that the body can synthesise proteins, where does this take place?

Protein synthesis occurs in the liver. The liver is responsible for producing:

- Albumin
- Clotting factors
- Purine and pyrimidine bases
- α_1 acid glycoprotein
- α_1-anti-trypsin
- C-reactive protein.

How are proteins catabolised?

The liver plays a very important role not only in protein synthesis but also in protein catabolism. Proteins are first digested into amino acids. Excess amino acids are metabolised by deamination or transamination.

Deamination is the removal of the amino (NH_2) group leaving a carbon skeleton. These carbon skeletons can then enter other pathways such as the TCA cycle.

Transamination is where the amino group is transferred from one amino acid to another amino acid. This allows excess amino acids to be converted into compounds which can then be used to make energy by gluconeogenesis or fat synthesis. For example the transfer of an amino group from alanine to α-ketoglutarate will produce pyruvate and glutamate. Pyruvate can then be oxidised to acetyl CoA and enter the TCA cycle to produce energy.

What happens to the amino groups which are cleaved from amino acids?

The removal of the amino group from excess amino acids occurs predominantly within the liver and the kidneys. In the kidneys the amino group dissociates into ammonia and is excreted in the urine. In the liver the amino group is combined with carbon dioxide to produce carbamyl phosphate. Carbamyl phosphate enters the urea cycle, also called the ornithine cycle, and contributes to the formation of urea. The formation of one molecule of urea requires the energy from three molecules of ATP. Approximately 30 g of urea is produced every day.

What do you know about creatine?

Creatine is a protein found in muscle, the brain and in the blood. It is synthesised in the liver from methionine, glycine and arginine. In the muscle creatine is phosphorylated and contains high-energy phosphoryl bonds which can be used for the generation of ATP from ADP. When muscles contract the energy for the first few seconds of the contraction is supplied by ATP which is generated from phosphorylated creatine. Creatine kinase is the enzyme required to phosphorylate creatine, and is used as a marker of skeletal muscle damage after trauma, myocardial infarction or extreme exercise.

Immunology

1.7.1. Immunology – Rebecca A Leslie

What do you understand by the term *immunity*?

Immunity refers to the host's ability to defend against infection. It is a defence mechanism.

What are the basic components of the immune system?

The main facts that the examiners are trying to ascertain by asking this question are the two different types of immunity, acquired and innate. State the two types and then give a brief description of each. They can ask a more in-depth question if they want to.

There are two types of immunity: innate immunity and acquired immunity.

Innate immunity is a non-specific, rapid response which does not require previous exposure to the offending organism.

Acquired immunity requires previous exposure to the offending agent for an efficient response. Acquired immunity can be further sub-classified into humoral and cellular immunity.

Tell me more about the innate immune response

The innate immune response is also known as the non-specific immune response and provides the first line of defence against invading bacteria.

The three most important components of innate immunity are the anatomical barriers which prevent microorganisms from gaining access to the body, tissue bactericides including complement, and the ability to undergo inflammatory and phagocytic responses.

Examples of anatomical barriers include the skin, mucous membranes, mucus which traps bacteria, acidic gastric juice which kills microorganisms and the normal bowel flora which prevents invading bacteria from colonising.

If an invading microorganism manages to penetrate these normal anatomical barriers, it will meet a hostile environment. This is because all internal tissues contain bactericidal substances such as lysosomes that destroy invading organisms. Lysosomes are also present in mucus, saliva, tears and sweat.

Dr Podcast Scripts for the Primary FRCA, ed. Rebecca A. Leslie, Emily K. Johnson and Alexander P. L. Goodwin.   Published by Cambridge University Press. © R. A. Leslie, E. K. Johnson and A. P. L. Goodwin 2011.

If the invading organism still manages to survive despite these mechanisms, then special cells are rapidly activated. These cells include leucocytes and macrophages which engulf and kill foreign organisms. Bacterial invasion is also challenged by the activation of complement in blood and tissues and the initiation of an inflammatory response.

You mentioned leucocytes. Can you tell me more about these cells?

There are many different types of leucocytes including neutrophils, monocytes, basophils, eosinophils and lymphocytes.

Neutrophils make up 60–70% of leucocytes and are responsible for phagocytosis and inflammatory mediator release.

Monocytes act in the blood like macrophages act in the tissues, therefore they phagocytose invading agents in the blood.

Basophils are the circulatory equivalent to mast cells.

Eosinophils protect against helminths and parasites by releasing toxic proteins on to the surface of their cells.

Lymphocytes are generally involved with acquired immunity with the exception of natural killer cells which bind and kill both tumour cells and cells infected by viruses.

What initiates the inflammatory response?

The inflammatory response is triggered by pathogen invasion or tissue injury. An invaded or damaged tissue releases several proteins that lead to a cascade of events which produces inflammation. One of these proteins is kallikrein which is an enzyme which converts high molecular weight kininogen into bradykinin. Another protein released by damaged tissue is cyclo-oxygenase 2 which catalyses the conversion of arachidonic acid in to local signalling molecules called eiocosanoids, of which the most important inflammatory mediator is prostaglandin.

Mast cells and macrophages, which are present in the damaged tissues, also release the inflammatory factors histamine, and cytokines of which interleukin-1β and tumour necrosis factor (TNF) are the most important.

Bradykinin, prostaglandin, histamine and the cytokines are the prime mediators of an acute inflammatory response. Collectively these mediators cause dilation of blood vessels in the surrounding area, which causes redness and a localised increase in temperature. The mediators also cause the capillary walls to become more leaky which results in oedema and loss of plasma proteins from the intra-vascular compartment. They also sensitise nociceptors to cause pain.

In an inflammatory reaction the leucocytes we mentioned earlier are also attracted to the site of tissue damage and invading microorganisms are phagocytosed.

What do you know about acquired immunity?

Adaptive immunity is a tailored response to destroy invading organisms by recognising specific antigens and targeting them with corresponding anti-bodies. There are two different types of acquired immunity, cellular immunity and humral immunity.

Tell me about cellular immunity

Cellular immunity is provided by T lymphocytes. Lymphocytes are white blood cells which are produced in the bone marrow. Lymphocytes continuously re-circulate between the blood and the lymphoid tissue so that they can find invading organisms wherever they enter the body. T lymphocytes all carry cell surface receptors which recognise antigens, however each cell can only recognise one antigen. As a result there are well over 100 million different types of lymphocytes circulating which recognise the commonly encountered antigens.

When a new antigen enters the body it will eventually come in contact with an antigen-presenting cell such as a macrophage, dendritic cells or B lymphocytes. These cells internalise the antigen by endocytosis and after processing it, present it on their outer surface to the steady flow of lymphocyte cells. Macrophages are able to act as antigen-presenting cells because they have major histocompatibility complex (MHC) antigens on their surface. This allows them to recognise the antigen, endocytose and process the antigenic material before binding the processed antigen material to the major histocompatibility complex II molecules on the surface of the cell.

Helper T lymphocytes which contain the surface glycoprotein CD4 recognise major histocompatibility complex II on antigen-presenting cells. The T helper cells then release cytokines which activate cytotoxic cells such as B lymphocytes and more macrophages.

Cytotoxic T lymphocytes express the surface glycoprotein CD8 and interact with major histocompatibility complex I on antigen-presenting cells. The activated cytotoxic T cells will kill any infected cells that they encounter.

Activation of B lymphocytes result in the production of memory cells which will enable a much faster response to be made if the antigen is ever encountered again. Similarly a subpopulation of stimulated T helper cells will become T memory cells. Activation of B lymphocytes also leads to the formation of plasma cells which produce anti-bodies which leads to humoral immunity.

What do you mean by humoral immunity?

Humoral immunity is mediated by anti-bodies which are produced by plasma cells in response to an encounter with an antigen.

When anti-bodies bind to the specific antigen there are several possible outcomes. An inactive complex may be formed which is then phagocytosed, the anti-bodies may act as an opsonin and facilitate phagocytosis by macrophages and neutrophils or the anti-body–antigen complex may activate the complement system.

What are the different types of anti-bodies?

Don't simply name the different types of anti-bodies, show off your knowledge by describing and drawing the typical immunoglobulin molecule, see Figure 1.7.1a.

Anti-bodies exist in several forms, immunoglobulin G which is the most common, immunoglobulin A, immunoglobulin M, immunoglobulin D and immunoglobulin E.

The typical immunoglobulin molecule is composed of four peptide chains, two heavy chains and two light chains. The chains are linked together by disulphide bonds.

The different types of immunoglobulins and therefore the difference in physical characteristics and properties are due to differences in the heavy peptide chains.

Each light and heavy chain has a constant region at the carboxyl end of the peptide chain and a variable region at the amino end. There is considerable variation in the amino acid sequence of the variable region and this forms the antigen-binding site.

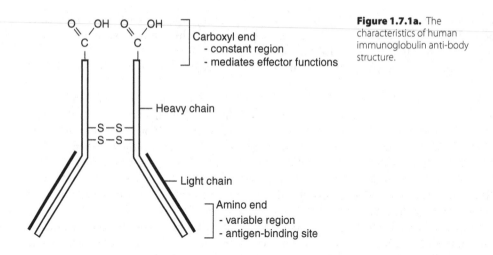

Figure 1.7.1a. The characteristics of human immunoglobulin anti-body structure.

Carboxyl end
- constant region
- mediates effector functions

Heavy chain

Light chain

Amino end
- variable region
- antigen-binding site

What is the secondary immune response?

On secondary exposure to an antigen there is an accelerated immunological response, which is called the secondary immune response. Large amounts of anti-bodies are formed in only 1–2 days, compared to the 5 days it takes in a primary response. This is due to the activities of specific memory B cells and memory T cells which were formed during the primary immune response. These memory cells, when stimulated by a homologous antigen, "remember" having previously seen the antigen and are able to rapidly divide and differentiate into effector cells. Stimulating memory cells to rapidly produce very high (effective) levels of persistent circulating anti-bodies is the basis for giving regular "booster"-type vaccinations to humans and pets.

What are the differences between innate and acquired immunity?

The innate and acquired immune responses both function to protect against invading organisms, but they differ in a number of ways. Firstly the innate immune system is constitutively present and reacts immediately to infection. In contrast the acquired immune response to an invading organism takes some time to develop.

Also the innate immune system is not specific in its response and reacts equally well to a variety of organisms, whereas the acquired immune system is antigen-specific and reacts only with the organism that induced the response.

Another difference between innate and acquired immunity is that the acquired immune system exhibits immunological memory. Therefore it "remembers" that it has encountered an antigen and reacts more rapidly on subsequent exposure to the same organism. The innate immune system does not possess a memory.

What is the complement system?

Don't be scared by this question; be reassured that the examiners are equally unlikely to be able to describe in great detail every stage of the complement system. However it is important that you have a basic knowledge of complements and are aware of the two different pathways involved in their activation.

Complement consists of a group of approximately 25 serum proteins which are important in the control of inflammation. Complement proteins are present in the circulation in an inactive form. The activation of complement occurs in a sequential manner with each activated component catalysing the activation of the next component. This results in an amplification of the response.

There are two different complement pathways, the classical pathway and the alternative pathway. Both of these pathways go on to activate the common or membrane attack pathway.

The classical pathway is initiated by antigen–anti-body complexes, whilst the alternative pathway is continuously and spontaneously activated by insoluble polysaccharides and non-self cells. Through a number of steps both of these pathways produce complement C3. When activated C3 produces C3a and C3b. C3b goes on to cleave C5 into C5a and C5b. The formed C5b then combines with C6, C7, C8 and C9 to produce a membrane attach complex that damages cell membranes.

What are the functions of complement?

In summary the complement system coats bacteria and immune complexes, activates phagocytosis and destroys target cells.

The different components of the complement system have different functions:

- The C3a and C5a fragments are responsible for releasing toxins which cause smooth muscle contraction, histamine release and increased vascular permeability and therefore inflammation.
- Complements C1, C2 and C3 are responsible for opsonisation, which is the coating of bacteria so that they can attract and bind to phagocytic cells so they can be easily ingested.
- The membrane attack complex disrupts the cell membrane phospholipids to cause cell death.

Chapter

2.1

Pharmacological principles

2.1.1. Pharmacokinetics – Rebecca A Leslie

What do you mean by the term *pharmacokinetics*?

Pharmacokinetics is the way the body handles the drug. There are four different aspects of pharmacokinetics: absorption, distribution, metabolism and excretion.

A variety of routes can be used to administer drugs. Which routes are you aware of?

This is a surprisingly simple question. Do not try and make it more difficult than it is.
Routes commonly used by anaesthetists to administer drugs include oral, intra-venous, intra-muscular, inhalational, sublingual, rectal, transdermal, epidural and intra-thecal.

What is bioavailability?

Bioavailability is the fraction of the administered drug reaching the systemic circulation, compared with the amount if the same dose of the drug was given intra-venously. The bioavailability for a drug given intra-venously is therefore always 100%.

How can bioavailability be measured?

This question will be easier to answer if you are able to draw a simple graph, see Figure 2.1.1a.
Bioavailability can be measured by plotting the plasma concentration of the test dose and the intra-venous doses against time. The area under the curve (AUC) for both the test dose and the intra-venous dose must then be calculated. The bioavailability is the ratio of area under the curve of the test dose divided by the area under the curve for the intra-venous dose.

$$\text{Bioavailabilty} = \frac{\text{AUC test dose}}{\text{AUC IV dose}}.$$

Dr Podcast Scripts for the Primary FRCA, ed. Rebecca A. Leslie, Emily K. Johnson and Alexander P. L. Goodwin.   Published by Cambridge University Press. © R. A. Leslie, E. K. Johnson and A. P. L. Goodwin 2011.

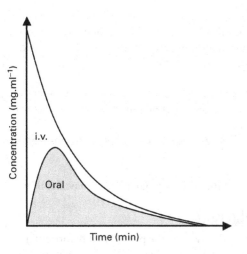

Figure 2.1.1a. Bioavailability. Reproduced with permission from Cross, M. and Plunkett, E. 2008. *Physics, Pharmacology and Physiology for Anaesthetists: Key Concepts for the FRCA.* Cambridge: Cambridge University Press. © M. Cross and E. Plunkett 2008.

What factors influence bioavailability?

Remember to start by classifying your answer.

Several factors can influence bioavailability such as the route of administration, pharmaceutical preparation, physicochemical interactions, patient factors and pharmacokinetic factors.

Route of administration

By definition intra-venous administration has a bioavailability of 100%, whilst the bioavailability of sublingual, transdermal, subcutaneous and oral route is much lower. In general the oral route has the lowest bioavailability.

Pharmaceutical preparation

If a drug has large particle size or significant protein binding then there will be delayed absorption compared to a drug which is presented with small particle size or limited protein binding.

Physicochemical interactions

Physicochemical interactions can potentially modify the action of, or inactivate drugs, for example, the absorption of tetracyclines is reduced by concurrent administration of milk.

Patient factors

It is also important to take into consideration various patient factors which may affect the absorption of drugs. Coeliacs disease and other congenital or acquired malabsorption syndromes will affect the absorption of drugs.

Trauma and drugs such as opiates will also delay gastric transit time, slowing absorption.

Pharmacokinetic factors

First-pass metabolism is an important pharmacokinetic factor that affects bioavailability.

What do you mean by first-pass metabolism?

When a drug is absorbed from the gut it passes to the liver via the portal tract before entering the systemic circulation. First-pass metabolism is the metabolism of the drug before it has reached the systemic circulation. It can occur in the bowel wall or in the hepatocytes of the liver.

As a result of first-pass metabolism an adequate plasma concentration may not be achieved when a drug is given orally at the same dose as is needed when given intra-venously.

Drugs which induce hepatic enzymes, such as rifampicin, phenytoin and phenobarbitone, will increase the metabolism of other drugs by the liver and as a result increase the first-pass metabolism and reduce the bioavailability. Conversely, drugs which inhibit hepatic enzymes, such as cimetidine and amiodarone, will reduce first-pass metabolism. As a result this reduces the amount of the drug metabolised in the liver and therefore increases the amount of the drug reaching the systemic circulation, the bioavailability.

What is the hepatic extraction ratio?

The hepatic extraction ratio is the fraction of drug removed from the blood by the liver on each pass through the liver. It depends on three factors:

- Hepatic blood flow
- The uptake into the hepatocyte
- The enzyme metabolic capacity.

Drugs with a high extraction ratio include propranolol, opiates and lignocaine.

Which routes of administration avoid first-pass metabolism?

If a drug is administered as a sublingual, buccal, nasal, rectal or transdermal preparation they avoid first-pass metabolism.

Which drugs can be administered transdermally and what are the advantages of this route of administration?

Drugs can be given via the transdermal route either for their topical effects, such as local anaesthetics (EMLA) and steroids, or can be given to avoid first-pass metabolism. Fentanyl, nitrates, hyoscine and oestrogen preparations are all drugs which can be given transdermally.

Transdermal formulations are produced to ensure a slow, constant release of drug. This provides a steady plasma concentration without significant peaks and troughs.

Transdermal preparations can also be helpful when the oral route is not tolerated or compliance is a problem.

What factors influence transdermal absorption?

The lipid bilayers of the stratum corneum prevent the absorption of polar substances and only highly lipid-soluble drugs can be absorbed transdermally.

The site of application is important for transdermal absorption, and it must have a good blood supply.

The concentration of the drug and the contact surface area will also affect transdermal absorption.

What are the advantages and disadvantages of intra-muscular drug administration?

Intra-muscular drug administration has a bioavailability that approaches 100% and has a much more rapid speed of onset than oral administration. The rate of absorption will depend heavily on the regional perfusion at the site of the intra-muscular injection. The deltoid, gluteus and quadriceps have a good blood supply so are often used for intra-muscular injections. However, poorly perfused sites will delay absorption and the patient may receive a second dose before the first has been absorbed. If the perfusion is then restored the patient will receive a large bolus, and levels may rise to the toxic range. Intra-muscular injections are painful and unpleasant for the patient. In addition they may cause a local abscess, haematoma or inadvertent intra-venous administration.

Describe the effect of particle size on inhalational drug administration.

You may not be expecting a question like this, but don't let your mind go blank. Just think about the different drugs we administer via the inhalational route, and why we do so.

Drugs which are administered by inhalation can have local or systemic effects. The size of the particle dictates whether the drug will make it as far as the alveolus or stay in the upper airways. If a drug reaches the alveoli then it will be absorbed and will cause systemic effects. If the drug stays in the upper airways, then the drug will only cause local effects. Droplets of less than 1 micron in diameter, which can be produced by a nebuliser, will reach the alveoli, any particles larger than this will only reach the airway mucosa from the larynx to the bronchioles.

The airways are the intended site of action of inhaled or nebulised bronchodilators. However drugs given for a local effect may be absorbed and cause unwanted systemic effects. For example the cushingoid side effects of chronic inhaled steroids, or a tachycardia and hypokalaemia from high doses of β 2-agonists.

What determines how a drug is distributed in the body?

The distribution of a drug throughout the body depends on how well it can cross cell membranes; this in turn is influenced by lipid solubility, protein binding, ionisation and molecular size.

If a drug is highly lipid soluble then it is freely able to pass through cell membranes and as a result is often extensively distributed throughout the body. Drugs which can freely pass out of the plasma are initially distributed to tissues with the highest blood flow, such as brain, lung, kidney, thyroid and adrenals, then to tissues with moderate blood flow such as muscle, and finally the drug is distributed to tissues with poor blood flow such as fat.

Protein binding acts to hold the drug within the circulation and prevent movement into tissues. Warfarin is an example of a drug which is extensively protein bound and consequently remains in the plasma.

Polarity is also important in the distribution of drugs throughout the body. Polar drugs are unable to pass through cell membranes unless there are fenestrations within the cell membrane. Non-depolarising muscle relaxants are polar so have a very limited distribution. They are able to pass into muscles through fenestrations in the cell membrane but otherwise are confined to the plasma.

Large molecules are also unable to leave the plasma as they are too large to pass between cells.

What is a pro-drug?

Drug metabolism normally reduces the activity of a drug; however, some drugs are in an inactive form until they undergo metabolism when they become an active moiety. These drugs are called pro-drugs.

The definition of a pro-drug is a drug that has no inherent activity but can be converted by the body into an active drug. Enalapril and diamorphine are pro-drugs that we commonly use.

How are drugs metabolised?

Although you will not be expected to know the different stages of drug metabolism in detail it is important that you are able to give a broad overview of the processes involved.

There are two phases of metabolism, phase 1, the non-synthetic phase, and phase 2, the synthetic phase. Most drugs first undergo phase 1 metabolism before undergoing phase 2 metabolism. However, some drugs are metabolised by phase 2 reactions only.

Phase 1 reactions include oxidation, reduction and hydrolysis. The majority of phase 1 reactions are catalysed by a group of enzymes in the liver called cytochrome P450.

Some exceptions to normal phase 1 metabolism by cytochrome P450 in the liver include:

- Adrenaline, noradrenaline and dopamine are metabolised by an enzyme called mitochondrial enzyme monoamine oxidase.
- Alcohol is metabolised by alcohol dehydrogenase.
- Atracurium undergoes Hoffmann degradation in a pH- and temperature-dependent manner in plasma.
- Esters are broken down by non-specific esterases in plasma.
- GTN which is inactivated by the gastric mucosa.
- Angiotensin-converting enzyme inhibitors, which are metabolised in the lung.

Phase 2, or the synthetic phase, increases the water solubility of the metabolites in order to allow the drug to be excreted in the urine or the bile. Phase 2 reactions include glucuronidation, sulphation, acetylation, methylation and glycination.

What is the difference between elimination and excretion?

Think this through carefully before answering. It is the type of question where, even though you know the answer, you may confuse yourself.

Elimination is the removal of the drug from the plasma; therefore it includes distribution and metabolism.

Excretion is the removal of the drug from the body.

Where are the main sites of drug excretion?

Drugs are chiefly excreted in the bile and in the urine. Breast milk and tears also excrete small quantities of some drugs.

In general drugs with a high molecular weight are too large to be filtered or secreted by the kidney so are preferentially excreted in the bile, whereas drugs with a small molecular weight are excreted in the urine.

There are three processes by which drugs are excreted in the urine. Firstly, drugs which are small, poorly lipid soluble and are not protein bound are filtered at the glomerulus and pass into the glomerular ultrafiltrate and consequently the urine. The second method is by active transport in the proximal convoluted tubule. Here drugs are secreted into the urine against their concentration gradients using energy consuming processes. The third method is the diffusion of drugs down their concentration gradient in the distal convoluted tubule. Basic drugs are preferentially excreted in acidic urine as this increases the amount present in an ionised form where they are unable to be reabsorbed. Conversely, acidic drugs are preferentially excreted in alkaline urine.

In biliary excretion, the drugs are secreted from the hepatocyte into the biliary canaliculus against their concentration gradient. It is an energy consuming process.

What consideration do you need to take in a patient with renal disease?

In patients with renal disease caution must be taken when administering drugs that are normally excreted via the renal tract as they may accumulate. If a drugs clearance is entirely renal, a single dose of the drug in a patient with renal impairment may have a significantly prolonged effect. If it is imperative to give a drug that is excreted by the renal system to a patient with renal impairment a dose alteration must be made.

Firstly you must consider the volume of distribution. If the volume of distribution is normal then the loading dose should be the same as you would give a patient in health. However if the volume of distribution is increased, as it often is in patients with renal impairment due to fluid retention, then the loading dose may need to be higher than for patients without renal impairment.

In both situations repeated doses and the frequency of the doses must be reduced.

What investigations would be helpful in determining the dose reduction in renal impairment?

The creatinine clearance is useful in estimating the dose reduction required for a given degree of renal impairment. The new dose is determined using the formula:

Reduced dose = Usual dose × impaired clearance/normal clearance.

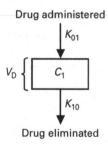

Drug administered

V_D { C_1 }

Drug eliminated

> The terminology for the so-called 'central' compartment is C_1. There are various rate constants that should be included in the diagram: K_{01} is the rate constant for a drug moving from the outside of the body (compartment 0) to the central compartment (compartment 1); K_{10} is the rate constant of elimination from C_1 to C_0. Single-compartment models do not occur physiologically.

Figure 2.1.1b. One-compartment model. Reproduced with permission from Cross, M. and Plunkett, E. 2008. *Physics, Pharmacology and Physiology for Anaesthetists: Key Concepts for the FRCA.* Cambridge: Cambridge University Press. © M. Cross and E. Plunkett 2008.

Is there a similar formula for working out drug alterations for patients with hepatic impairment?

No, there is no single measure of hepatic function compared with the creatinine clearance for renal impairment.

There are several different tests we use to measure liver function; there are the tests which measure synthetic function such as the INR and albumin and tests which measure inflammatory damage such as aminotransaminase.

What do you understand by the compartment model for drug distribution?

The compartment model works on the principle that the body is divided into a number of hypothetical compartments, with each compartment different in size and different in the transfer rate for each drug. The compartment models are used to help understand the changes in plasma concentration over time. We often talk about one, two and three compartment models.

What do you mean by a one-compartment model?

You should draw a diagram whilst explaining the principle, see Figure 2.1.1b.

A one-compartment model makes the assumption that when a drug is administered it is all evenly dispersed within one body compartment. The drug is then eliminated from this one compartment in an exponential manner. In reality a one-compartment model is an over simplification and never occurs in clinical practice.

What do you mean by an exponential?

Keep your answer to basic mathematics. When talking about exponential functions you must mention and draw exponential growth and decay curves. Try and give examples of when both occur in nature.

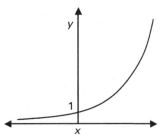

The curve is asymptotic to the x axis. At negative values of x, the slope is shallow but the gradient increases sharply when x is positive. The curve intercepts the y axis at 1 because any number to the power 0 (as in e^0) equals 1. Most importantly, the value of y at any point equals the slope of the graph at that point.

Figure 2.1.1c. Basic positive exponential. Reproduced with permission from Cross, M. and Plunkett, E. 2008. *Physics, Pharmacology and Physiology for Anaesthetists: Key Concepts for the FRCA.* Cambridge: Cambridge University Press. © M. Cross and E. Plunkett 2008.

Exponential functions occur commonly when looking at the behaviour of physiological systems. Exponential functions take the form $y = e^x$, where e is a fixed base, and could be any positive real number. Exponential functions are characterised by the fact that their rate of growth is proportional to their value.

If $y = e^x$ is plotted you get a non-linear curve which rises rapidly at an increasing rate, and where the gradient of the curve is proportional to the height of the curve. This curve is called an exponential growth curve, see Figure 2.1.1c. This is seen in the early stages of growth in bacterial and cell cultures. The exponential growth will only remain until availability of the food supply limits the growth.

If $y = e^{-x}$ is plotted you produce a falling curve where the gradient is again proportional to the height of the curve, see Figure 2.1.1d. This curve is called the exponential decay curve and it occurs in drug washout curves where the concentration of the drug that remains in the bloodstream is proportional to the rate of drug excreted from the body.

What is the volume of distribution of a drug?

The volume of distribution is the apparent volume into which the drug disperses. It reflects the distribution of the drug throughout the body.

What are the factors which affect the volume of distribution?

The volume of distribution is affected by the lipid solubility of the drug. Drugs which are highly lipid soluble have a large volume of distribution, while drugs that are extremely lipid insoluble have a very small volume of distribution as they are unable to leave the blood. The volume of distribution is also influenced by the degree of plasma protein binding, the amount of tissue protein binding and the regional blood flow to the tissues.

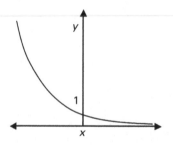

The x axis is again an asymptote and the line crosses the y axis at 1. This time the curve climbs to infinity as x becomes more negative. This is because −x is now becoming more positive. The curve is simply a mirror image, around the y axis, of the positive exponential curve seen above.

Figure 2.1.1d. Basic negative exponential. Reproduced with permission from Cross, M. and Plunkett, E. 2008. *Physics, Pharmacology and Physiology for Anaesthetists: Key Concepts for the FRCA.* Cambridge: Cambridge University Press. © M. Cross and E. Plunkett 2008.

In a single-compartment model, how can you calculate the volume of distribution?

The volume of distribution does not necessarily correspond to a physiological or an anatomical volume so it cannot be measured clinically. It can however be calculated simply from knowledge of the dose administered and the plasma concentration occurring immediately after administration.

Volume of distribution = Dose/Plasma concentration at time zero.

What is the clearance of a drug?

Clearance is used to describe the amount of plasma cleared of the drug per unit time. The normal units are ml per minute.

Using the clearance how can you calculate the actual rate of elimination?

The actual rate of elimination of a drug depends not only on how much plasma is cleared of the drug per minute but also what the plasma concentration of the drug is at a given time.

Rate of elimination = Clearance × Plasma concentration.

What is the elimination half-life?

The half-life describes the relationship between plasma concentration and time. The half-life is the time taken for the plasma concentration to drop by 50% of its initial value, see Figure 2.1.1e.

After four half-lives the concentration has fallen by 93.7% and by five half-lives the plasma concentration has dropped 96.8% of its original concentration.

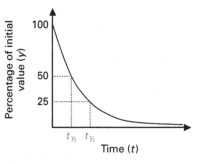

This curve needs to be drawn accurately in order to demonstrate the principle. After drawing and labelling the axes, mark the key values on the y axis as shown. Your curve must pass through each value at an equal time interval on the x axis. To ensure this, plot equal time periods on the x axis as shown, before drawing the curve. Join the points with a smooth curve that is asymptotic to the x axis. This will enable you to describe the nature of an exponential decline accurately as well as to demonstrate easily the meaning of half life.

Figure 2.1.1e. Graphical representation of half-life. Reproduced with permission from Cross, M. and Plunkett, E. 2008. *Physics, Pharmacology and Physiology for Anaesthetists: Key Concepts for the FRCA.* Cambridge: Cambridge University Press. © M. Cross and E. Plunkett 2008.

How is a time constant different to the half-life?

First define what a time constant is and then state how it is different from a half-life.

The time constant is the time it would take for the plasma concentration to drop to zero if the initial rate of elimination continued, see Figure 2.1.1f. It is extrapolated from the curve of a graph plotting plasma concentration against time. We know that in reality the initial rate of elimination does not continue but decreases in an exponential manner, therefore after one time constant the plasma concentration has actually only fallen to 36.8% of its initial concentration. After the second time constant this reduced concentration drops by a further 36.8%, which is 13.5% of the initial value.

Therefore a time constant is the time taken for the drug plasma concentration to drop to 36.8% of its initial value, while in contrast the half-life is the time taken for the plasma drug concentration to drop by 50% of its original value. The half-life is equal to 0.693 times the time constant.

If you require a certain plasma concentration for a drug to be therapeutic how do you calculate a suitable loading dose?

In a one-compartment model, in addition to knowledge of the desired plasma concentration you need to know the volume of distribution in order to calculate the loading dose. Imagine you know the volume of fluid the drug will enter and you know what plasma concentration you want, a simple multiplication of these two values tells you how much drug you need to give.

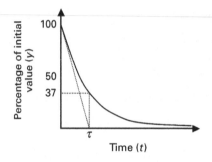

This curve should be a graphical representation of the first and second definitions of the time constant as given above. After drawing and labelling the axes, mark the key points on the *y* axis as shown. Draw a straight line falling from 100 to baseline at a time interval of your choosing. Label this time interval τ. Mark a point on the graph where a vertical line from this point crosses 37% on the *y* axis. Finally draw the curve starting as a tangent to your original straight line and falling away smoothly as shown. Make sure it passes through the 37% point accurately. A well-drawn curve will demonstrate the time constant principle clearly.

Figure 2.1.1f. Graphic representation of a time constant. Reproduced with permission from Cross, M. and Plunkett, E. 2008. *Physics, Pharmacology and Physiology for Anaesthetists: Key Concepts for the FRCA.* Cambridge: Cambridge University Press. © M. Cross and E. Plunkett 2008.

Therefore:

Loading dose = Plasma concentration × Volume of distribution.

How do you calculate the amount needed to maintain the plasma concentration?

To maintain that plasma level (after a loading dose), you need to continuously replace the amount of drug which is removed from the body per minute. Therefore to maintain a steady state the rate of infusion needs to equal the rate of elimination.

So, we already know that:

Rate of elimination = Clearance × Plasma concentration.

We also know that to maintain plasma concentration:

Rate of infusion = Rate of elimination.

Therefore:

Rate of infusion = Clearance × Plasma concentration.

If no loading dose is given how long will it take for the infusion dose to reach steady state?

If no loading dose is given and the rate of infusion started as determined by the above equation, it will take five half-lives or three time constants to reach steady state. In other

Drug administered

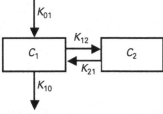

Drug eliminated

> A second (peripheral) compartment can now be added, which may mathematically represent the less vascular tissues of the body. All the rate constants that were in the previous model still apply but in addition you must indicate that there are additional constants relating to this new compartment. The terminology is the same; K_{12} represents drug distribution from C_1 to C_2 and K_{21} represents drug redistribution back into C_1. Demonstrate in your diagram that elimination occurs only from C_1 no matter how many other compartments are present.

Figure 2.1.1g. Two-compartment model. Reproduced with permission from Cross, M. and Plunkett, E. 2008. *Physics, Pharmacology and Physiology for Anaesthetists: Key Concepts for the FRCA.* Cambridge: Cambridge University Press. © M. Cross and E. Plunkett 2008.

words it will take five half-lives before the drug is continuously within the therapeutic range.

Why can some drugs be given as repeated doses whilst others must be given as an infusion?

If a drug has a wide therapeutic range without causing toxicity then it can be given by repeated doses. The first dose should bring the plasma concentration up into the therapeutic range. The plasma concentration will then gradually drop over time, according to its half-life. At the minimum therapeutic concentration the next dose should be given to bring the plasma concentration back well into the therapeutic range. After one half-life, the plasma concentration will be half the initial concentration. As long as this concentration is still within the therapeutic range then the dose frequency can equal the elimination half-life.

Some drugs have a very narrow therapeutic range with the risk of toxicity high, for these drugs it is not possible for them to be given as repeated doses and they must be given as an infusion.

What is the two-compartment model?

Demonstrate good understanding by drawing a diagram, see Figure 2.1.1g.

The two-compartment model has two distinct compartments, the central compartment which represents the plasma, and the peripheral compartment which represents the tissues. The drug enters (K_{01}) and is eliminated (K_{10}) from the central compartment. From the central compartment the drug is redistributed into the peripheral compartment (K_{12}); however, it cannot be eliminated directly from this compartment and must first return to the central compartment (K_{21}) for elimination.

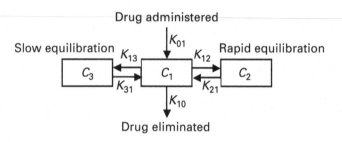

Drug administered

Slow equilibration K_{13} K_{01} K_{12} Rapid equilibration

C_3 C_1 C_2

K_{31} K_{21}

K_{10}

Drug eliminated

> A third compartment can now be added that mathematically represents the least vascular tissues of the body. All the rate constants that were in the previous model still apply but in addition you must indicate that there are additional constants relating to this new compartment. The terminology is the same. Demonstrate in your diagram that elimination occurs only from C_1 no matter how many other compartments are present. Most anaesthetic drugs are accurately modelled in this way. Remember that the compartments are not representing precise physiological regions of the body. Instead they are designed to model areas of the body that share similar properties in terms of rates of equilibration with the central compartment. Your diagram should show, however, that one of the peripheral compartment models is slowly equilibrating tissues while the other models tissues that are equilibrating more rapidly.

Figure 2.1.1h. Three-compartment model. Reproduced with permission from Cross, M. and Plunkett, E. 2008. *Physics, Pharmacology and Physiology for Anaesthetists: Key Concepts for the FRCA.* Cambridge: Cambridge University Press. © M. Cross and E. Plunkett 2008.

When a drug is given into the central compartment, there is a rapid decline in concentration due to distribution into the peripheral compartment. This process will continue until equilibrium between the two compartments is reached. Next there is a slower decline as the drug is eliminated from the body. During this time the drug is redistributed down a concentration gradient from the peripheral compartment back into the plasma for elimination. This phase is called terminal elimination.

Analysis of the time-log plasma concentration curves show that two exponential processes are involved, one for distribution and one for terminal elimination. The slope of these curves represents the rate constant for each of the two processes.

The reciprocal of the rate constant is the time constant, from which we can derive the distribution half-life and the terminal elimination half-life.

How is this different from the three-compartment model?

Like with the two-compartment model the three-compartment model consists of a central compartment into which the drug is infused and from which excretion can occur. In addition there are two further compartments with which the drug can be exchanged. The second compartment generally accounts for the well-perfused tissues, whilst the third compartment consists of the poorly perfused tissues, see Figure 2.1.1h. As a result the pharmacokinetics of the second compartment is much faster than the third.

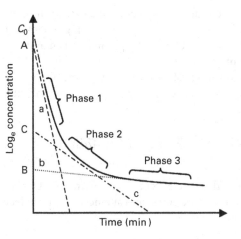

Figure 2.1.1i. Concentration versus time. Reproduced with permission from Cross, M. and Plunkett, E. 2008. *Physics, Pharmacology and Physiology for Anaesthetists: Key Concepts for the FRCA.* Cambridge: Cambridge University Press. © M. Cross and E. Plunkett 2008.

> Draw and label the axes as before. This time draw a tri-exponential decline. Draw a tangent to phase 3 (line b) as before giving a y intercept at B. Next draw a tangent to phase 2 (line c) that would occur if line b were subtracted from the original tri-exponential decline. Show that this line intercepts the y axis at C. Finally draw a tangent to phase 1 (line a), which would occur if lines b and c were subtracted from the original tri-exponential decline. Show that this intercepts the y axis at A. As before, A + B + C should equal C_0. Line a represents distribution to rapidly equilibrating tissues and line c represents distribution to slowly equilibrating tissues. Line b always represents elimination from the body.

Analysis of the time–log plasma concentration curves will now show three exponential processes; phase 1 for distribution into the second compartment, phase 2 for distribution into the third compartment and the phase 3 for terminal elimination, see Figure 2.1.1i.

Most of our anaesthetic agents represent a three-compartment model, where they initially enter the plasma, before being redistributed into muscle and then later into fat.

What is the context-sensitive half-life?

When an infusion is given, it initially passes into the central compartment (the plasma), it is then quickly moved into the second compartment, and more slowly into the third compartment.

When the infusion is stopped the drug will continue to move down a concentration gradient into the second and third compartments. In addition the drug will be metabolised and excreted from the central compartment. The drug will continue to be redistributed into the second and third compartments until equilibrium occurs among all three compartments.

When equilibrium is reached the only way of removing the drug from the plasma is by metabolism and excretion, as the drug cannot move against a concentration gradient into the tissues.

Metabolism causes a reduction in plasma concentration and hence reduces the drug concentration in the central compartment. This will cause a reverse concentration gradient and the drug is re-distributed from the peripheral tissues back into the plasma. This maintains the plasma concentration well beyond the end of the infusion.

The time taken for the drug concentration to fall by half at the end of an infusion which was designed to maintain a constant concentration is called the context-sensitive half-life. The context is the length of the infusion.

How do the plasma concentration and the effect site concentration change during an infusion?

At induction the plasma concentration is greater than the effect site concentration. During maintenance the plasma and effect site concentrations are equal, and at emergence the effect site concentration is greater than the plasma concentration.

Are you aware of any drugs that have a fairly constant context-sensitive half-life?

Remifentanil is a fentanyl derivative that unlike most anaesthetic agents has a relatively constant context-sensitive half-life over a wide range of infusion durations. This means that a patient can be maintained on a remifentanil infusion for a long period of time without the drug accumulating. When the infusion is stopped the clinical effects will rapidly disappear. This means that the patient can be given prolonged infusions of remifentanil for analgesia during surgery but will wake up rapidly when it is no longer needed.

What does TIVA stand for, and what are its advantages?

TIVA stands for total intra-venous anaesthetic. It is where only intra-venous anaesthetic agents are used to provide anaesthesia.

If TIVA is used, you avoid using volatile agents and therefore avoid their complications, which include post-operative nausea and vomiting, distension of fluid filled spaces, post-operative diffusion hypoxaemia and the production of fluoride ions. TIVA can also be used when inhaled agents should be avoided such as in patients at risk of malignant hyperthermia, or when it may be difficult to administer volatile agents, such as during bronchoscopy.

Tell me about target controlled infusions (TCI)?

The target controlled infusion system uses a computer-controlled infusion pump that allows the anaesthetist to select a target blood concentration required for a certain effect, such as sedation or anaesthesia. The microprocessor is pre-programmed with the pharmacokinetic model specific for that drug, such as the three-compartment model of propofol pharmacokinetics. The pump continuously calculates the distribution and elimination of the intra-venous anaesthetic agent, and successively adjusts the infusion rate to maintain a predicted plasma drug concentration.

The anaesthetist initially inputs the desired induction and maintenance target plasma concentrations, and the TCI pump will then work out the dose that needs to be given to maintain the target levels. If it is a highly stimulating point of surgery a new target plasma concentration can be entered and a small bolus is automatically delivered to the patient. Equally, if a lower plasma concentration level is set the infusion will automatically stop for a short period of time to allow the level to drop to the desired new concentration, at which point the infusion will restart at a slower rate.

The TCI pumps will also inform you of the decrement time, which is an estimate of the time it will take for the patient to wake up if the infusion is stops at that point.

What do you mean by first- and zero-order kinetics?

These terms are used to describe the elimination of drugs from the body.

In first-order kinetics a constant proportion of the drug is removed per unit time, so the rate of elimination is proportional to the amount of the drug present in the body. The majority of drugs are eliminated in this way as there is a relative excess of enzymes compared with the substrate.

Zero-order kinetics is where a constant amount of the drug is eliminated per unit time, so despite the plasma concentration of the drug the same amount is eliminated per unit time. This is often called saturation kinetics, because the enzymes become saturated and cannot be influenced by substrate concentration. Several drugs at high doses will convert to zero-order kinetics, including phenytoin, salicylates, theophylline and thiopentone.

Describe the graphs that depict first- and zero-order kinetics

If time is plotted on the x axis with plasma concentration on the y axis the graph for first-order kinetics will be a negative exponential curve whilst that for zero-order kinetics will show a linear relationship.

2.1.2. Pharmacodynamics – Rebecca A Leslie

What do you understand by the term pharmacodynamics?

Pharmacodynamics looks at what effects a drug has on the body and the mechanism of drug action.

How do drugs exert their effects?

Try and keep your answer simple. Leave the examiners opportunity to ask you more details on specific areas if they choose to.

There are three main ways in which drugs produce their effects:

- The physiochemical properties of the drug
- Enzyme inhibition
- Receptor activation.

Can you tell me some examples where the action of the drug is due to the physiochemical properties?

Give examples of drugs that we frequently use in anaesthetics or intensive care.

Antacids exert their effects by altering the pH and neutralising gastric acid.

Mannitol, when given intra-venously, will alter plasma osmolarity. This produces an osmotic diuresis by drawing water from the tissues into the intra-vascular compartment.

Activated charcoal has a large surface area to mass ratio so is used to adsorb ingested poisons and drugs.

Chelating agents, such as penicillamine, are used to reduce the concentration of metallic ions within the body. Dicobalt edentate is used to chelate cyanide ions and is used in cyanide poisoning or sodium nitroprusside toxicity.

What is an enzyme?

An enzyme is a biological protein which catalyses chemical reactions but remains unchanged itself. They are often highly specific for a given substrate and are sensitive to pH and temperature.

Can you give examples of drugs that work by interacting with enzymes?

The majority of drugs that act on enzymes inhibit their action. Enzyme inhibition produces two effects. Firstly the concentration of the substrate that is normally metabolised by the enzyme is increased, and secondly the product of the reaction is decreased.

Aspirin works by inhibiting platelet cyclo-oxygenase. This prevents the production of thromboxane A2 and therefore prevents thromboxane-induced platelet aggregation and vasoconstriction.

Angiotensin-converting enzyme (ACE) inhibitors prevent the conversion of angiotensin I into II, and in addition this prevents the breakdown of bradykinin. The therapeutic effects of ACE inhibitors, when used in heart failure and hypertension, are due to the reduction in angiotensin II levels. However the common side effect of an intractable cough is due to the raised levels of bradykinin.

Another example of a drug that works by interacting with an enzyme is neostigmine, which causes reversible inhibition of acetyl cholinesterase.

What is a ligand?

A ligand is any substance that is able to bind to a specific site on a receptor.

What is a receptor?

A receptor is a specific protein molecule that is usually located in the cell membrane and contains a specific ligand binding site. Binding of an extra-cellular molecule initiates biochemical events within the cell.

Do all ligands initiate a response when they bind to the receptor?

No, not all pharmaceutical ligands are designed to produce a response when they bind to a receptor. In addition some ligands may bind to more than one receptor and have a different mechanism of action at each receptor. An example of this is the ionotropic effects of γ-aminobutyric acid (GABA) at GABA/A and the metabotrophic actions of GABA at GABA/B receptors.

How would you classify different receptors?

Receptors can be classified depending on their mechanism of action. There are receptors which cause altered ion permeability, receptors whose actions result from intermediate messenger production and receptors that regulate gene transcription.

Tell me more about receptors that alter ion permeability, and give examples of drugs that work in this way

Given that both acetylcholine and GABA receptors work by altering ion permeability it is crucial that you know about it in detail.

Receptors that alter ion permeability tend to be cell membrane spanning complexes, which have the potential to form a channel through the membrane. When a ligand binds to the receptor the channel opens, which allows the passage of ions down their concentration gradient. This occurs at the neuromuscular junction. Binding of two acetylcholine molecules to the two α-subunits of the acetylcholine receptor causes the formation of an ion channel. There is subsequently a rapid increase in the passage of sodium through this channel that causes membrane depolarisation.

In a similar manner when benzodiazepines bind to GABA/A receptors, a channel is formed that causes an increase in the passage of chloride ions into the cell. This leads to hyperpolarisation of the neurone. Note that benzodiazepines do not bind to the same site as the natural ligand GABA, but to the α-subunit of the receptor.

Can you give me an example of a drug that exerts its affect by reducing ion permeability?

Yes, ketamine acting on the NMDA receptor is an example of a drug that reduces the ion permeability of the receptor it acts on.

When glutamate and glycine bind to the NMDA receptor an ion channel forms, and the receptor is activated. Calcium ions are then able to pass through the cell membrane and electrical signals conducted. However when ketamine binds to the NMDA receptor it acts as an antagonist, closing the ion channel and preventing the passage of calcium ions.

You mentioned that some drugs work by producing an intermediate messenger. Which intermediate messengers are you aware of?

There are several different intermediate messengers that are used to bring about an intracellular change from an extra-cellular stimulus. These include the G-protein coupled receptor system, tyrosine kinase systems and the guanylyl cyclase system.

Can you give me examples of ligands that activate these intermediate messengers?

The β-agonists act via G-protein coupled adrenoceptors in the heart to increase the levels of cyclic AMP and cause positive inotropy. Opiates also act at G-protein coupled receptors.

Insulin and growth factor act via tyrosine kinase receptors to cause their intra-cellular effects.

Atrial natriuretic peptide and nitric oxide exert their effects by increasing the levels of the intermediate messenger cyclic guanylyl cyclase.

What do you know about the G-protein coupled receptor?

Listen carefully to this question, they are asking about the G-protein coupled receptor, not about G-proteins themselves. Always answer the question.

G-protein coupled receptors are membrane-bound proteins with a serpentine structure that traverse the cell membrane seven times. The ligand binds to the extra-cellular side of the receptor and as a result activates a G-protein on the cytosolic side of the receptor, which activate intermediate messengers to bring about the intra-cellular change. This type of receptor interaction is called metabotropic.

As well as transmitting the stimulus across the cell membrane, the G-protein system provides amplification. This is because intra-cellular messengers may be reused after an initial stimulus, so the ligand affecting the reaction may have a continued action. Consequently drugs acting at G-protein coupled receptors can be incredibly potent.

What are G-proteins?

You will be expected to have good basic knowledge of how G-proteins work.

G-proteins are heterotrimeric proteins that mediate the intra-cellular changes from an external stimulus. G-proteins consist of three subunits; α, β and γ. They are called G-proteins because the α-subunit can bind both guanylate diphosphate (GDP) and guanylate triphosphate (GTP).

In the inactive form the α-subunit binds GDP. When a ligand binds and activates the G-protein coupled receptor the GDP is exchanged for GTP. The α-GTP subunit then dissociates from the β-γ dimer and either activates or inhibits the effector intra-cellular protein. This protein is normally cyclic AMP but is occasionally phospholipase C.

After activating the effector protein the α-subunit acts like GTPase and breaks down the GTP to regenerate the inactive α-GDP subunit. This in turn rejoins the β- and γ-subunits to recreate the heterotrimeric protein complex.

What are the different types of G-proteins called?

There are three main types of G-proteins, G_S, G_i and G_q proteins. It is a difference in the α-subunit that makes these G-proteins different.

G_S proteins have α-subunits that stimulate adenylyl cyclase therefore increasing the amount of cyclic AMP. The cAMP is then responsible for the biochemical effect, and may cause protein synthesis, gene activation or changes in permeability. In contrast G_i proteins have α-subunits that inhibit adenylyl cyclase so reduce levels of intra-cellular cAMP.

G_q has α-subunits that activate phospholipase C. Phospholipase C controls the breakdown of phosphoinositides to form inositol triphosphate (IP_3) and diacylglycerol (DAG). IP_3 causes calcium release from the endoplasmic reticulum, which then cause membrane hyperpolarisation or enzyme release. DAG causes activation of protein kinase C, which results in biochemical effects specific to the nature of the cell.

Can you give me some examples of G-protein interactions?

The α 1-adrenergic agonists bind to G_q protein-linked receptors activating phospholipase C, which leads to an increased production of inositol triphophate and diacylglycerol.

The α 2-adrenergic agonists and opiates bind to G_i proteins to reduce the activity of adenylyl cylase, reducing levels of cAMP and hence neurotransmission.

The β 1-adrenergic receptors interact with G_S proteins to increase the cellular level of cAMP and increased cardiac contraction.

How do phosphodiesterase inhibitors work?

cAMP formed by G-proteins is broken down by phosphodiesterases, therefore phosphodiesterase inhibitors prevent the breakdown of cAMP and its action is subsequently prolonged. This is why drugs such as aminophylline and milrinone have inotropic properties.

Tell me about the insulin receptor

The insulin receptor is made up of two α- and two β-subunits. They are located within the cell membrane, but only the β-subunits traverse the whole cell membrane. When insulin binds to the α-subunits, it causes the addition of a phosphate group to the tyrosine residues, which are within the cell on the β-subunit. This activates further phosphorylation of other target proteins, which then produce the intra-cellular effects. One of these intra-cellular effects is the increase in glucose transporter (Glut4) molecules on the cell membrane of muscle and adipose tissue resulting in the increased uptake of glucose from the blood into the tissues.

Tell me about receptors that regulate gene transcription

Steroid and thyroid hormones act on receptors that regulate gene transcription. The receptors are within the cytoplasm. When a steroid binds to the receptor the receptor–steroid complex moves into the nucleus and acts on DNA transcriptase to alter the production of cellular proteins.

2.1.3. Drug interactions – Emily K Johnson

Tell me about drug interactions

Define and classify.
Drug interactions occur when the patient's response to a drug is modified by the action of another drug. For example the action of one drug may be increased or decreased by the action of a second drug.

Drug interactions can be classified into pharmaceutical incompatibility between drugs, pharmacokinetic interactions and pharmacodynamic interactions.

Tell me more about the different types of drug interactions giving examples of each type

Pharmaceutical incompatibility is when two drugs are chemically or physically incompatible. For example if two drugs are mixed and one complexes with the other and inactivates it. These types of interactions can occur outside the body, for example if thiopentone and suxamethonium are mixed in the same syringe they form a complex. Pharmaceutical incompatibilities can also occur inside the body and can be used to benefit the patient. For example in heavy metal poisoning the metals can be chelated by chemicals and removed from the GI tract or the circulation. An example of this would be penicillamine used in heavy metal poisoning or Wilson's disease where copper is deposited in the body. Drugs can also react with plastic syringes and may therefore require special administration sets, such as paraldehyde, which requires a glass syringe for administration.

Pharmacokinetic interactions occur when the absorption, distribution, metabolism or excretion of a drug is modified by the presence of another drug.

Examples of interactions involving drug absorption are activated charcoal being given to absorb certain toxic compounds in the stomach in poisoning cases, preventing absorption. Also, giving prokinetics such as metoclopramide alters the whole GI tract function. This could increase the absorption of coadministered oral analgesics or other oral medications. Giving agents such as muscarinic antagonists to inhibit gastric emptying can have the opposite effect, slowing the absorption of orally administered drugs.

Drug distribution can be altered in many ways. Any agent reducing cardiac output can reduce the speed of an absorbed drug reaching its site of action. For example β-blockers reduce cardiac output and therefore suxamethonium will take longer to reach the neuromuscular junctions and take effect. Many drugs compete for plasma protein binding sites. This causes problems only with highly protein bound drugs when their enzyme systems are close to saturation. An example is phenytoin which is 90% protein bound. When a co-administered drug, such as a sulphonamide, displaces phenytoin from the plasma proteins its free level rises. Due to its readily saturated enzyme system, its metabolism cannot increase accordingly so levels of the active drug rise.

Metabolism terminates the actions of many drugs and commonly occurs in the liver. Phase 1 reactions, oxidation, reduction or hydrolysis often involve the cytochrome P450 enzyme system. Many drugs induce or inhibit the enzymes in this system and therefore influence the metabolism of other drugs. For example induction of these enzymes by rifampicin can result in failure of oral contraceptives or increased metabolism and failure of anti-coagulants. Inhibition of these enzymes by cimetidine can result in reduced metabolism and increased activity of many drugs, for example warfarin.

Excretion can also be modified, for example by changing urinary pH elimination of weak acids and bases can be influenced. Sodium bicarbonate will increase urinary pH enhancing excretion of aspirin, a weak acid.

Pharmacodynamic interactions occur when two drugs interact at or near the site of action. They can be direct if the two drugs have the same receptor mechanism or indirect if they have different receptor mechanisms.

An example of a direct interaction would be flumazenil reversing the effect of benzodiazepines. It is a competitive antagonist and therefore competes for and occupies the same receptor, displacing the agonist but not causing the same effect. Another example is naloxone reversing the effects of opioids.

An example of an indirect interaction is the use of neostigmine in the reversal of nondepolarising muscle relaxants. Neostigmine inhibits acetylcholinesterase so there is more acetylcholine present in the synaptic cleft. This competes with the non-depolarising muscle relaxant for the binding sites on the nicotinic receptor. Another example is the two inotropic agents adrenaline and enoximone. Adrenaline acts via a G-protein coupled receptor to increase levels of cAMP and enoximone acts by inhibiting phosphodiesterase intracellularly which also increases levels of cAMP. Therefore these two agents interact indirectly to increase cAMP and improve contractility.

What is the cytochrome P450 system?

Questions about cytochrome P450 often come up in MCQs and structured oral examinations. It is a topic you need to know well and you should be able to list the inducers and inhibitors of the enzyme.

Cytochrome P450 is a family of proteins in the smooth endoplasmic reticulum of hepatocytes. They are enzymes that mediate oxidation and reduction of many drugs. There are many isoforms of the enzyme, seven of which are the most important in human drug metabolism. The isoform often involved in drug interactions is CYP 3A4.

What factors induce the cytochrome P450 enzyme system?

Several factors can induce cytochrome P450 resulting in the increased metabolism of drugs and therefore decreasing their actions.

Drugs inducing the system are barbiturates, phenytoin, carbamazepine, griseofulvin and rifampicin. Chronic alcohol consumption induces the enzymes. Polycyclic hydrocarbons from tobacco and grilled meats induce some isoforms of the enzyme. Broccoli induces one isoform of the enzyme.

What factors inhibit the cytochrome P450 enzyme system?

Many drugs inhibit cytochrome P450, resulting in decreased metabolism and increased plasma concentrations of concurrently used drugs. Imidazole derivatives including ketoconazole, itraconazole, omeprazole, cimetidine and etomidate all inhibit by combining with haem. Other drugs inhibiting the system are macrolide antibiotics, most anti-depressants, HIV protease inhibitors, cyclosporine and amiodarone. Grapefruit juice also inhibits an isoform of the enzyme.

Define summation and give an example

Summation is when the action of two drugs is additive. An example is the effect of premedication with a benzodiazepine such as midazolam and then propofol given at induction of anaesthesia. When used in combination with midazolam, the dose of propofol required to achieve the same level of anaesthesia is lower.

Define synergism and give an example

Synergism is when the combined action of two drugs is greater than the action that would be expected from summation alone. An example is the combination of sulphonamide antibiotics and trimethoprim. When given alone both drugs are bacteriostatic but if given together they are bactericidal. Clonidine and opiates is a further example of synergism.

Define potentiation and give an example

Potentiation is when one drug increases the effect of another drug. An example is the potentiation of non-depolarising neuromuscular blockade by magnesium.

What is an isobologram?

You could be shown an isobologram in an OSCE or structured oral examination situation and asked to interpret it.

An isobologram is a graph describing the combined effect of two drugs (Figure 2.1.3a). It can be used to study the interactions between two drugs. The fractional concentrations of each drug would be represented on the x and y axis and a straight line showing an inversely proportional relationship represents a purely additive effect between the drugs. A non-linear

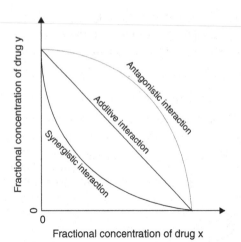

Figure 2.1.3a. Isobologram.

relationship represents some form of interaction with a concave curve representing synergism and a convex curve representing antagonism.

2.1.4. Agonists and antagonists – Rebecca A Leslie

What do you understand by the terms *affinity* and *intrinsic activity*?

Affinity is how avidly the drug binds to its receptor, or how well the key fits in the lock.

Intrinsic activity, also known as efficacy, is a measure of the magnitude of the effect that the drug produces after it has bound to the receptor.

What is potency?

Potency is a measure of the quantity of a drug needed in order to produce the maximal effect. If a large dose is required to produce maximal effect a drug is not very potent, however if a small dose produces the maximal effect a drug is considered to be potent.

How can we compare the potency of two different drugs?

We can compare the potency of two different drugs by using either the median effective concentration (EC_{50}) or the median effective dose (ED_{50}).

Describe what you mean by the terms EC_{50} and the ED_{50}

The median effective concentration or EC_{50} is the concentration of a drug that produces a specific response that is exactly half-way between baseline and maximum.

The median effective dose or ED_{50} is the dose of a drug that induces a specific response in exactly 50% of the population who take it.

What is an agonist?

Give a simple clear definition using the terms they have just asked you to describe.

An agonist is a drug that has significant affinity for its receptor and has full intrinsic activity. Therefore when it binds to the receptor it produces a maximum response that the receptor is capable of mediating, this is described as having an intrinsic activity of 1.

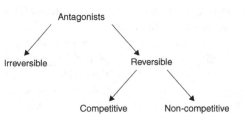

Figure 2.1.4a. Classification of antagonists.

What is a partial agonist?

Again give a clear definition and if possible give an example of a partial agonist to show the depth of your understanding and the clinical relevance.

A partial agonist is a drug that has significant receptor affinity but only partial intrinsic activity. So unlike with a true agonist, when the drug binds to the receptor a maximum response is never mediated despite an increase in the dose of the drug. It is therefore said to have an intrinsic activity of between 0 and 1. An example of a partial agonist is buprenorphine acting at the μ-receptor.

Partial agonists can act as either agonists or antagonists depending on the circumstances.

If used alone they are agonists because they produce a response, even if it is not the maximum response that a true agonist would produce. They also act as agonists if they are used alongside a low dose of a true agonist. However, if they are used in conjunction with high doses of a true agonist for the same receptor, the partial agonist will act as a competitive antagonist. This is because they will compete with the true agonist for the receptor, preventing the true agonist from having full occupancy and therefore preventing a maximal response.

So just to recap, the distinguishing feature of a partial agonist is that it fails to produce a maximal effect even at very high doses when all the receptors are occupied.

What is an inverse agonist?

An inverse agonist is a drug that has significant receptor affinity and intrinsic activity, but it exerts an opposite effect to the endogenous agonist.

What is an antagonist?

An antagonist has significant receptor affinity but has no intrinsic activity. So when a drug binds to the receptor no response is mediated. Antagonists are therefore described as having an intrinsic activity of 0.

What different types of antagonists do you know about?

Remember to classify your answer. Different types of antagonists can be confusing so have a clear structure in your head. It may help to write down the classification as you are describing it so as not to get confused, see Figure 2.1.4a. Then move on to describe each type in turn.

Antagonists can be classified as reversible or irreversible.

Reversible antagonists can be further sub-classified as competitive or non-competitive.

Reversible competitive antagonists compete for the same receptor as the agonist. This means that the effect of the antagonist can be overcome by increasing the dose of the agonist. Examples of competitive antagonists include the non-depolarising muscle relaxants, which compete for the nicotinic receptor of the neuromuscular junction, and β-blockers which compete with adrenaline at the β-adrenergic receptor sites in the heart.

Reversible non-competitive antagonists prevent receptor activation through conformational distortion of the receptor rather than binding to the same site as the agonist or altering binding of the agonist. Because they are non-competitive their action cannot be overcome by increasing the concentration of the agonist. An example of a reversible, non-competitive antagonist is ketamine, which antagonises glutamate at the NMDA receptors.

Irreversible antagonists bind irreversibly to the receptor or at a distant site and prevent the agonist from binding to its receptor. With irreversible antagonism increasing the agonist dose will not overcome the blockade because the antagonist has bound irreversibly. An example is phenoxybenzamine, which binds irreversibly to α-adrenoceptors antagonizing the effect of catecholamines.

What is the difference between a competitive antagonist and an inverse agonist?

An inverse agonist will exert its own physiological effect, the opposite to the agonist, when it binds with the receptor whereas a competitive antagonist has no direct effect of its own and simply stops the endogenous agonist exerting its effect.

What is the dose–response curve?

Do not wait to be told to draw the graph, draw it whilst you describe it. Try to avoid drawing the diagram in silence before describing it, as the examiners are not going to appreciate long pauses of silence.

The dose–response curve is a graph with the concentration of the drug on the x axis and the response on the y axis, see Figure 2.1.4b. It is hyperbolic in shape. The shape of this curve shows that initially as the drug concentration increases and the receptor occupancy increases, so accordingly the response increases dramatically. However, when the number of empty receptors decreases, the effect of increasing the drug dose has a smaller effect on the response elicited, so the slope of the curve flattens out completely at 100%.

On a dose–response curve when the dose of the agonist is zero, the response will always be zero. In addition the maximum response will always be 100%. The EC_{50} value, which is the concentration of the drug which when achieved will produce a response half way between the baseline and maximum response.

What is a log-dose response curve? What is its advantages?

The log-dose response curve is a semi-logarithmic plot. The curve is plotted using a logarithmic scale for the dose on the x axis and response on the y axis, see Figure 2.1.4c.

Unlike the hyperbolic shape of the dose–response curve this produces the classical sigmoid shape curve. The hyperbolic shape of the dose–response curve makes it difficult to identify the maximum response, and also makes it hard to make comparisons with other agonists and antagonists. In contrast when using the log-dose response curve, the steep part of the curve is approximately linear. This makes the assessment of the relationship between dose and response easier to understand. The ED_{50} value is on the steep, linear part of this curve.

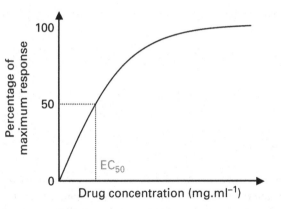

This graph will have been produced from a functional assay in the laboratory on a single subject and is concerned with drug potency. Demonstrate that the EC_{50} is as shown.

Figure 2.1.4b. Dose–response curves. Reproduced with permission from Cross, M. and Plunkett, E. 2008. *Physics, Pharmacology and Physiology for Anaesthetists: Key Concepts for the FRCA.* Cambridge: Cambridge University Press. © M. Cross and E. Plunkett 2008.

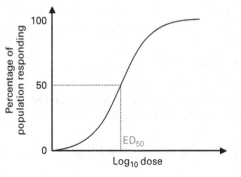

The curve is sigmoid as the x axis is now logarithmic. Ensure the middle third of the curve is linear and demonstrate the ED_{50} as shown. Make this your reference curve for a full agonist and use it to compare with other drugs as described below.

Figure 2.1.4c. Log-dose response curve. Reproduced with permission from Cross, M. and Plunkett, E. 2008. *Physics, Pharmacology and Physiology for Anaesthetists: Key Concepts for the FRCA.* Cambridge: Cambridge University Press. © M. Cross and E. Plunkett 2008.

How would the curve for a drug with a lower potency compare to a drug with a higher potency?

The potency of the drug will cause a parallel shift of the curve to the left or the right. A more potent drug will shift the curve to the left, because lower concentrations are required

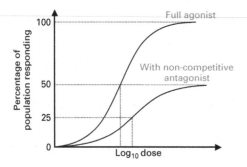

Because a non-competitive antagonist alters the shape of the receptor, the agonist cannot bind at all. The usual sigmoid curve is displaced down and to the right in a similar manner to the graph of agonist versus partial agonist drawn above. Increasing the dose of agonist does not improve response as receptor sites are no longer available for binding.

Figure 2.1.4d. Non-competitive antagonist curves. Reproduced with permission from Cross, M. and Plunkett, E. 2008. *Physics, Pharmacology and Physiology for Anaesthetists: Key Concepts for the FRCA.* Cambridge: Cambridge University Press. © M. Cross and E. Plunkett 2008.

to produce the response. A drug with less potency will move the curve to the right as higher concentration is required to produce the same response. The maximum response of both of the drugs will be the same, so the height of the curves is identical.

What else would make the curve move to the right?

If a competitive antagonist is given alongside a full agonist this will also cause a parallel shift of the curve to the right. This is because a higher concentration of the agonist is then required to produce the full response because it is competing with the antagonist.

What would happen to the shape of a curve if a non-competitive antagonist was given?

If a non-competitive antagonist is given, such as ketamine at the NMDA receptor, the log-dose curve will again move to the right, however in addition, the maximum achievable response is reduced. This is because when a non-competitive antagonist is given, even increasing the dose of the agonist will not overcome the effects of the antagonist. Therefore the maximum response can never be achieved, see Figure 2.1.4d.

What would happen to the shape of the curve if the drug was a partial agonist?

If a partial agonist is given there is no parallel shift in the curve however it will be impossible to elicit the maximum response despite high drug doses, so the height of the curve would be smaller, see Figure 2.1.4e.

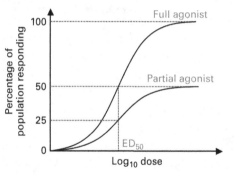

Draw a standard log-dose versus response curve as before and label it 'full agonist'. Next draw a second sigmoid curve that does not rise so far on the y axis. The inability to reach 100% population response automatically makes this representative of a partial agonist as it lacks efficacy. The next thing to consider is potency. The ED_{50} is taken as the point that lies half way between baseline and the maximum population response. For a full agonist, this is always half of 100%, but for a partial agonist it is half whatever the maximum is. In this instance, the maximum population response is 50% and so the ED_{50} is read at 25%. In this plot, both the agonist and partial agonist are equally potent as they share the same ED_{50}.

Figure 2.1.4e. Partial agonist curves. Reproduced with permission from Cross, M. and Plunkett, E. 2008. *Physics, Pharmacology and Physiology for Anaesthetists: Key Concepts for the FRCA.* Cambridge: Cambridge University Press. © M. Cross and E. Plunkett 2008.

What is the dose ratio?

The dose ratio is the term used to describe the extent of the rightward shift of the log-dose response curve in the presence of a competitive antagonist. It is used to determine the factor by which the dose of the agonist must be increased to produce a maximal response in the presence of the competitive antagonist.

$$\text{Dose ratio} = \frac{\text{Dose of agonist in presence of inhibitor}}{\text{Dose of agonist in absence of inhibitor}}.$$

2.1.5. Isomerism – Rebecca A Leslie

What are isomers?

This is a common question, and it is important to have a succinct answer. Most people know what isomers are but are unable to give a good definition, make sure you can.

Isomers are chemical compounds which have the same molecular formula and therefore the same molecular weight, but a different structural arrangement.

As a result of the different structural arrangement they have different physical or chemical properties.

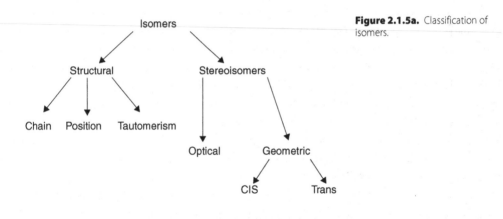

Figure 2.1.5a. Classification of isomers.

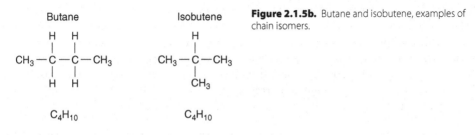

Figure 2.1.5b. Butane and isobutene, examples of chain isomers.

What are the different types of isomers?

Regardless of how well they know it, it is common for candidates to get confused about the different types of isomers in the exam. Think it through carefully before answering. In addition you may find it helpful to write down the different classes and their sub-divisions as you are explaining it, see Figure 2.1.5a.

There are two main classes of isomers; structural isomers and stereoisomers.

Structural isomers have identical chemical formulae, but a different order of atomic bonds, therefore they have different chemical structures. Depending on the degree of structural similarities between the two isomers their pharmacological effect may range from identical to markedly different. Structural isomers can be further sub-classified as chain structural isomers, position structural isomers and dynamic structural isomers also called tautomerism.

Stereoisomers have both the same atoms and the same bond structure as each other but they have a different three-dimensional configuration. Stereoisomers can be sub-classified as optical stereoisomers and geometric stereoisomers.

Can you tell me more about the different types of structural isomers?

The three different types of structural isomers are chain structural isomers, position structural isomers and dynamic structural isomers.

Chain isomers are compounds where the carbon chain alters but the function groups remain the same. Butane and isobutene are an example of chain structural isomers, see Figure 2.1.5b.

Isoflurane

```
      F    H  F
      |    |  |
H — C — O — C — C — F
      |    |  |
      F    Cl F
```

Enflurane

```
      F    F  H
      |    |  |
H — C — O — C — C — F
      |    |  |
      F    F  Cl
```

Figure 2.1.5c. Isoflurane and enflurane, examples of position isomers.

Position structural isomers in contrast to chain structural isomers have the same basic chain structure but the functional groups are in different positions. Isoflurane and enflurane are examples of position structural isomers, see Figure 2.1.5c.

Dynamic structural isomers or tautomerism is the term given when a molecule exists in two different forms, often depending on the physical environment. For example midazolam is ionised at pH 4 but changes structure by forming a seven-membered unionised ring at physiological pH, rendering it lipid soluble.

Can you give some examples of stereoisomers?

As I mentioned earlier there are two types of stereoisomers: geometric and optical.

Geometric isomers have the same chemical constituents and the same covalent bonds but a difference in the spatial arrangement of atoms. Geometric isomers occur when a molecule has two dissimilar groups attached to two atoms that are in turn linked either by a double bond or a ring structure. If the two groups of atoms are on the same side of the covalent bond or ring then this arrangement is called *cis*. However, if the atoms are on opposite sides of the covalent bond or ring then this is called trans.

Mivacurium contains three geometric isomers, the majority of the solution is the *trans–trans* isomer, a third is the *trans–cis* isomer and only 6% is the *cis–cis* isomer. Atracurium has 10 stereoisomers, of which *cis*-atracurium is one.

Optical isomers are molecules that appear to be mirror images of each other and could not be superimposed. They contain at least one chiral centre.

What is a chiral centre?

A chiral centre is a central atom (normally a carbon atom or a quaternary nitrogen) that is surrounded by four different chemical groups. The different groups are arranged around the central atom. One group extends vertically from the central atom whilst the other three groups point to the vertices of a tetrahedron. This configuration means that there are two possible arrangements of the atoms, which are mirror images of each other and therefore cannot be superimposed. This is often described as the property of "handedness", and in fact the word chiral originates from the Greek word for hand. The right hand is a mirror image of the left hand, yet they cannot be superimposed.

All optical stereoisomers are optically active, which means that they will rotate a plane of polarised light. One isomer will rotate the light to the left whilst the other will rotate it to the right. Another name for optical stereoisomers is enantiomers.

Optical stereoisomers have the same pharmacochemical properties such as boiling point, density and colour, so if the drug action depends on these pharmacochemical properties then all the enantiomers can be expected to have similar actions. However if the action of the drug depends on binding to a receptor then the conformational differences of the enantiomers will lead to marked differences in the activity of the different optical isomers.

How are different optical stereoisomers named?

Optical stereoisomers were previously named according to which way they rotated a plane of polarised light, dextrorotatory to the right, and laevorotatory to the left.

This naming system has now been replaced by the absolute arrangement of the atoms of the four groups surrounding the central atom. It requires knowledge about the atomic numbers of the atoms. Firstly the atom of the lowest atomic number is identified and the observer imagines this lies behind the plane of the page. The other three atoms now lie on this plane and their atomic numbers identified. If their atomic numbers descend in a clockwise fashion then there are labelled R or rectus, if they descend in an anti-clockwise manner then they are labelled S for sinister.

What is a racemic mixture?

A racemic solution is one that contains equal proportions of different enantiomers. Examples of racemic mixtures that we use frequently in anaesthetics include the volatile agents with the exception of sevoflurane, bupivicaine and atropine.

In racemic mixtures even though there are equal proportions of two different enantiomers, one of the enantiomers may be responsible for all the side effects whilst the other enantiomer may confer the majority of the activity of the drug.

What is an enantiopure preparation?

This is a preparation of a drug that only contains one enantiomer. In general the sinister, or S form has a better pharmacokinetic and pharmacodynamic profile than the rectus, or R form. Recently S-bupivicaine, S-ropivicaine and S-ketamine have become widely available and have a much better side effect profile than the forms that contain the R isomer as well.

What are diastereoisomers?

Diastereoisomers are compounds that contain more than one chiral centre, so there are multiple stereoisomers. These isomers are not mirror images of each other, therefore cannot be called enantiomers.

Atracurium contains four chiral centres, two of which are carbon atoms whilst the other two are quaternary nitrogen atoms. As a result atracurium contains 10 different three-dimensional structures, one of which is *cis*-atracurium.

Do physiological enantiomers exist?

In the body compounds with a chiral centre normally exist as single isomers. This is because the enzymes involved in their production normally only produce one conformation. For example, naturally occurring carbohydrates are dextrorotatory, so they rotate light to the right. Glucose is an example of this as it exists naturally in the body as D-glucose, which is the dextrorotatory enantiomer, interestingly this is why it is often called dextrose.

Chapter

2.2

Intra-venous anaesthetic agents

2.2.1. Propofol and thiopentone – Joy M Sanders

What are the properties of an ideal intra-venous anaesthetic agent?

Physical

- Soluble in water
- Stable in solution
- No reconstitution before use
- Stable in the presence of air and light
- Long shelf-life at room temperature
- Not supportive of bacterial growth
- Compatible with other drugs and fluids
- No additives
- Inexpensive.

Pharmacokinetic

- Rapid onset of action
- High oil/water solubility
- Non-cumulative with infusion
- Rapid and predictable recovery
- Completely metabolised to inactive and non-toxic substances
- Safe to use in renal or hepatic impairment.

Pharmacodynamic

- No pain on injection
- Safe following extravasation or inadvertent intra-arterial injection
- No adverse drug reactions
- Smooth induction of anaesthesia in one arm–brain circulation time
- Analgesic, anti-emetic and anti-epileptic properties

Dr Podcast Scripts for the Primary FRCA, ed. Rebecca A. Leslie, Emily K. Johnson and Alexander P. L. Goodwin.   Published by Cambridge University Press. © R. A. Leslie, E. K. Johnson and A. P. L. Goodwin 2011.

- Muscle relaxation
- No emergence phenomena
- No increase in cerebral blood flow, intra-cranial pressure or intra-ocular pressure
- Reduces cerebral metabolic rate ($CMRO_2$)
- Minimal cardiovascular depression or stimulation
- Minimal respiratory depression
- No histamine release or bronchospasm
- No impairment of corticosteroid synthesis
- Safe in pregnancy and paediatrics
- Not teratogenic.

No currently available agent fulfils all these criteria. The concept however remains useful as a benchmark for assessing new agents.

What is the ideal agent for total intra-venous anaesthesia (TIVA) and explain why?

The ideal agent for TIVA would be short acting with a short half-life to decrease the risk of accumulation and prolonged recovery. It would also provide a smooth and rapid induction, have a high metabolic clearance and rapid elimination. Propofol is an ideal agent in this respect, as it confers these properties. Its pharmacological profile and linear pharmacokinetics allow it to be given by infusion, whilst still providing good recovery characteristics. It can be used together with alfentanil, fentanyl or remifentanil.

During a propofol infusion, the peripheral compartments are steadily loaded. With increasing duration of the infusion, more peripheral loading will occur such that, in time, there will be a greater load of propofol to redistribute from the peripheral compartments back into the central compartment. This maintains the propofol concentration in the plasma and consequently, its duration of action. The pharmacokinetics of propofol are predictable; as the infusion starts to load the second and third compartments, they approach steady state, and the final rate of infusion falls to match the rate of drug excretion. During prolonged infusion, the context-sensitive half-life increases. However, if the infusion has been carefully titrated or used in low dose in combination with a remifentanil infusion, wake up may still be relatively fast. Context-sensitive half-life is approximately 20 minutes after 2 hours' infusion, 30 minutes after 6 hours' infusion and 50 minutes after 9 hours' infusion. It should be remembered that there are pharmacokinetic variations between patients therefore the infusion must still be titrated to effect.

Propofol TIVA is particularly useful in neuroanaesthesia. In addition to the advantageous properties already mentioned, it does not impair autoregulation or cause any increase in cerebral blood flow, cerebral metabolic rate for oxygen or intra-cranial pressure.

Can you draw the structures of propofol and thiopentone?

Propofol is a substituted stable phenolic compound: 2,6-di-isopropylphenol, see Figure 2.2.1a.

Thiopentone is a sulphur analogue of the oxybarbiturate pentobarbitone: 5-ethyl, 5'-methyl butyl thiobarbituric acid, see Figure 2.2.1b.

Intravenous agents

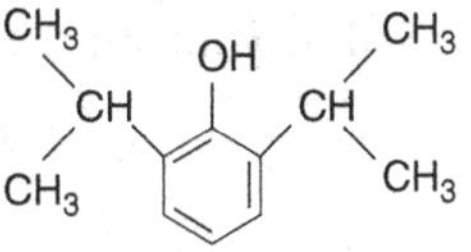

Figure 2.2.1a. Structure of propofol.

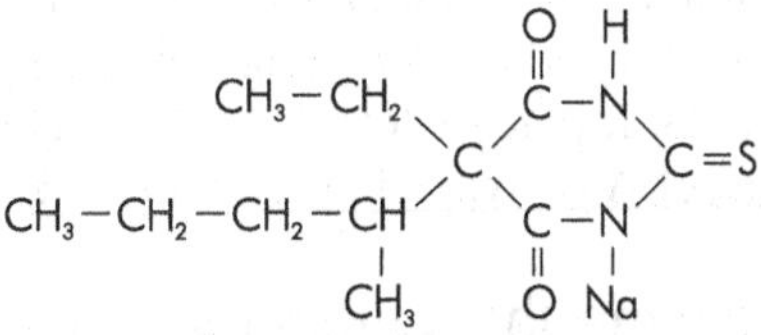

Figure 2.2.1b. Structure of thiopentone. Reproduced with permission from Smith, T., Pinnock, C. and Lin, T. 2009. *Fundamentals of Anaesthesia.* Cambridge: Cambridge University Press. © Cambridge University Press 2009.

What is in a thiopentone ampoule?

Sodium thiopentone is supplied in a rubber topped bottle, as a pale yellow powder of 5-ethyl, 5'-methyl butyl thiobarbituric acid, containing 6% anhydrous sodium carbonate (a base). The gaseous environment within the bottle is nitrogen which prevents oxidation. The sodium carbonate prevents CO_2 in the air from forming free acid that would react with the thiopentone. The sodium ion replaces the hydrogen ion that associates C1 and C2 of the base compound (see above).

The powder is readily soluble in water producing a 2.5% (2.5 g/100 ml) solution with a pH of 11. All salts of weak acids are alkaline in solution. At pH 11, having a pKa = 7.6 it is almost entirely (99.9%) ionised. However, once in the blood the pH falls towards 7.4 at which 61% of the drug is unionised. This unionised portion is the more lipid-soluble and readily crosses the blood–brain barrier into the lipid-rich brain tissue, where it exerts its effect.

What properties does the S atom confer to thiopentone?

Thiopentone is a thiobarbiturate and is the sulphur analogue of pentobarbitone, an oxy-barbiturate. Thiobarbiturates have a fast onset of action and a relatively short duration of action and recovery period. These properties make thiopentone a useful anaesthetic induction agent, inducing anaesthesia in one arm–brain circulation time of intra-venous injection. They are highly lipid soluble and rapidly cross the blood–brain barrier to penetrate the brain.

What molecule is formed when the S atom is replaced by an O atom?

Substituting the sulphur atom on C2 in thiobarbiturates with oxygen produces an oxybarbi-turate (e.g. phenobarbitone). Oxybarbiturates are the basic form of barbiturates. It is believed that the GABA-A receptor has a binding site for these drugs, which have a slow onset and long duration of action. They are useful hypnotics and sedative agents but are too slow to be used as induction agents.

Where in the CNS do propofol and thiopentone act?

Thiopentone acts on the β-subunits of the GABA-A receptors in the CNS. It causes an increase in the duration of opening of the chloride channels, resulting in hyperpolarisation and neuronal inhibition. The mechanism of action of propofol is less clear but is thought to involve reduced opening times of the sodium channels in the neuronal membranes of the CNS. It potentiates glycine and GABA (inhibitory neurotransmitters) and may inhibit the NMDA subtype of the glutamate receptor.

Tell me about propofol

Propofol is the most commonly used induction agent in the UK. It is also used in TIVA, for sedation in intensive care and during regional anaesthesia. Propofol is 2,6-di-isopropyl phenol, a phenol derivative. Due to its low solubility in water it is formulated as a white isotonic oil-in-water emulsion containing 1% or 2% propofol in 10% soya bean oil, 2.25% glycerol, 1.2% purified egg phosphatide, sodium hydroxide and water. The emulsion has a pH of 6–8.5 and a pKa of 11. At the physiological pH of 7.4, most of the drug is unionised, and therefore active. It is given intra-venously at a dose of 1.5–2.5 mg/kg for induction and as an infusion of 4–12 mg/kg/hr for maintenance of anaesthesia.

Describe the pharmacokinetics of propofol

Pharmacokinetics is the study of what the body does to a drug. It concerns the absorption, distribution, metabolism and elimination of drugs.

Absorption

- Propofol is only licensed for use via the intra-venous route and therefore has 100% bioavailability.

Distribution

- Propofol is 98% protein bound in the plasma.
- The volume of distribution is 4 L/kg.
- The distribution half-life is 1–2 minutes, resulting in a very short duration of anaesthesia after a bolus dose of the drug.

Metabolism

- Propofol is rapidly metabolised in the liver, mainly to inactive glucuronide, and sulphate and glucuronide conjugates of the hydroxylated metabolite via cytochrome P450. Extra-hepatic mechanisms may also contribute. Its metabolism is unaffected by renal and hepatic disease.

Excretion

- The metabolites are excreted in the urine, with 0.3% being excreted unchanged. The clearance is 30–60 ml/kg/min and the terminal elimination half-life is 5–12 hours. Clearance is reduced in renal failure. It does not accumulate under normal conditions.

Can you compare and contrast propofol and thiopentone?

Physical

Propofol is an alkyl phenol derivative. It is a white, isotonic, neutral aqueous emulsion in 10% soybean oil, 1.2% purified egg phosphatide, 2.25% glycerol and sodium hydroxide.

Thiopentone on the other hand, is a thiobarbiturate. It is presented as a hygroscopic yellow powder of sodium thiopentone with 6% sodium bicarbonate, reconstituted with water to 2.5% solution. The dose of propofol is 1.5–2.5 mg/kg as an intra-venous bolus for induction of anaesthesia, 4–12 mg/kg/hr as an infusion for maintenance of anaesthesia and 0.3–4 mg/kg as an infusion for sedation. The dose of thiopentone is 4–6 mg/kg as an intra-venous bolus for induction of anaesthesia.

Propofol has a molecular weight of 178 and a pH of 6–8.5. It has a pKa in water of 11 so at this pH it is almost entirely unionised. Of the drug, 98% is protein bound. In contrast, thiopentone has a molecular weight of 264, its solution has a pH of 10.5, a pKa of 7.6, at which it is almost entirely ionised. However, once in the blood the pH falls towards 7.4 at which 61% of the drug is unionised so is more lipid soluble and can readily penetrate the brain. Of the drug, 60–80% is reversibly bound to protein (mainly albumin) and is therefore non-diffusible and inactive.

Pharmacokinetics

Propofol and thiopentone have a rapid onset of action and recovery, although late recovery with thiopentone is delayed. Both propofol and thiopentone induce anaesthesia in one brain–arm circulation time. Propofol has a distribution half-life of 1–2 minutes, resulting in a brief duration of anaesthesia following bolus administration of the drug. Consciousness is lost in approximately 30 seconds and waking occurs approximately 10 minutes after a single dose. Thiopentone lasts for 5–15 minutes. Propofol is non-cumulative when infused (under normal conditions), making it an ideal agent for total intra-venous anaesthesia. Thiopentone on the other hand is cumulative with repeated administration. Propofol has a volume of distribution of 4 L/kg and a clearance of 30–60 ml/min/kg. Thiopentone has a volume of distribution of 2.5 L/kg and a clearance of 3.5 ml/min/kg. Owing to the high clearance of propofol, plasma levels fall more rapidly than those of thiopentone following the initial distribution phase. The elimination half-life of propofol is 5–12 hours, whereas it is longer with thiopentone, at 6–15 hours. Both drugs are metabolised in the liver, propofol by oxidation and thiopentone by conjugation. Propofol is metabolised to 2,6-diisopropylphenol glucuronide and 2,6-di-isopropylquinol glucuronide, whereas thiopentone is metabolised to thiopental carboxylic acid, hydroxy-thiopental and pentobarbital. Both agents are eliminated in the urine, less than 1% unchanged.

Pharmacodynamics

Central nervous system

Both propofol and thiopentone reduce intra-cranial pressure, cerebral perfusion pressure and cerebral metabolic rate of oxygen consumption. Both drugs are anti-convulsants, but conversely there is a small risk of convulsions when propofol is used in epileptic patients. Excitatory movements are common with propofol.

Cardiovascular system

Both agents cause reduction in systemic vascular resistance, cardiac output and consequently, blood pressure. Vasodilatation with propofol occurs secondary to propofol-stimulated production and release of nitric oxide. Propofol has variable effects on heart rate, occasionally causing reflex tachycardia but more usually causes bradycardia. Thiopentone on the other hand causes a compensatory tachycardia.

Respiratory system

Both agents cause respiratory depression and a reduced response to hypercapnia. A greater suppression of laryngeal reflexes is seen with propofol, which assists in the placement of laryngeal mask airways. Thiopentone may cause laryngospasm or bronchoconstriction.

Renal/hepatic

Renal and hepatic function are unaffected by propofol, whereas thiopentone causes a decrease in renal plasma flow, an increase in anti-diuretic hormone release and consequently a decrease in urine output. Thiopentone has no effect on hepatic function and is used in hepatic encephalopathy.

Gastrointestinal

Propofol possibly has an anti-emetic effect that may be mediated by antagonism of dopamine D_2 receptors. Thiopentone can cause splanchnic vasoconstriction.

Other

Thiopentone has no effect on the pregnant uterus and is used routinely in obstetrics. Propofol is not licensed in pregnancy, as there is high placental transfer and associated neonatal depression. In addition, the safety for prolonged propofol infusion in the paediatric population is questioned. It can lead to hyperlipidaemia, metabolic acidosis, myocardial failure and death.

Propofol causes pain on injection. Thiopentone causes tissue damage with extravasation, and arterial constriction and thrombosis with intra-arterial injection. Thiopentone is contraindicated in porphyria, whereas propofol appears to be safe.

2.2.2. Etomidate and ketamine – Joy M Sanders

What is etomidate?

Etomidate is a carboxylated imidazole derivative and an ester.

What does an ampoule of etomidate contain?

It contains a clear colourless solution of 20 mg of etomidate in 10 ml (i.e. 2 mg/ml or a 0.2% solution) of 35% propylene glycol in water. It has been formulated in propylene glycol to improve the stability of the solution. The pH of the aqueous solution is 8.1.

What are the side effects of etomidate?

Etomidate certainly does have some favourable properties, but due to its side effect profile, it has only a limited place in anaesthetic practice.

Central nervous system

During induction of anaesthesia, etomidate may cause involuntary muscle movements, hypertonus and tremor. A fifth of patients demonstrate generalised epileptiform electroencephalograph (EEG) activity following its use.

Respiratory system

Transient coughing and hiccupping are common.

Gastrointestinal

Etomidate is emetogenic and increases the incidence of postoperative nausea and vomiting.

Metabolic/other

Etomidate is a potent inhibitor of steroidogenesis in the adrenal cortex. Adrenal 11 β-hydroxylase and 17 α-hydroxylase enzymes are inhibited, which catalyse many of the reactions in the biosynthetic pathways from cholesterol to hydrocortisone. This results in a reduction in cortisol and aldosterone synthesis for 24 hours following its administration. This effect has been seen after single bolus doses and after infusions. The use of etomidate infusions for the sedation of critically ill patients is associated with increased mortality.

Pain on injection is experienced in 25% to 50% of patients. Etomidate has significant anti-platelet activities. Venous thrombosis may also occur. Etomidate may precipitate a porphyric crisis in patients with porphyria.

Why is it painful on injection?

A total of 25–50% of patients who receive the drug experience pain on injection, which is thought to be due to the propylene glycol solvent. The incidence of this is reduced by the addition of lignocaine. However, the newer preparation etomidate-lipuro, which is a lipid emulsion, appears to be less irritant.

Tell me about ketamine

Uses

Ketamine is used for the induction of anaesthesia, traditionally in high risk, shocked patients. It may also be used for maintenance of anaesthesia in burns, trauma and radiotherapy patients, because it usefully preserves airway reflexes. For the same reasons, it is used in "field" anaesthesia. It has local anaesthetic properties and has been used in spinal and epidural anaesthesia. It can be beneficial in the treatment of some forms of neuropathic pain and in the management of severe unresponsive asthma.

Chemical properties

Ketamine is a phencyclidine derivative. It is presented as a colourless solution containing 10, 50 or 100 mg/ml of ketamine hydrochloride with 1 in 10 000 benzethonium chloride as a preservative. Ketamine has a pH of 3.5–5.5 and a pKa of 7.5.

The ketamine preparation in common use is a racemic mixture of the S(+) and the R(−) isomer. These both have similar pharmacokinetic profiles although the S(+) isomer is 2–4 times as potent as the R(−) isomer. The S(+) isomer is also less psychoactive and has a faster recovery phase.

Mode of action

It is a non-competitive antagonist of the L-glutamate NMDA receptor in the CNS. Glutamate is the major excitatory neurotransmitter in the brain. It also interacts with opioid receptors, acting as an antagonist at μ-receptors and a partial agonist at κ-(OP2) and δ-(OP1) receptors.

Dose

For induction, the IV dose is 1–2 mg/kg administered over a period of 60 seconds. The onset of action occurs within 30 seconds and duration of action is 5–10 minutes. Supplemental IV doses of 0.5 mg/kg can be given. The intra-muscular (IM) dose is 10 mg/kg, with an onset of action of 2–8 minutes and duration of action of 10–20 minutes. For sedation the dose is 2 mg/kg IM or 10-mg increments intra-venously. Ketamine is also effective when given via the oral, epidural, intra-thecal, rectal or nasal routes.

Pharmacokinetics

Ketamine is well absorbed when given orally or intra-muscularly and has an oral bioavailability of 20%. It is only 25% protein bound. The volume of distribution is 3 L/kg and the distribution half-life is 11 minutes. Recovery is therefore mainly due to redistribution from brain to peripheral tissues. It is metabolised in the liver to weakly active metabolites, namely nor-ketamine, which has 30% of the potency of the parent compound. This is further metabolised to conjugates and is excreted in the urine. The clearance is 17 ml/kg/min and the elimination half-life is approximately 3 hours.

Pharmacodynamics

Cardiovascular system

Ketamine causes an increase in heart rate, blood pressure, central venous pressure and cardiac output as a result of an increase in sympathetic tone and blockade of noradrenaline uptake by sympathetic nerve endings. It is contraindicated in severe ischaemic heart disease and hypertension.

Respiratory system

Ketamine is a respiratory stimulant. It causes relative preservation of laryngeal reflexes and bronchodilatation via a direct action and sympathomimetic effects.

Central nervous system

Ketamine produces a state of dissociative anaesthesia, which is a combination of profound analgesia with light sleep. The cerebral blood flow, cerebral metabolic rate and intra-ocular pressure are all increased. It may cause vivid dreams and emergence phenomena such as hallucinations. These are less common in the young and the elderly and may be reduced if the patient is left undisturbed in the recovery period or by pre-medication with benzodiazepines.

Gastrointestinal/genitourinary

There is an increased incidence of post-operative nausea and vomiting. Salivation is also increased and anti-sialogogue pre-medication is recommended prior to its use. Ketamine increases uterine tone.

Other

Pain on injection, especially when using the IM route, may be reduced by adding lignocaine.

Inhalational anaesthetic agents

2.3.1. Inhalational agents – Joy M Sanders

What are the properties of an ideal inhalational agent?

Physical

- Liquid at room temperature
- High saturated vapour pressure (SVP) (for easy vaporisation)
- Low latent heat of vaporisation
- Low specific heat capacity
- Chemically stable in light and heat
- Inert when in contact with metal, rubber and soda lime
- Not flammable or explosive
- Long shelf-life
- Inexpensive
- No additives or preservatives
- Environmentally friendly
- Non-irritant, pleasant smell.

Pharmacokinetic

- Low blood:gas partition coefficient, i.e., fast effects
- High oil:gas partition coefficient, low minimum alveolar concentration (MAC)
- Minimal metabolism, no fluoride ion production
- Excretion via the lungs.

Pharmacodynamic

Central nervous system

- Smooth, rapid induction
- Only affects the CNS
- Rapidly reversible anaesthetic effects
- No increase in cerebral blood flow or intra-cranial pressure

Dr Podcast Scripts for the Primary FRCA, ed. Rebecca A. Leslie, Emily K. Johnson and Alexander P. L. Goodwin.   Published by Cambridge University Press. © R. A. Leslie, E. K. Johnson and A. P. L. Goodwin 2011.

- Some analgesic properties
- Not epileptogenic.

Cardiovascular system
- No cardiovascular depression
- No sensitisation of myocardium to catecholamines
- No decrease in coronary flow.

Respiratory system
- No breath-holding, laryngospasm, coughing, increase in secretions
- Bronchodilatation
- No respiratory depression.

Musculoskeletal
- Skeletal muscle relaxation
- Non-trigger for malignant hyperthermia.

Gastrointestinal
- Anti-emetic.

Renal/hepatic/haem
- No adverse renal/hepatic/haematological effects
- No decrease in renal or hepatic blood flow.

Other
- No effects on gravid uterus
- Not teratogenic/carcinogenic
- No interactions.

While the agents in use today demonstrate many favourable characteristics, no single agent has all the desirable properties mentioned.

Which properties of an inhalational agent determine the onset and potency?

- The onset is determined by the blood:gas partition coefficient. The lower the blood:gas solubility, the faster the onset of action.
- The potency is determined by the oil:gas partition coefficient. The higher the oil:gas partition coefficient, the more potent the agent.

What is the significance of the blood:gas partition coefficient?

The blood:gas partition coefficient is the ratio of the amount of anaesthetic in blood to that in gas when the two phases are of equal volume and in equilibrium with each other at 37°C.

There is a paradoxical association between the blood:gas partition coefficient and the speed of induction of inhalational agents. Poorly soluble inhalational agents exert a high partial pressure in the blood and therefore have a faster onset of action. Conversely, highly

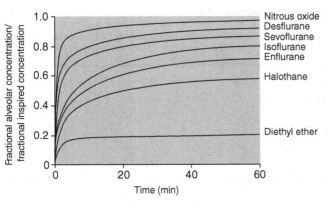

Nitrous oxide
Desflurane
Sevoflurane
Isoflurane
Enflurane

Halothane

Diethyl ether

Figure 2.3.1a. Wash-in curves for inhalational anaesthetic agents. Reproduced with permission from Smith, T., Pinnock, C. and Lin, T. 2009. *Fundamentals of Anaesthesia.* Cambridge: Cambridge University Press. © Cambridge University Press 2009.

soluble agents will rapidly enter the blood but will only exert a low partial pressure and therefore will have a slower onset of action. The anaesthetic effects are related to the partial pressure in the blood and consequently in the brain, and not to the absolute amount present.

In ascending order, the blood:gas partition coefficients of the inhalational agents are xenon (0.17), desflurane (0.42), nitrous oxide (0.47), sevoflurane (0.68), isoflurane (1.4), enflurane (1.9) and halothane (2.3).

The onset of action of an agent is not only related to the blood:gas partition coefficient, but is also influenced by the MAC, and other factors such as alveolar ventilation and respiratory irritability. For example, desflurane, whilst having a low blood:gas partition coefficient of around 0.4, is of limited use as an agent for gaseous induction due to its profound ability to irritate the respiratory tract. Also of note is that an agent associated with a rapid speed of onset of anaesthesia will have a rapid recovery.

Draw a graph to represent the relationship between the inspired concentration and the alveolar concentration for different inhalational agents

After prolonged administration of inhalational agents, the partial pressure of agent within the alveoli equilibrates with that in the arterial blood and subsequently the brain (Figure 2.3.1a). This is steady state, but for most inhalational agents this is rarely achieved as the process takes many hours. The time taken to reach steady state, or a ratio of alveolar concentration to inspired concentration of 1 varies between the different agents and depends on their blood:gas partition coefficient. Agents with a low partition coefficient, such as desflurane, reach equilibrium more quickly than agents with a high blood:gas partition coefficient.

What factors influence the speed at which inhalational agents approach equilibrium?

The rate at which inhalational agents approach equilibrium is determined by factors relating to the physiology of the patient and factors specific to the agents themselves.

A high inspired concentration of the agent results in a rapid increase in the partial pressure of agent in the alveoli and, consequently, a rapid onset of action. Similarly, if the alveolar ventilation is increased, the alveolar partial pressure of agent will increase faster leading to a

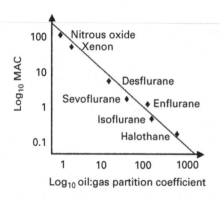

Figure 2.3.1b. Meyer-Overton hypothesis. Reproduced with permission from Cross, M. and Plunkett, E. 2008. *Physics, Pharmacology and Physiology for Anaesthetists: Key Concepts for the FRCA.* Cambridge: Cambridge University Press. © M. Cross and E. Plunkett 2008.

more rapid induction of anaesthesia. However, if the functional residual capacity is large, the inspired concentration of agent is essentially diluted which has the opposite effect in reducing the rate of onset of anaesthesia. The cardiac output also influences the kinetics of volatile agents. When the cardiac output is low, there is more time for the partial pressure of volatile agent in the alveoli to equilibrate with that of the arterial blood, and so increasing the onset of action. On the other hand, the concentration gradient between the alveolus and the blood is maintained in situations where the cardiac output is increased, resulting in a slower rise in alveolar partial pressure.

Other factors that influence the speed of equilibration of inhalational agents include the concentration effect and the second gas effect. The basis of these mechanisms can be explained by the fact that nitrous oxide is 20 times more soluble in blood than oxygen or nitrogen. If a high concentration of nitrous oxide is introduced into the alveoli, there will be a rapid rate of uptake into the pulmonary capillaries. This results in a reduction in the volume of the alveoli, as nitrous oxide is extracted faster than nitrogen enters the alveolus in the opposite direction. Consequently, the fractional concentration of any gases left in the alveoli will be increased. This is known as the **concentration effect**.

When inhalational agents are coadministered with high concentrations of nitrous oxide, this concentration effect will result in a higher alveolar partial pressure of inhalational agent. In addition to this, the extraction of alveolar gas also results in augmented ventilation, as tracheal gas containing inhalational agent is drawn into the alveoli. These mechanisms will increase the rate of equilibration of the alveolar fraction to inspired fraction ratio of inhalational agent and so will increase its onset of action. This is what is meant by the **second gas effect**.

What is the significance of the oil:gas partition coefficient?

Inhalational agents act in different ways at the level of the central nervous system. Direct interaction with the neuronal cell membrane is very possible, but indirect action via second messenger production is also likely. The high correlation between lipid solubility and anaesthetic potency suggests that inhalational agents have a hydrophobic site of action. The Meyer Overton hypothesis describes the correlation between lipid solubility (oil:gas partition coefficient) and potency (MAC) (see Figure 2.3.1b) and suggests that anaesthesia occurs when a sufficient number of inhalational agent molecules dissolve in the lipid bilayer of the neuronal cell membrane. If the hypothesis were true however, the product of the oil:gas partition coefficient and MAC would be constant. This does not seem to be the case, particularly with the newer inhalational agents. Also, many substances with high lipid solubility have no anaesthetic effect, and some larger molecules with high lipid solubility are less potent. Isoflurane and enflurane are structural isomers and have similar oil:gas partition coefficients. However, the MAC for isoflurane (1.17) is only approximately 70% of that for enflurane (1.68). Therefore it would appear that there are other factors influencing anaesthetic potency.

How does isoflurane/sevoflurane/desflurane comply with the criteria for an "ideal inhalational agent"?

Isoflurane

Isoflurane is a liquid at room temperature and is chemically stable in light. It has an SVP of 32 kPa at 20°C. It is inert when in contact with metal but is readily soluble in rubber. It is not flammable in normal anaesthetic concentrations and contains no stabilisers or preservatives. It is also relatively cheap. However, it does have a pungent smell, which may cause upper airway irritability, coughing and breath-holding, so is rarely used for inhalational inductions. It may react with dry soda lime producing carbon monoxide. With regard to pharmacokinetics, it has a blood:gas partition coefficient of 1.4, an oil:gas partition coefficient of 98 and a low MAC of 1.17. Only 0.2% is metabolised and none of the products have been linked to toxicity. It is safe in pregnancy.

Sevoflurane

Sevoflurane is also a liquid at room temperature and is stable in light. It has an SVP of 22 kPa at 20°C. It has a low solubility in rubber and plastics. It is non-flammable and the commercial preparation contains no additives or stabilisers. However, in contrast to isoflurane, it is non-irritant to the airways and has a pleasant odour, which makes it a good agent for inhalational inductions. It also has a low blood:gas partition coefficient of 0.7 and a relatively low MAC (of 2). Due to this marked insolubility in blood, it produces a rapid induction and emergence from anaesthesia. However it is relatively expensive and is unstable in the presence of moist soda lime, producing small amounts of a potentially toxic substance called compound A. It undergoes hepatic metabolism to a greater extent than all the other commonly used inhalational agents (at 3–5%), but little or no renal metabolism.

Desflurane

Desflurane is a liquid at room temperature and should be protected from light. It has a boiling point of 23.5°C and an SVP of 89 kPa at 20°C, which makes it extremely volatile and therefore unsuitable for administration via a conventional vaporiser. Desflurane is administered by the electronic TEC 6 vaporiser which heats the liquid to 39°C at an SVP of 200 kPa. It contains no additives and is flammable at a concentration of 17%. It has a low oil:gas partition coefficient of 29 and a high MAC of 6.6. Its low blood:gas partition coefficient of 0.47 allows rapid alteration in the depth of anaesthesia and a fast recovery. However, like isoflurane, it has a pungent odour that causes coughing and breath-holding and can also cause excessive secretions and apnoea, so is not an ideal agent for induction of anaesthesia. Due to its $-CHF_2$ groups, it may react with dry soda lime in a similar manner to isoflurane producing carbon monoxide. Only 0.02% of an administered dose is metabolised so its potential to produce toxic effects is minimal.

Pharmacodynamics

With regard to their pharmacodynamics, all these agents cause dose-dependent respiratory depression with a decrease in tidal volume and variable agent-specific effects on respiratory rate. They all cause bronchodilatation. All have effects on the cardiovascular system, but none so significant as to prevent their use. Isoflurane and desflurane cause a decrease in SVR and MAP, an increase in heart rate and a reasonably well-maintained cardiac output. Sevoflurane causes dose-dependent cardiovascular depression with reduced SVR, MAP and contractility. All these agents decrease cerebral vascular resistance and cerebral metabolic rate and increase cerebral blood flow and potentially intra-cranial pressure. None are epileptogenic (unlike enflurane). All cause does-dependent relaxation of the uterus and are potential triggers for malignant hyperthermia.

What is your favourite inhalation agent?

Here, we will use the example of sevoflurane.

Can you draw its chemical structure? (Figure 2.3.1c)

How is this agent metabolised?

Approximately 3–5% of absorbed sevoflurane undergoes hepatic metabolism by cytochrome P450 (isoform 2E1), producing hexafluorisopropanol and inorganic fluoride ions.

What type of compound is compound A?

It is a vinyl ester. Its chemical structure is $CH_2F\text{-}O\text{-}C(CF_3)=CF_2$

What are its effects on man?

Dose-dependent renal, hepatic and cerebral damage has been seen in rats but never in man, despite countless administrations.

Why is it nephrotoxic to animals but not humans?

Animal studies in rats have found that the lethal concentration of Compound A is 300–400 ppm after exposure to sevoflurane for 3 hours. A nephrotoxicity threshold of 150–200 ppm in humans has been inferred from results of such studies. The compound A concentrations found clinically in humans are considerably less than those that cause toxicity in animals, with maximum concentrations of less than 30 ppm after 5 hours, even at low flow rates. Furthermore, these levels are not associated with deranged renal function tests.

Which compounds form carbon monoxide with dry soda lime, and why?

Carbon monoxide (CO) production has occurred when inhalational agents containing the –CHF$_2$ group are passed over dry warm soda lime or baralyme. This was established following reports of CO release from circle systems that had been left with dry gas circulating over the weekend period. The inhalational agents implicated include isoflurane, enflurane and desflurane.

Desflurane

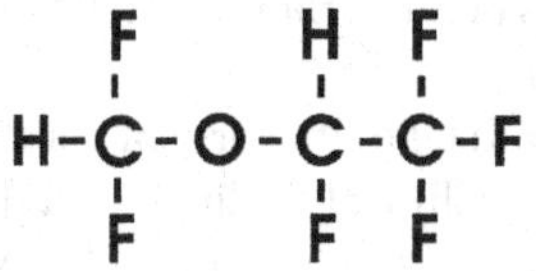

$$\text{H}-\overset{\overset{\displaystyle F}{|}}{\underset{\underset{\displaystyle F}{|}}{C}}-\text{O}-\overset{\overset{\displaystyle H}{|}}{\underset{\underset{\displaystyle F}{|}}{C}}-\overset{\overset{\displaystyle F}{|}}{\underset{\underset{\displaystyle F}{|}}{C}}-\text{F}$$

Enflurane

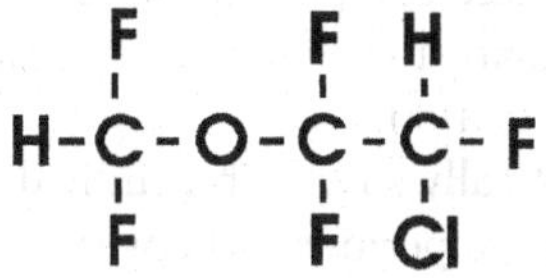

$$\text{H}-\overset{\overset{\displaystyle F}{|}}{\underset{\underset{\displaystyle F}{|}}{C}}-\text{O}-\overset{\overset{\displaystyle F}{|}}{\underset{\underset{\displaystyle F}{|}}{C}}-\overset{\overset{\displaystyle H}{|}}{\underset{\underset{\displaystyle Cl}{|}}{C}}-\text{F}$$

Halothane

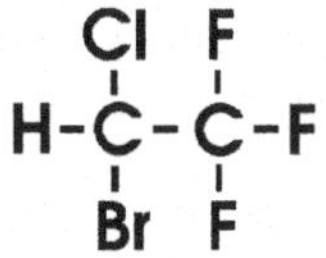

$$\text{H}-\overset{\overset{\displaystyle Cl}{|}}{\underset{\underset{\displaystyle Br}{|}}{C}}-\overset{\overset{\displaystyle F}{|}}{\underset{\underset{\displaystyle F}{|}}{C}}-\text{F}$$

Isoflurane

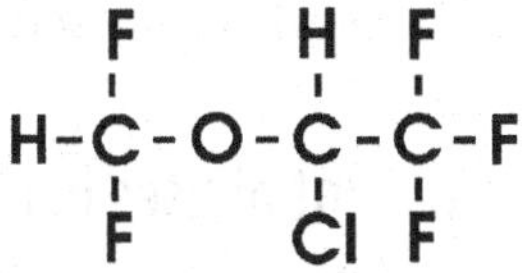

$$\text{H}-\overset{\overset{\displaystyle F}{|}}{\underset{\underset{\displaystyle F}{|}}{C}}-\text{O}-\overset{\overset{\displaystyle H}{|}}{\underset{\underset{\displaystyle Cl}{|}}{C}}-\overset{\overset{\displaystyle F}{|}}{\underset{\underset{\displaystyle F}{|}}{C}}-\text{F}$$

Sevoflurane

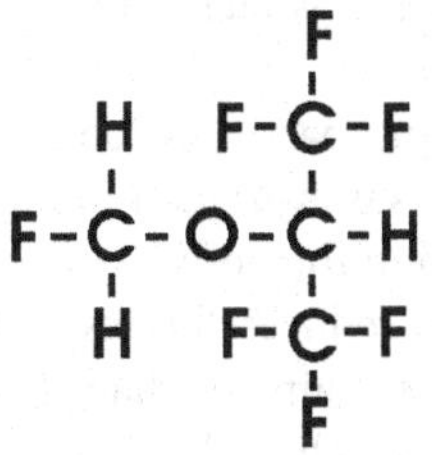

$$\text{F}-\overset{\overset{\displaystyle H}{|}}{\underset{\underset{\displaystyle H}{|}}{C}}-\text{O}-\overset{\overset{\displaystyle F-\overset{\overset{\displaystyle F}{|}}{C}-F}{|}}{\underset{\underset{\displaystyle F-\overset{|}{C}-F}{|}}{C}}-\text{H}$$

Figure 2.3.1c. Chemical structure of sevoflurane. Reproduced with permission from Smith, T., Pinnock, C. and Lin, T. 2009. *Fundamentals of Anaesthesia*. Cambridge: Cambridge University Press. © Cambridge University Press 2009.

Nitrous oxide

$$\text{N}=\text{N}=\text{O} \qquad \text{N}\equiv\text{N}-\text{O}$$

Two forms coexist as a resonant hybrid

What causes halothane hepatitis?

There are two types of hepatic damage observed with the use of halothane, both of which appear to be unrelated.

Type 1 (or mild) hepatotoxicity is self-limiting, often subclinical and has an incidence of 25–30% following administration of halothane. It is associated with mild transient increases in hepatic transaminases and altered post-operative drug metabolism. It is probably caused by **reductive** (anaerobic) metabolism of halothane as a result of hepatic hypoxia. It does not occur with the use of other inhalational agents because they are metabolised to a lesser extent than halothane and via different mechanisms.

Type 2 hepatotoxicity is very uncommon and takes the form of massive centrilobular liver cell necrosis leading to fulminant liver failure. Clinical findings include jaundice, fever and markedly elevated hepatic transaminase levels. It has a high mortality, which varies between 30% and 70%. The mechanism appears to be immune mediated and initially involves **oxidative** metabolism of halothane to an intermediate compound called trifluoroacetyl chloride (TFA). This may act as a hapten, binding covalently to hepatic proteins and forming a hapten-protein complex which induces anti-body formation.

Type 2 hepatotoxicity may occur in genetically susceptible individuals and is seen after repeated exposure to halothane with short time periods in between exposures. Other risk factors include obesity, hypoxaemia, female sex and middle age. It is a diagnosis of exclusion and all other causes of hepatic damage must be sought.

The Committee on Safety of Medicines in 1986 recommended that halothane should be avoided if:

- History of previous adverse reactions to halothane
- Previous exposure within 3 months, unless there is an overriding clinical indication for its use
- History of unexplained jaundice or pyrexia after previous exposure to halothane.

What do you know about xenon and its potential uses in anaesthesia?

In many ways xenon is the anaesthetic agent of the future. It is an inert odourless noble gas manufactured by the fractional distillation of air. It has no occupational or environmental hazards and makes up 0.000087% of the earth's atmosphere (0.87 ppm). It is not flammable and does not support combustion.

It has a MAC of 71% and a very low blood:gas partition coefficient of 0.14, resulting in an extremely rapid onset and offset of action. It is non-irritant to the respiratory tract and is compatible with soda lime. It is not metabolised in the body and is eliminated via the lungs.

Unlike the other inhalational agents, xenon reduces the respiratory rate and increases tidal volume and consequently minute volume remains unchanged. It has a higher density and viscosity than nitrous oxide but this appears to have little clinical significance. Even in high concentrations, it does not appear to cause diffusion hypoxia, unlike nitrous oxide. However, it does appear to be associated with post-operative nausea and vomiting.

Xenon is very cardiostable, with no myocardial sensitisation to catecholamines and unaltered contractility.

It produces unconsciousness and has significant analgesic properties. It also causes a degree of muscle relaxation at concentrations over 60%. It is not a trigger for malignant hyperthermia. However, xenon does increase cerebral blood flow and it is therefore not recommended for use in neuroanaesthesia. It can be used to enhance CT brain images, and radiolabelled xenon may be used to measure organ blood flow and ventilation in V/Q scanning.

Its use has unfortunately been limited by its massive cost of production, which is 2000-fold greater than that of nitrous oxide. In addition, there are no appropriately designed anaesthetics machines available for use with xenon, there is difficulty in monitoring its inspired and expired concentrations, and there is still a lack of experience in its use.

What do you know about helium?

Helium is a light, inert gas. It is present in air and in natural gas, from which it is extracted. It is supplied as 100% helium in brown cylinders at 137 bar. It is also available as heliox, which is 79% helium and 21% oxygen, presented in brown bodied cylinders with brown and white quartered shoulders, at the same pressure. It does not support combustion.

Helium's most useful property is that it has a lower density than oxygen, nitrogen and air. Therefore, if flow is turbulent, the velocity will be higher when heliox is used. For example, in upper airway obstruction, heliox reduces the work of breathing and increases alveolar oxygen supply. It is less useful in lower airway obstruction, such as asthma, because peripheral flow is mainly laminar and therefore depends on viscosity (which is greater for heliox than for nitrogen/oxygen mixtures). However it may be of some benefit where flow is turbulent. Helium oxygen mixtures are also useful in deep sea diving to avoid nitrogen narcosis. The characteristic high pitched voice associated with breathing these mixtures is due to their lower density which produces higher frequency vocal sounds. Helium can also be used to measure lung volumes because of its very low solubility.

2.3.2. MAC – Joy M Sanders

Define MAC

MAC is the minimum alveolar concentration of inhalational anaesthetic agent at sea level (1 atmosphere) and in 100% oxygen, at which 50% of un-premedicated subjects will fail to respond to a standard midline incision.

MAC is therefore the ED_{50}, or the effective dose in 50% of subjects. In the other 50% of subjects, MAC may be higher or lower. When considering the concentration of anaesthetic that would prevent response to a stimulus in 95% of subjects, it is referred to as the MAC95 (which is actually more useful).

MAC is inversely related to potency, i.e., an agent with a high MAC has a low potency. When MAC is plotted on a graph against the oil:gas partition coefficient (a measure of lipid solubility) using log scales, the relationship is linear (see figure 2.3.1b). MAC can be used to compare the potencies of different inhalational agents.

The alveolar concentration of inhalational agents (or their MAC) can be estimated by measuring the end-tidal concentration. Rapid cerebral blood flow means that equilibrium between alveolar and brain concentrations occurs rapidly, and once equilibrium is reached the actual concentrations in the alveoli and brain tissue are virtually equal. Therefore MAC is a useful guide to clinical dosage.

MAC of different agents used simultaneously are additive. In other words, if a patient receives 0.5 MAC of one agent (e.g. sevoflurane) and 0.5 MAC of another agent (e.g. nitrous oxide) they will receive a total of 1 MAC.

MAC is normally distributed and therefore not all patients will be unresponsive to a "standard surgical stimulus". Equally, some patients will be unresponsive with less than 1 MAC. MAC relates to movement and not awareness. The alveolar concentration of volatile anaesthetic required to prevent awareness is less than the concentration to prevent movement.

There are two other terms in use, namely "MAC-BAR" and "MAC awake". "MAC-BAR" (Blocks Adrenergic Response) is defined as the minimum alveolar concentration of inhalational agent at which the increase in heart rate or blood pressure (or both) as a result of skin incision is prevented in 50% of subjects.

"MAC awake" is defined as the minimum alveolar concentration of inhalational agent at which 50% of subjects no longer respond appropriately to command when concentrations of agent are gradually increased from the awake state. This term can also be used when referring to the alveolar concentration at which 50% of subjects respond appropriately when emerging from anaesthesia (in the absence of other CNS depressant drugs). This is sometimes expressed as a ratio of MAC awake:MAC and is approximately 0.3–0.5 for most of the inhalational agents in use. It has been suggested that MAC awake is the minimum alveolar concentration required to prevent awareness during general anaesthesia although this is not widely accepted.

What factors affect MAC?

MAC can be increased and decreased by different factors.

MAC is *decreased* by:

- Increasing age (10% for every 10 years)
- Hypovolaemia
- Hypothermia
- Hypoxia
- Hypocapnia
- Hyponatraemia
- Hypothyroidism
- Anaemia
- Pregnancy
- Acute alcohol consumption
- Drugs which suppress the central nervous system (e.g. opioids, benzodiazepines)
- Other drugs: e.g. clonidine, lidocaine, nitrous oxide.

MAC is *increased* by:

- Decreasing age
- Hyperthermia
- Hypercapnia
- Hypernatraemia
- Thyrotoxicosis
- Chronic alcohol and opioid abuse
- Severe anxiety
- Sympathoadrenal stimulation
- Increases in ambient pressure.

It is *unaffected* by gender, weight, height and duration of anaesthesia.

What are the MAC values and oil:gas partition coefficients of inhalational agents that you use?

This answer requires knowledge of the table of physical properties of volatile agents that you just have to learn prior to the exam, see Table 2.3.2a. It's best to learn the values for all anaesthetic agents, including halothane, nitrous oxide and xenon, although in a structured oral

Table 2.3.2a. Physical properties of commonly used volatile agents

Inhalational agent	MAC (%vol.)	Oil:gas partition coefficient
Halothane	0.75	224
Isoflurane	1.15	98
Enflurane	1.68	98
Sevoflurane	2.0	53
Desflurane	6.60	19
Xenon	71	1.9
Nitrous oxide	105	1.4

examination you're likely to be asked about agents that you commonly use (which may of course include nitrous oxide).

The agents with lower MAC values have higher oil:gas partition coefficients, and those with higher MAC values have lower oil:gas partition coefficients.

2.3.3. Nitrous oxide – Emily K Johnson

What are the uses of nitrous oxide?

Define and keep your answer concise.

Nitrous oxide is an inorganic gas with a number of uses. It is used as adjunct to general anaesthetic, as an analgesic during labour or other painful procedures and it can also be used for cryotherapy.

Do you know when it was first used and by whom?

This is unlikely to be a pass–fail question but a bit of background knowledge can only impress the examiners!

Joseph Priestley, an English chemist, first produced nitrous oxide in 1772. Humphrey Davy investigated it further in 1799. He wrote a book about it and noted its analgesic properties. It was first used for dental extractions in 1844 by Wells but due to the discovery of chloroform it was not used much again until 1863 when it was reintroduced by Colton.

How is nitrous oxide manufactured?

Nitrous oxide is manufactured by heating ammonium nitrate to 250°C. The equation showing this reaction is:

$$NH_4NO_3 \rightarrow N_2O + 2H_2O$$

The temperature must be carefully controlled or a number of contaminants may be produced during the process. These contaminants are ammonia, nitrogen, nitric oxide, nitrogen dioxide and HNO_3. If inhaled these are irritant to the airways initially but cause pulmonary oedema several hours later and may go on to cause destructive pulmonary fibrosis after 2 to 3 weeks.

The contaminants are actively removed in the manufacture of nitrous oxide by passage through scrubbers, water and caustic soda.

How is nitrous oxide stored?

Nitrous oxide is stored in French blue cylinders as a liquid with its vapour on top. In hospitals nitrous oxide is kept in large cylinders in two manifolds. The gauge pressure is 4400 kPa, which does not represent the cylinder content until all the remaining nitrous oxide is in the gaseous phase only. Liquid is less compressible than gas so the cylinder should only be partially filled.

What is the filling ratio?

The filling ratio is the weight of fluid in the cylinder divided by the weight of water required to fill the cylinder. For nitrous oxide in the UK it is 0.75 but in hotter climates it is 0.67 to avoid explosions.

Tell me the physical properties of nitrous oxide

Nitrous oxide is a colourless gas with a sweet smell. It is non-flammable but does support combustion. It has a molecular weight of 44, a boiling point of $-88°C$, a critical temperature of $36.5°C$ and a critical pressure of 72 bar. It has a MAC of 105%, the oil:gas solubility coefficient is 1.4 and the blood:gas solubility coefficient is 0.47.

What are the advantages of nitrous oxide?

Nitrous oxide has several advantages. It is a potent analgesic and offers better pain relief in labour than pethidine. It is a weak anaesthetic and in concentrations of above 80% will render most subjects unconscious. It only has a MAC of 105% but in combination with its analgesic properties it reduces the MAC of other volatile anaesthetics and is a useful carrier gas for the more potent anaesthetics. Due to the low blood:gas partition coefficient of nitrous oxide of 0.47 it has a rapid onset and equilibration. Due to this rapid uptake from the alveoli it increases the alveolar concentration of other agents therefore accelerating the induction of anaesthesia via the second gas effect.

What are the disadvantages of nitrous oxide?

Nitrous oxide has several disadvantages. It has a very high diffusing capacity, 25 times that of nitrogen. This means in non-compliant air-filled cavities such as the middle ear, it will increase the pressure rapidly by diffusing into the cavity. In compliant air-filled cavities such as pneumothoraces or bowel, it will diffuse in and increase the volume. For example after 4 hours of breathing 66% N_2O the bowel cavity will have expanded by 200%.

Another disadvantage of nitrous oxide is its emetic effect. This is caused by a combination of its effect on opioid receptors, its sympathomimetic effects as well as its effects of bowel distension. Nitrous oxide also has toxic effects, which include bone marrow suppression and neurotoxicity. Due to the second gas effect it causes diffusion hypoxia; however, this doesn't normally present a significant clinical problem as it can be resolved with supplemental oxygen.

Nitrous oxide, in common with volatile agents, causes respiratory depression with an increased rate to compensate for a reduced tidal volume. It is also negatively inotropic and can exacerbate any ischaemic heart disease.

Nitrous oxide makes up 1% of the global greenhouse gases so pollution is another disadvantage.

How can the analgesic effects of nitrous oxide be explained?

Nitrous oxide may exert its analgesic effects in several ways. It acts on opioid receptors and has the potency of morphine for a short time. It may act also by modulation of endorphins and encephalins within the central nervous system, possibly through its stimulatory effect on dopaminergic neurones, which may then cause release of these endogenous opioid peptides. This would explain why it is possible to partially antagonise the effects of nitrous oxide with naloxone.

It is thought nitrous oxide may activate a supra-spinal descending pain inhibition system releasing encephalins from interneurones in the substantia gelatinosa of the spinal cord. These encephalins inhibit pain transmission by substance P synapses.

What is entonox?

Entonox is a 50:50 mixture of nitrous oxide and oxygen.

Tell me more about the storage, properties and uses of entonox

Entonox is used for analgesia in labour and during other painful procedures. It is stored in French blue cylinders with white and blue shoulders at a pressure of 13 700 kPa. The critical temperature of nitrous oxide is 36.5°C but in the mixture with oxygen this is lowered to −5.5°C. This is called the pseudocritical temperature. Therefore below this temperature liquefaction and separation occur, resulting in a mixture of nitrous oxide with approximately 20% dissolved oxygen and a gas mixture of a high concentration of oxygen above the liquid. This is potentially dangerous as the oxygen is drawn off first, then the remaining dissolved oxygen comes out of solution and eventually a hypoxic mixture is delivered, which is close to 100% nitrous oxide. This separation is most likely to occur at a pressure of 117 bar. When the delivery is via a pipeline at 4 bar the pseudocritical temperature is less than −30°C. To prevent these problems from occurring cylinders should be stored horizontally, to increase the area for diffusion, and at temperatures above 5°C. A dip tube can also be used in the cylinders with its tip ending in the liquid phase causing this to be used first preventing delivery of less than 20% oxygen.

What is the Poynting effect?

The Poynting effect refers to the bubbling of oxygen through liquid nitrous oxide, with vaporisation of the liquid to form the gaseous mixture of entonox. The two gases dissolve into each other and behave differently as a mixture than you would expect from knowing their individual properties.

Explain the concentration effect

The concentration effect is the greater rate of increase in the alveolar concentration when compared to the inspired concentration of nitrous oxide, when high concentrations are inspired. This effect is only applicable to nitrous oxide because only nitrous oxide gets used in sufficiently high concentrations to demonstrate it. The principle underlying the concentration effect is the large gradient generated by high concentrations of nitrous oxide because of its ability to diffuse so rapidly. As it fills the alveoli large amounts rapidly diffuse into the pulmonary capillaries therefore drawing gas from the conducting airways into the alveoli to keep the volume constant. Ventilation is increased to supply this extra volume. This causes the alveolar concentrations to change more rapidly when the nitrous concentrations are higher.

Explain the second gas effect

The second gas effect is due to the concentration effect. Another gas such as oxygen or a volatile agent used alongside high concentrations of nitrous oxide will be concentrated in the alveolus for two reasons, firstly due to the rapid uptake of nitrous oxide and secondly due to the increased ventilation. The result is that induction time is shorter due to increased concentrations of volatile agents and there are also increased oxygen levels.

Explain diffusion hypoxia

Diffusion hypoxia is the reverse of the second gas effect. At the end of anaesthesia when the patient ceases to inhale nitrous oxide as the anaesthetic gases are turned off the volume of nitrous oxide diffusing from the blood into the alveolus is greater than the volume of the gas diffusing from the alveolus to the blood. This results in a dilution of the oxygen in the alveolus and potential hypoxia. However, if the patient is switched onto 100% oxygen at the end of the anaesthetic this does not have an impact. It would be clinically important if the patient was switched onto air at the end of anaesthesia.

What do you know about the toxic effects of nitrous oxide?

Nitrous oxide inhibits the enzyme methionine synthetase. This enzyme is responsible for the synthesis of methionine, thymidine and tetrahydrofolate. It does this by oxidising the cobalt atom in vitamin B12 and vitamin B12 is a co-factor for the enzyme. These effects have been shown to occur after 40 minutes of breathing nitrous oxide. Methionine is a precursor of myelin and low levels of methionine can cause subacute degeneration of the cord in B12 deficiency, and dorsal column impairment acutely. Tetrahydrofolate is an important nucleotide in DNA synthesis and this is why nitrous oxide can lead to megaloblastic anaemia in B12 and folate deficiency.

Nitrous oxide is thought to be teratogenic, although this has been proven only in rats. This may be due to its effects on methionine synthetase in combination with its α-adrenoceptor agonism, which has been associated with developmental disorders such as situs inversus. The toxic effects may be reversed with folinic acid, which provides another source of tetrahydrofolate.

Neuromuscular blocking agents and anti-cholinesterases

2.4.1. Neuromuscular blocking drugs – Rebecca A Leslie

What is the neuromuscular junction?

It is imperative you know this topic inside out, which is why we have included an overview in this section. Ideally draw a diagram as you are describing the neuromuscular junction, remembering to label all the important features.

The neuromuscular junction forms a connection between the motor neurone and a skeletal muscle fibre. The neurotransmitter at this junction is acetylcholine.

The terminal axon of the fast Aα motor neurone lies in a groove situated in the middle of the surface of the single muscle fibre that it is innervating. In most muscles a single terminal axon innervates a single muscle fibre. However in some muscles such as intra-ocular, intrinsic laryngeal and some facial muscle fibres innervation is by multiple slower Aγ motor fibres.

The post-synaptic membrane is folded to form peaks and troughs on its surface. The membrane over the peaks contains acetylcholine receptors whilst within the troughs the enzyme acetylcholinesterase is present.

When an action potential arrives at the terminal axon the depolarisation causes an influx of calcium ions. The calcium ions combine with proteins present to facilitate the fusion of synaptic vesicles, containing acetylcholine, with the pre-synaptic membrane.

Following the release of acetylcholine into the synaptic cleft it binds to the acetylcholine receptors present on the peaks of the post-synaptic membrane. The central ion channel of the receptor opens allowing the movements of ions across the membrane. The movement of these ions allows the generation of a miniature end-plate potential. The summation of several end-plate potentials continues until the threshold potential is reached. At this point voltage-gated sodium channels open causing rapid depolarisation of the cell membrane. This depolarisation spreads throughout the muscle fibre and eventually reaches the sarcoplasmic reticulum causing calcium release and muscle contraction.

How is acetylcholine broken down?

Acetylcholine is broken down by the acetyl-cholinesterase present within the troughs of the post-synaptic membrane. Acetyl-cholinesterase binds to either the ester group of the

Dr Podcast Scripts for the Primary FRCA, ed. Rebecca A. Leslie, Emily K. Johnson and Alexander P. L. Goodwin.   Published by Cambridge University Press. © R. A. Leslie, E. K. Johnson and A. P. L. Goodwin 2011.

acetylcholine molecule or the quaternary ammonium group. The choline is removed and recycled whilst the acetylated enzyme is hydrolysed to acetic acid.

How would you classify drugs which produce neuromuscular blockade?

When asked this question it is tempting to jump in and describe depolarising and non-depolarising muscle relaxants but remember there are other ways to block the neuromuscular junction, which become obvious if you know the physiology of the neuromuscular junction.

The passage of neuronal transmission to skeletal muscle can be blocked in a number of ways that can be classified according to their mechanism of action into these four groups:

- Prevent acetylcholine synthesis
- Prevent acetylcholine release
- Deplete acetylcholine stores
- Block the acetylcholine receptor.

Acetylcholine is formed by the combination of choline and acetyl CoA in a reaction that is catalysed by the enzyme choline acetyl transferase. Acetylcholine is synthesised within the axoplasm of the motor neurone and is transported to the terminal axon where it is stored in synaptic vesicles.

Choline is derived from the diet and is recycled from the breakdown of other acetylcholine molecules. Hemicholinium is an example of a drug which prevents acetylcholine synthesis. It is a synthetic compound which prevents the uptake of choline into the cholinergic nerve endings hence reducing acetylcholine synthesis.

Magnesium ions and aminoglycosides inhibit calcium entry into the synaptic terminal, and by doing so prevent the release of acetylcholine. In contrast botulinum toxin binds irreversibly to the nicotinic nerve terminals to prevent acetylcholine release.

The tetanus toxin is an example of a toxin which depletes acetylcholine stores rendering the muscle paralysed.

Neuromuscular blocking drugs which block the acetylcholine receptor fall into two categories depending upon their mode of action; non-depolarising and depolarising.

Tell me about depolarising neuromuscular blockade

This topic is covered in a lot more detail in the Suxamethonium section, see section 2.4.2.

The only depolarising drug in routine clinical use in the UK is suxamethonium (succinylcholine).

Suxamethonium in molecular structure is essentially two acetylcholine molecules joined by an ester linkage. It is used to produce rapid and profound muscle relaxation facilitating intubation of the trachea, to produce paralysis for very short surgical procedures and to modify the effect of seizures following electro-convulsive therapy. It is presented as a colourless solution of the chloride salt at a concentration of 50 mg/ml and should be stored at 4°C to prevent deterioration. Suxamethonium solutions are destroyed by an alkaline pH and therefore should not be mixed with thiopentone.

The mechanism of action of suxamethonium is by reversibly binding to the acetylcholine receptors present on the post-synaptic membrane, causing depolarisation of the membrane. Due to the mechanism of breakdown of suxamethonium the depolarisation is prolonged and creates a membrane potential, which will not allow generation of further action potentials and hence muscle relaxation.

Suxamethonium is broken down by plasma cholinesterase (butyrylcholinesterase), which is present within the plasma but not the neuromuscular junction. The lack of plasma cholinesterase within the neuromuscular junction explains the prolonged duration of action of suxamethonium at the acetylcholine receptor. The hydrolysis of suxamethonium by plasma cholinesterase produces a weakly active metabolite, succinylmonocholine, and choline, which is further hydrolysed by plasma cholinesterase to succinic acid and choline. Following administration of a dose of suxamethonium only approximately 20% of it reaches the neuromuscular junction. Due to the rapid metabolism of suxamethonium only between 2 and 10% is excreted in the urine.

How do non-depolarising muscle relaxants work?

Non-depolarising muscle relaxants are competitive antagonists at the neuromuscular junction. They bind to the α-subunit of the nicotinic receptor on the post-junctional membrane.

How would you classify non-depolarising muscle relaxants?

Non-depolarising muscle relaxants can be classified as:

- Aminosteroidal compounds. Examples include vecuronium, rocuronium and pancuronium.
- Benzylquinoliniums. Examples include atracurium, mivacurium and tubocurarine.

They can be further classified according to their duration of action. Mivacurium is a very short acting non-depolarising muscle relaxant, whilst atracurium and rocuronium are intermediate acting and pancuronium is a long acting muscle relaxant.

How are the non-depolarising neuromuscular blockers metabolised?

Non-depolarising muscle relaxants are metabolised in two different ways. Some, such as mivacurium and atracurium are hydrolysed in the plasma, whilst others like rocuronium and vecuronium are metabolised to varying degrees in the liver. The un-metabolised fraction of the drug is excreted in the urine or the bile.

Tell me more about how atracurium is metabolised

Atracurium is metabolised by two metabolic pathways: ester hydrolysis and Hoffmann elimination.

At body pH and temperature atracurium undergoes spontaneous degradation into laudanosine and a quaternary monoacrylate in a process called Hoffmann elimination. Both acidosis and hypothermia will slow down Hoffmann elimination.

Ester hydrolysis accounts for up to 60% of the metabolism of atracurium and occurs as a result of non-specific esterases which are unrelated to plasma cholinesterases. Ester hydrolysis results in the production of laudanosine, a quaternary alcohol and a quaternary acid. Unlike Hoffmann elimination, ester hydrolysis is accelerated in acidosis, however in the clinical range of pH this is unlikely to make a dramatic difference.

Is laudanosine an active metabolite?

No, laudanosine has no neuromuscular blocking properties. It is a tertiary amine and has a half-life of between 2 and 3 hours. Concerns were made about the effects of laudanosine after it was found that at very high plasma concentrations the EEG of anaesthetised dogs demonstrated epileptiform changes, however even after several days' infusion of atracurium in humans the plasma concentration never reaches these levels.

What are the side effects of atracurium?

Atracurium has the propensity to cause histamine release. This can either be localised or systemic.

Systemic histamine release can affect both the cardiovascular and respiratory system, leading to hypotension and bronchospasm.

Atracurium is also associated with critical illness myopathy.

What is *cis*-atracurium?

Atracurium is a mixture of 10 stereoisomers because the atracurium molecule has four chiral molecules. The *cis*-atracurium is one of the stereoisomers. It has a more favourable side-effect profile and its potential for histamine release is extremely low.

How does the dose of *cis*-atracurium compare to the dose of atracurium?

The *cis*-atracurium is 3–4 times more potent than atracurium. The intubating dose of *cis*-atracurium is only 0.2 mg/kg, whereas the intubating dose of atracurium is approximately 0.5 mg/kg. As a result, the speed of onset of *cis*-atracurium is slower than atracurium. However the onset time can be improved by giving a larger dose as the potential to cause histamine release is very low.

What is the intubating dose of rocuronium?

The intubating dose of rocuronium is 0.6 mg/kg, and intubating conditions are reached within approximately 100–120 seconds. If a dose of 1 mg/kg is given then intubating conditions can be reached within 60 seconds.

What are the side effects of the aminosteroidal neuromuscular blockers?

Remember to discuss drug side effects system by system, in this case the most important systems are central nervous system, cardiovascular system and the respiratory system.

The aminosteroidal neuromuscular blocking agents have no effect on the central nervous system and do not increase intra-cranial or intra-occular pressure.

Vecuronium and rocuronium have very limited cardiovascular effects. In contrast pancuronium causes a tachycardia due to vagolytic effects.

All the aminosteroidal agents cause respiratory paralysis, but unlike the benzylquinoliniums they do not cause histamine-induced bronchospasm.

How do anti-biotics modify the action of non-depolarising neuromuscular blockers?

Aminoglycosides and tetracyclines prolong the muscle relaxation produced by non-depolarising agents. This is thought to be as a result of the antibiotics competing with calcium and thus prevent the release of acetylcholine.

Which other drugs modify the action of non-depolarising neuromuscular blockers?

Drugs which prolong the neuromuscular blockade include volatile agents, lithium, local anaesthetics and calcium channel antagonists.

Volatile agents reduce the neurotransmitter release at the neuromuscular junction by depressing the somatic reflexes in the central nervous system and as a result prolong the block. Calcium channel antagonists reduce the calcium influx into the nerve terminal and hence reduce acetylcholine release whilst lithium blocks sodium channels. At low doses local anaesthetics also block sodium channels and can prolong the neuromuscular blockade.

Which physiological factors influence neuromuscular blockade?

Hypothermia, hypermagnesaemia, hypokalaemia and acidosis all prolong the neuromuscular block.

Hypothermia reduces the metabolism of the muscle relaxants, magnesium reduces acetylcholine release by competing with calcium, and reduced levels of potassium makes the resting potential more negative.

What are the properties of an ideal neuromuscular blocker?

It is important you have a good classification for answering questions about the ideal properties of a specific type of drug. This will then lend itself to all the different drugs and make answering the questions significantly easier. I think the easiest classification is division into the physical properties, the pharmacokinetic properties and the pharmacodynamic properties.

The ideal properties of a muscle relaxant can be divided into the physical properties, the pharmacokinetic properties and the pharmacodynamic properties.

The physical properties of an ideal neuromuscular blocking agent are that it is cheap, water soluble and has a long shelf-life with no special storage requirements.

The pharmacokinetic properties of an ideal muscle relaxant are that it has a short duration of action with a predictable reversal that it is non-cumulative so can be given as an infusion when necessary, that it is completely metabolised into non-active metabolites and its metabolism is not affected by hepatic or renal failure.

The pharmacodynamic properties of an ideal neuromuscular blocking agent include a rapid onset of action, high potency and no cardiovascular or respiratory side effects. It must also be safe to use in children and during pregnancy and ideally have a non-depolarising mechanism of action.

2.4.2. Suxamethonium – Caroline SG Janes

Suxamethonium is a very common structured oral examination topic and examiners will expect good knowledge of this drug and will be very unforgiving if you cannot provide it. We recommend you study the podcasts on the neuromuscular junction and neuromuscular monitoring prior to this podcast.

What class of drug is suxamethonium?

A depolarising neuromuscular blocker.

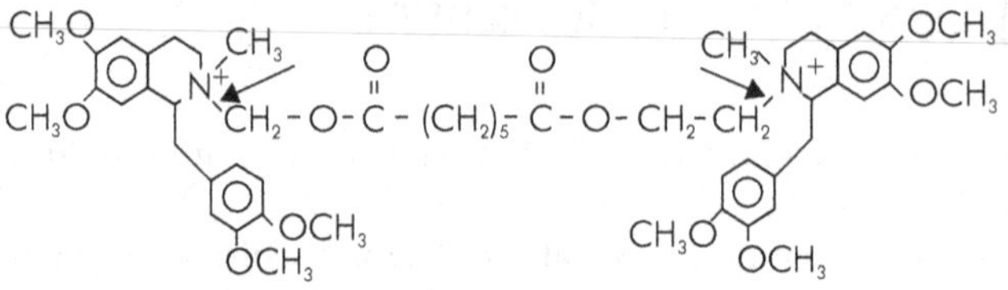

Atracurium

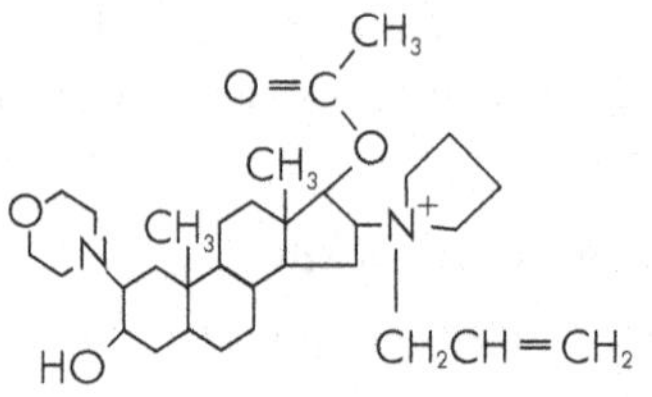

Rocuronium

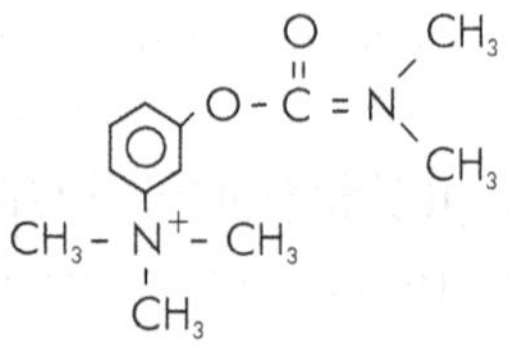

Neostigmine

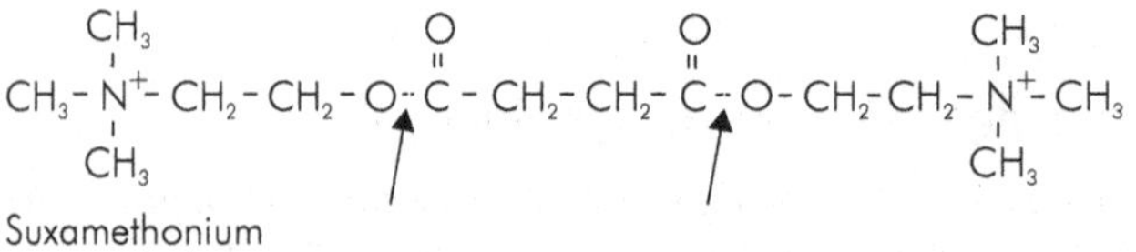

Suxamethonium

Figure 2.4.2a. Structure of suxamethonium. Reproduced with permission from Smith, T., Pinnock, C. and Lin, T. 2009. *Fundamentals of Anaesthesia*. Cambridge: Cambridge University Press. © Cambridge University Press 2009.

What is the structure of suxamethonium?

Suxamethonium is made up of two molecules of acetylcholine (ACh) joined by an acetyl group bond, see Figure 2.4.2a. Each ACh molecule contains an ester bond.

Tell me about the presentation and uses of suxamethonium

It is an odourless, colourless solution that should be stored at 4°C. In the UK it is available as a chloride in 2-ml ampoules of 50 mg/ml, the dosage is 1–2 mg intra-venously. It is used predominantly in rapid sequence induction and for short surgical procedures.

What is the mechanism of action and kinetics of suxamethonium?

Suxamethonium acts on the nicotinic ACh receptor present on the post-synaptic membrane of the neuromuscular junction. It causes depolarisation and subsequent prevention of transmission of further action potentials.

It has a short duration of action of 3–5 minutes and is hydrolysed by plasma cholinesterase to succinic acid and choline. Only 10% is excreted in the urine.

What are the characteristics of a partial depolarising block?

A depolarising block is also described as a phase I block. It is characterised by equal but reduced twitch height with train of four count and with single pulse stimulation, and it causes a sustained but reduced tetanic contraction with no fade or post-tetanic potentiation, see Figure 3.2.3b.

Following administration of large doses of suxamethonium a phase II block may occur whereby features of non-depolarising blockade gradually replace that of depolarising blockade. The mechanism of phase II block is uncertain but may involve pre- or post-junctional receptor modulation.

Please list the side effects of suxamethonium

Remember the magic number eight and make sure you start with the commonest side effects first, don't jump in with malignant hyperthermia or the examiner may stop you and take you down a path you would rather avoid.

1. Myalgia; this is most common in young females.
2. Cardiac arrhythmias; the main arrhythmia is a bradycardia, which is usually sinus or nodal but can also be ventricular in origin; bradycardia occurs most commonly in paediatrics and with a second dose.
3. Hyperkalaemia; in normal individuals a transient increase of 0.5 mmol/L occurs which rapidly resolves, this however may be enough to cause cardiac arrest in patients with high levels to start with and in renal failure.
4. Increased intra-ocular pressure; this can increase by approximately 10–15 mmHg but only transiently. Suxamethonium should therefore be used cautiously in open eye injuries. Concurrent administration of thiopentone offsets this rise.
5. Intra-gastric pressure; this rises by approximately 10 cmH$_2$O but is offset by an increase in the lower oesophageal sphincter tone.
6. Anaphylaxis.
7. Suxamethonium apnoea.
8. Malignant hyperpyrexia (MH).

What are the contra-indications of suxamethonium?

If you know the side effects of suxamethonium you can more or less work out the contra-indications.

It is contraindicated in patients with raised potassium levels, severe muscle trauma, a history of malignant hyperpyrexia or suxamethonium apnoea. In patients with burns of more than 10% or spinal cord trauma it should be avoided from approximately 24 hours to 18 months after the injury. Its use should also be avoided in patients with muscle disease if at all possible.

What is malignant hyperthermia or MH?

This is an open question which might tempt you to tell the examiner everything you know about MH, try to resist listing lots of random facts and keep to the basics – if the examiner wants more details he/she can ask you for it.

MH is a life-threatening, autosomal dominant condition that occurs only in susceptible individuals and is triggered by volatile anaesthetics or suxamethonium. It results from uncontrolled skeletal muscle metabolism. It is important to be able to recognise and treat it promptly as if left untreated it can quickly progress to circulatory collapse and death.

What are the features of MH?

The classic features of MH are masseter spasm and muscle rigidity, a rising temperature of more than 2°C per hour and a rising end-tidal carbon dioxide. However, the first symptom of MH may just be an unexplained tachycardia so it's important to have a high index of suspicion. As oxygen demand outstrips supply the oxygen saturations will start to fall.

Blood results typically show elevated levels of serum calcium, potassium, creatine kinase and myoglobin and as the disease progresses a metabolic acidosis develops often followed by acute renal failure.

How is MH managed?

The triggering agent should be withdrawn immediately. Dantrolene is the only definitive treatment and should be given as soon as possible. Supportive treatment should include correction of acidosis, aggressive cooling, respiratory support with 100% oxygen and hyperventilation and inotropic support. Hyperkalaemia should be corrected. Acute renal failure and disseminated intra-vascular coagulation should be treated as necessary. The patient should be transferred to intensive care and treated until there is complete resolution of symptoms. Anaesthesia should be maintained throughout.

What is dantrolene and how does it work?

Dantrolene is a muscle relaxant that works by uncoupling the excitation–contraction process preventing calcium release from the sarcoplasmic reticulum in skeletal muscle. The dose in MH is 2–3 mg/kg repeated as necessary up to a maximum dose of 10 mg/kg. It is available as an orange powder in 20-mg vials containing mannitol and sodium hydroxide. Reconstitution requires 60 ml of water per vial and is very labourious due to its insolubility. Since its introduction the mortality of MH has reduced from 90% to 10%.

What is the pathophysiology of MH?

MH is caused by a mutation in the gene coding for the ryanodine receptor found on chromosome 19. The ryanodine receptor is located on the sarcoplasmic reticulum and plays a crucial role in calcium control.

What tests are available to confirm MH?

The caffeine-halothane contracture test is the standard in diagnosing MH. A biopsied piece of muscle is subjected to 2% halothane and caffeine and tension in the muscle is measured – contracture occurs in susceptible muscle. Patients are labelled susceptible, equivocal or non-susceptible. Tests should be carried out in all suspected cases and immediate relatives.

What is suxamethonium apnoea?

Suxamethonium apnoea occurs in genetically susceptible patients who have a decreased plasma pseudocholinesterase activity. In these individuals suxamethonium is not broken down and causes prolonged neuromuscular blockade and hence paralysis and apnoea. It can result from genetic variability or acquired conditions. Acquired deficiency results from liver or cardiac failure, renal disease, pregnancy, thyrotoxicosis, malnutrition, burns, following plasmaphoresis or drugs that inhibit cholinesterases.

Tell me more about genetic causes of suxamethonium apnoea?

Suxamethonium apnoea is caused by single amino acid substitutions in the genes coding for pseudocholinesterase activity, these are located on the E1 locus of chromosome 3. Several autosomal recessive alleles have been identified and the degree of enzymatic inhibition by dibucaine and fluoride has been used to describe the genetic variations. There are four alleles described: usual also known as normal (Eu), atypical also known as dibucaine-resistant (Ea), fluoride-resistant (Ef) and silent (Es). Ninety-six percent of the population are homozygous for the normal gene with full enzyme function and 0.001% are homozygote for the silent gene with no enzyme function. Dibucaine and fluoride numbers denote the percentage of inhibition – the higher the number the better the enzyme function.

An individual can be homozygote for any of these alleles or the alleles can exist in any heterozygous combination with each other. In homozygotes for the silent and atypical gene paralysis can last up to 4 hours, in homozygotes for the fluoride-resistant gene paralysis can last up to 2 hours. Heterozygotes with abnormal genes make up approximately 4% of the population and exhibit mildly prolonged paralysis of up to 10 minutes.

How would you manage a patient that may have a prolonged block following suxamethonium administration?

Anaesthesia and ventilatory support should be continued until the block wears off. This is usually done in intensive care. Alternatively fresh frozen plasma can be given as it contains plasma cholinesterase.

2.4.3. Anti-cholinesterases – Rebecca A Leslie

What types of acetylcholine receptors are there?

There are two types of acetylcholine receptors: nicotinic and muscarinic. Muscarinic receptors are G-protein coupled receptors that act via second messengers, whereas nicotinic receptors are ligand-gated ion channels.

Describe the structure of the nicotinic receptor

Your answer here should start with a diagram showing the structure of the nicotinic receptor, see Figure 1.4.1b. As you draw it give details of the different components as they are described here.

Nicotinic receptors are membrane proteins that are made up of five subunits. There are two α-, one β-, one ε- and one δ-subunit.

The acetylcholine binding sites are on the two α-subunits of the receptor. When one acetylcholine binds to the α-subunit it increases the affinity for acetylcholine at the other α-subunit. As acetylcholine binds to these binding sites they cause a conformational change that causes a central channel in the receptor to open. The channel then allows the passage of sodium ions and other cations through the cell membrane, which causes depolarisation and generates an action potential.

How is acetylcholine formed?

Acetylcholine is an acetyl ester of choline. It is synthesised in the cytoplasm of nerve endings from acetyl-coenzyme A and choline. The reaction is catalysed by the enzyme choline acetyl transferase.

$$\text{Acetyl CoA} + \text{Choline} \quad \xrightarrow{\text{Choline acetyl transferase}} \quad \text{Acetylcholine.}$$

Acetyl A is synthesised from pyruvate in the mitochondria of the axon terminals whilst choline is derived from the breakdown of acetylcholine and from the diet.

What happens to acetylcholine after its synthesis?

An active transport system moves acetylcholine into the synaptic vesicles, where it is stored until it is released in response to an action potential. Each vesicle contains 10 000 acetylcholine molecules, and approximately 200 vesicles are released after every action potential. Once the acetylcholine is released it enters into the synapse and binds to the post-synaptic acetylcholine receptors in order to propagate the action potential. After binding to the post-synaptic receptor the acetylcholine molecule is hydrolysed by acetylcholinesterase to form choline and acetate.

Tell me about the acetylcholinesterase enzyme. What are the binding sites called?

Acetylcholinesterase is the enzyme that breaks down acetylcholine.

It has an esteratic and an anionic binding site. The anionic site binds with the positively charged quarternary ammonium end, and the esteratic site binds to the acetate end.

Tell me about acetylcholinesterase inhibitors. What uses do they have in clinical practice?

Acetylcholinesterase inhibitors are also known as anti-cholinesterases. They antagonise the acetylcholinesterase enzyme at the neuromuscular junction, inhibiting the breakdown of acetylcholine. This increase in synaptic acetylcholine allows displacement of the neuromuscular blocking agents from the nicotinic receptor, and thus restores the transmission across the neuromuscular junction. Therefore one important use of acetylcholinesterase inhibitors is for the reversal of neuromuscular blockade during anaesthesia.

Acetylcholinesterase inhibitors are also useful in clinical practice in situations where there is not enough acetylcholine, such as myasthenia gravis. By giving an acetylcholinesterase inhibitor and preventing the breakdown of acetylcholine you can increase the action of the limited acetylcholine that is available.

What are some disadvantages of acetylcholinesterase inhibitors?

The effects of acetylcholinesterase inhibitors are not specific to the neuromuscular junction so the effects of increased acetylcholine concentrations are also seen at muscarinic receptors. This causes bradycardia, arrhythmias, bronchospasm, nausea, vomiting, increased gut motility and salivation. To prevent these side effects it is common to give an anti-cholinergic drug at the same time as giving an acetylcholinesterase inhibitor.

Can you classify the three different types of acetylcholinesterase inhibitors?

Acetylcholinesterase inhibitors can be classified according to their mechanism of action:

- **Competitive antagonism.** The only drug in this group is edrophonium, which is used to perform a diagnostic test for myasthenia gravis. It rapidly and transiently improves muscle power.
- **Formation of a carbamylated enzyme complex.** Examples include both neostigmine and pyridostigmine. These work by forming a carbamylated complex with acetylcholinesterase.
- **Irreversible inactivation of acetylcholinesterase.** Such as organophosphates, which due to their mechanism of action have no role in clinical practice but are used as insecticides and chemical weapons.

The first two groups are structurally similar and are both quartenary ammonium compounds.

How does neostigmine act to reverse neuromuscular block?

Neostigmine is an acetylcholinesterase inhibitor. It is used to increase acetylcholine concentrations at the neuromuscular junction by preventing its breakdown by acetylcholinesterase.

Neostigmine is a quarternary amine and is structurally similar to acetylcholine. It can therefore bind to aceylcholinesterase. The cationic part of neostigmine binds to the anionic site, and the terminal carbon atom binds to the esteratic site. The phenol group, which is the middle of the neostigmine molecule, breaks away leaving both binding sites of the aceylcholinesterase enzyme occupied by fragments.

This impairs the ability of aceylcholinesterase to metabolise acetylcholine, allowing acetylcholine to accumulate and displace the non-depolarising muscle relaxant, which has competitively bound to the acetylcholine receptor. In doing so, neuromuscular transmission is restored and paralysis is reversed.

How do organophosphates work and how can you treat organophosphate poisoning?

Organophosphorus compounds are extremely toxic and are used in insecticides and nerve gases.

Organophosphates phosphorylate the esteratic site of the acetylcholinesterase enzyme. This inhibits the actions of the enzyme. The enzyme complex is very stable unlike the carbamylated complex formed when neostigmine attaches to the acetylcholinesterase. This makes it resistant to hydrolysis.

Toxic effects include muscle weakness, polyneuropathy, respiratory failure and cholinergic crisis, which include both muscarinic and nicotinic effects.

In practice, treatment of organophosphate poisoning relies upon the production of new acetylcholinesterase enzyme. Supportive treatment is required in the interim and may include ventilation. Atropine can be given to counteract the muscarinic effects, and pralidoxime is a specific drug that promotes hydrolysis of the phosphorylated enzyme complex.

What do you know about sugammadex?

Sugammadex is a selective relaxant binding agent (SRBA) which is used for the reversal of neuromuscular blockade by aminosteroidal agents. It is a modified γ-cyclodextrin.

Cyclodextrins are oligosaccharides that have a tube-like structure. The tube has a lipophilic core and a water-soluble hydrophilic exterior. The γ-cyclodextrin has been modified from its natural form with the addition of eight glucopyranose units. These extensions increase the cavity size allowing greater encapsulation of rocuronium within the cavity.

When sugammadex is administered it rapidly encapsulates rocuronium molecules within its lipophilic core rendering it unavailable to bind to the acetylcholine receptor at the neuromuscular junction.

The kidneys rapidly excrete the rocuronium–sugammadex complex.

What are the advantages of sugammadex?

The main advantage of sugammadex is the reversal of neuromuscular blockade without having to rely on the inhibition of acetylcholinesterase. As a result its administration does not risk causing bradycardia, increased secretions, increased gastrointestinal motility and bronchospasm, which can occur if neostigmine's actions are unopposed at muscarinic receptors.

Secondly sugammadex can be administered individually and an anti-muscarinic agent such as glycopyrolate does not have to be co-administered. This reduces the risk of drug errors that can occur when administering two drugs simultaneously.

In addition, when fast onset and short duration of muscle relaxation is required there is now an alternative option to the use of suxamethonium, which has a number of undesirable side effects. When given at high doses rocuronium has a rapid onset of action and with sugammadex available it can be rapidly reversed, therefore, could be used as a potential alternative to suxamethonium.

Can sugammadex be used with other neuromuscular blocking agents other than rocuronium?

Sugammadex also has affinity for other aminosteroidal neuromuscular blocking agents such as vecuronium, however its affinity is lower than its affinity for rocuronium. Vecuronium is more potent than rocuronium, therefore fewer molecules are present at the neuromuscular junction for an equivalent blockade. Sugammadex encapsulates at a ratio of 1:1 and will reverse vecuronium despite the reduced affinity because there are fewer molecules to bind compared to rocuronium.

What are the disadvantages of sugammadex?

Sugammadex is currently very expensive and is not recommended in patients with severe renal impairment (GFR $<$ 30 ml/min). In addition, some commonly used drugs such as flucloxacillin and fusidic acid may displace rocuronium or vecuronium from the sugammadex molecule and reoccurrence of the block may occur.

Another disadvantage is that it may decrease progesterone levels in women taking the oral contraceptive pill, so women should act as though one pill has been missed after sugammadex administration.

Dysgeusia, a metal taste in the mouth, was the most commonly reported adverse event during the clinical trials.

What is the dose of sugammadex?

Neuromuscular monitoring is recommended for dose calculation prior to sugammadex administration. If there are two twitches during a train of four the dose of sugammadex is 2 mg/kg. If the neuromuscular blockade is more profound and there are only two twitches after a post-tetanic count then 4 mg/kg is required. If immediate reversal is required the dose of sugammadex is 16 mg/kg.

Sugammadex is supplied as 2-ml (200-mg) or 5-ml (500-mg) vials. It must be remembered that if rapid reversal is required then multiple vials will need to be used. For example in a 80-kg man requiring rapid reversal a dose of 1280 mg (16 mg/kg) is needed which equates to approximately 2.5 five-ml vials.

Local anaesthetics

2.5.1. Local anaesthetics – Emily K Johnson

This topic is common in the exam and you will be expected to have a thorough knowledge of the main local anaesthetic agents, their mode of action, pharmacological properties and side effects.

What are the main classes of local anaesthetics?

Define and classify.

Local anaesthetic drugs are compounds that produce temporary blockade of neuronal transmission when applied to a nerve fibre. They are classified into two main groups, the amides and the esters. Both groups consist of a lipophilic aromatic ring, a link and a hydrophilic amine.

You should be able to draw the basic structure of esters and amides and explain the difference. It would be advisable to be able to draw the basic structures of the commonly used local anaesthetic agents as this could also be asked.

Give examples of each class of local anaesthetics

Amides include lidocaine, prilocaine, bupivacaine, levo-bupivacaine and ropivacaine. This is the most commonly used group. Esters include cocaine, procaine and amethocaine.

What are the differences between esters and amides?

The differences between esters and amides can be divided into structural and functional differences.

The structural differences are the chemistry of the link between the aromatic ring and the amine, esters have an –O–CO– link whereas amides have a –NH–CO– link. (See Figure 2.5.1.a.)

The functional differences include their stability in solution; esters are relatively unstable in solution, whereas amides remain stable for up to 2 years.

They have different pharmacokinetic properties. Distribution varies as esters are minimally protein bound whereas amides are more extensively bound in the plasma. Metabolism

Dr Podcast Scripts for the Primary FRCA, ed. Rebecca A. Leslie, Emily K. Johnson and Alexander P. L. Goodwin.   Published by Cambridge University Press. © R. A. Leslie, E. K. Johnson and A. P. L. Goodwin 2011.

Aromatic ring Amide side chain **Figure 2.5.1a.** Basic structure of local anaesthetics.

Ester link:

Amide link:

differs as esters are rapidly hydrolysed by plasma cholinesterases to inactive compounds, resulting in a short elimination half-life. Amides are metabolised more slowly in the liver by amidases. Therefore they may accumulate in hepatic dysfunction. Esters have a higher incidence of allergy, which is associated with one of the metabolites, para-aminobenzoate.

How do local anaesthetics work?

Local anaesthetics work by entering the neurone and blocking inward sodium current at the voltage-gated sodium channels in the cell membrane. This prevents depolarisation and therefore stops action potential propagation. They block the sodium channels from the inside of the neurone and have a higher affinity for sodium channels in the open or inactivated state, as opposed to the resting state.

Local anaesthetics are weak bases and are mostly ionised at neutral pH because their pKa is above 7.4. The amount unionised depends on the pKa of the particular agent. The unionised portion of the local anaesthetic is lipid soluble and is therefore free to diffuse through the phospholipid membrane of the neurone. Once in the axoplasm of the neurone they are protonated and are preferentially attracted to open sodium channels. It is this ionised form that binds to the internal aspect of the sodium channel and blocks it.

The unionised portion of the drug is thought to dissolve in the phospholipids membrane causing the membrane to swell. This also results in inactivation of the sodium channels.

What is the significance of pKa?

It is almost inevitable you will be asked about pKa if the topic of local anaesthetics is asked. Make sure you understand it well and are able to explain it clearly.

The pKa is the pH at which half the drug is ionised and half is unionised. Local anaesthetics exist in equilibrium between ionised and unionised forms, it is their pKa and the pH of their surroundings that dictate the percentage ionised form compared to unionised form. The Henderson–Hasselbalch equation allows us to calculate the ratio of the two states.

You should be able to write out the Henderson–Hasselbalch equation and explain it. This requires practice so you don't get in a muddle!

For an acid $pH = pKa + \log\dfrac{\text{(ionized form)}}{\text{(unionized form)}}$.

For a base $pH = pKa + \log\dfrac{(\text{unionized form})}{(\text{ionized form})}$.

At a pH below its pKa, a greater proportion of a weak base will exist in its ionised form, whereas at a pH above its pKa a greater proportion of a weak base will be unionised. The pKa of lidocaine is 7.9, of bupivacaine is 8.1 and of cocaine is 8.6. Thus when local anaesthetics, which are weak bases, are introduced to physiological pH of 7.4, which is below their pKas, they are only partially unionised. The proportion of unionised drug is more the lower the pKa, therefore lidocaine has a higher proportion of unionised drug at physiological pH than bupivacaine and cocaine. This influences the speed of onset of action. As it is unionised drug that diffuses across the phospholipid membrane, the drugs with lower pKas have a quicker onset of action.

What is the significance of lipid solubility?

Lipid solubility is closely related to potency, the more lipid soluble, the more potent the agent. However in vivo there are many other factors influencing potency, such as tissue distribution and vasodilatation, which influence the amount of local anaesthetic available for action at the nerve cell membrane.

What is the significance of protein binding?

Protein binding is associated with the duration of action of local anaesthetics. Highly protein bound agents have longer duration of action. Duration of action is also influenced by vasodilatation, as is the drugs potency. (Vasodilatation will reduce potency and duration of action.) Generally local anaesthetics cause vasodilatation in low concentrations and vasoconstriction in high concentrations. Cocaine is the exception to this rule, as it produces vasoconstriction in all concentrations.

Compare and contrast bupivacaine and lidocaine. How does ropivacaine compare?

If you can draw the chemical structures of the agents in question then do so to help describe the structural differences between the agents (Figure 2.5.1b).

Bupivacaine and lidocaine are both amide local anaesthetics. Bupivacaine is more potent than lidocaine. The relative lipid solubility of bupivacaine is 1000, compared to 150 for lidocaine, which represents its greater potency. The toxic dose of bupivacaine is 2 mg/kg with or without adrenaline and the toxic plasma concentration is anything greater than 1.5 µg/ml, the toxic dose of lidocaine is 3 mg/kg without adrenaline and 7 mg/kg with adrenaline and the toxic plasma levels are greater than 5 µg/ml.

The duration of action of bupivacaine is longer than that of lidocaine. This is explained by the difference in plasma protein binding between the drugs. The higher the protein binding the longer the duration of action and bupivacaine is 95% protein bound compared to lidocaine which is 70% protein bound.

The elimination half-life is also shorter in lidocaine at 100 minutes compared to 160 minutes for bupivacaine.

The onset of action is quicker for lidocaine than bupivacaine (Table 2.5.1a). This property is reflected by the pKa. The pKa of lidocaine is 7.9, leaving 25% unionised at physiological pH

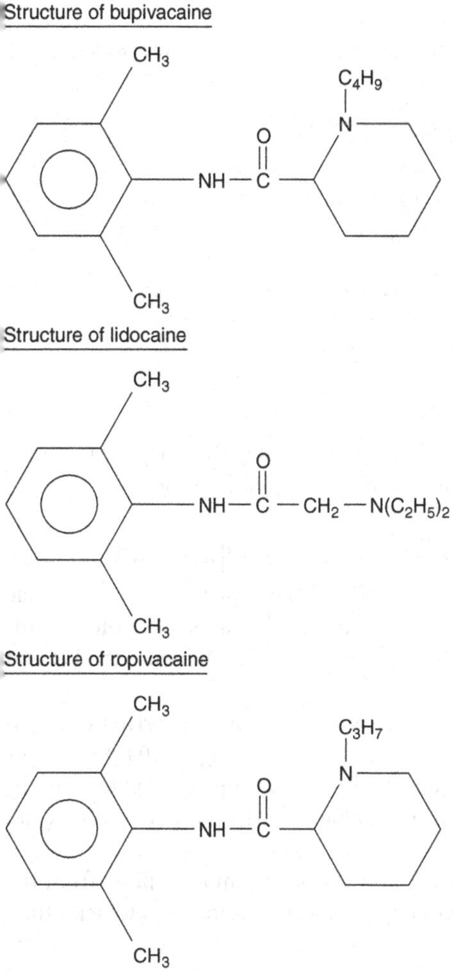

Structure of bupivacaine

Figure 2.5.1b. Structure of bupivacaine, lidocaine and ropivacaine.

Structure of bupivacaine

CH_3

C_4H_9

N

$NH-C$ (O)

CH_3

Structure of lidocaine

CH_3

$NH-C$ (O) $-CH_2-N(C_2H_5)_2$

CH_3

Structure of ropivacaine

CH_3

C_3H_7

N

$NH-C$ (O)

CH_3

compared to bupivacaine, which has pKa of 8.1, leaving only 15% unionised at physiological pH. This means more lidocaine is unionised to diffuse into the neurone and block the sodium channels.

Ropivacaine is another amide local anaesthetic. It is structurally different with a propyl group on its piperidine nitrogen instead of the butyl group in bupivacaine. It is present as the pure S-enantiomer, compared to bupivacaine which is a racemic mixture of the S- and R-enantiomer. Ropivacaine has a slightly reduced potency when compared to that of bupivacaine as its lipid solubility is lower than that of bupivacaine, but higher than that of lidocaine. It has a slower onset of action than lidocaine, similar to that of bupivacaine. The lower lipid solubility of ropivacaine compared to bupivacaine results in slower penetration of larger myelinated motor nerve fibres, producing a more discriminative block. This means ropivacaine should produce a slower onset, shorter duration and less dense motor block compared to bupivacaine. All other pharmacological properties of ropivacaine are similar to those of bupivacaine, except its toxic plasma concentration. Ropivacaine is much less cardiotoxic and

Table 2.5.1.a. Comparison between bupivacaine and lidocaine

Property	Bupivacaine	Lidocaine
Type of LA		
Relative potency (lipid solubility)	8 × more potent	1
Toxic dose	2 mg/kg	3 mg/kg
Toxic dose with adrenaline	2 mg/kg	7 mg/kg
Toxic plasma concentration	>1.5 μg/ml	>5 μg/ml
Protein binding (duration of action)	95%	70%
Elimination half-life	160 minutes	100 minutes
pKa (onset of action)	8.1	7.9
% unionised at pH 7.4 (onset of action)	15%	25%

has a toxic plasma concentration of greater than 4 μg/ml, compared with 1.5 μg/ml for bupivacaine. The dose of ropivacaine is 3 mg/kg compared to 2 mg/kg for bupivacaine.

Tell me more about the cardiac effects of lidocaine and bupivacaine

Both bupivacaine and lidocaine block sodium channels and cause phase 0 of the cardiac action potential to increase more slowly, delaying the arrival at the threshold potential for spontaneous depolarisation. They also prolong the refractory period. Therefore the PR and QRS intervals are prolonged.

Both drugs depress the myocardium but bupivacaine more so, it causes persistent depression of the myocardium and pacemaker cells. This is because it takes roughly 10 times longer to diffuse away from the sodium channels compared with lidocaine. This can lead to arrhythmias and ventricular fibrillation. Calcium and potassium channel disruption may also occur, again leading to arrhythmias.

Ropivacaine differs structurally to bupivacaine and it dissociates more rapidly from the cardiac sodium channels, producing less myocardial depression therefore less toxicity than bupivacaine.

Why do local anaesthetics not work in infected tissues?

Local anaesthetics are relatively ineffective in infected tissues because of the acid environment. The low pH of infected tissues further reduces the unionised fragment of local anaesthetics available to diffuse across the lipid membrane. In addition the inflammation in infected tissue causes vasodilatation and the increased blood supply results in faster removal of local anaesthetic from the site.

What are the concentrations of local anaesthetics used in spinal and epidural anaesthetics?

Local anaesthetic concentrations used in spinal and epidural anaesthesia vary. Generally in spinal anaesthetics 0.5% bupivacaine is used if a dense block is required. Epidural anaesthetics, particularly in labour, require analgesia but motor block is not required or wanted, therefore the concentrations used are lower. Common practice is to use a 0.1% bupivacaine infusion to achieve this. Higher concentrations can be used if analgesia is inadequate, for example 0.25% bupivacaine, or if epidural top up is required for caesarean section a dense block is needed and 0.5% bupivacaine or 1% lignocaine are commonly used, in doses up to 20 ml.

What is "heavy" marcain?

"Heavy" marcain is bupivacaine in solution with glucose 80 mg/ml. The glucose is added for subarachnoid blocks to increase the predictability of the blocks. The glucose increases the density of the solution above that of CSF, so gravity can be used to manipulate the level of the block.

What are the maximum doses of the commonly used local anaesthetics with and without adrenaline?

Maximum or toxic doses should be used as a guide to the maximum amount of local anaesthetic you can administer to a patient. However because the absorption of local anaesthetic varies depending on the site of injection, the agent used and the presence of vasoconstrictors the toxic dose without regard to the site of administration is unhelpful. For example the maximum dose for lignocaine is 3 mg/kg without adrenaline, so for a 70-kg person, using a 1% solution which contains 10 mg/ml, you could use a maximum of 28 ml. However if less than 10 mg, or 1 ml of the solution was to be inadvertently injected into the carotid or vertebral artery it could cause high levels in the brain and coma, apnoea and cardiac arrest.

Nevertheless, in practice we use the maximum doses as a guide. They are as follows: for lignocaine 3 mg/kg without adrenaline and 7 mg/kg with adrenaline, bupivacaine 2 mg/kg with or without adrenaline, ropivacaine 3 mg/kg with or without adrenaline, prilocaine 6 mg/kg without adrenaline, 9 mg/kg with adrenaline.

What are the features of local anaesthetic toxicity?

The features are dependent on the plasma levels of the local anaesthetic. They are divided into neurological and cardiac features.

Neurological features generally occur first. Initially the patient may complain of tingling around the lips and paraesthesia, light-headedness and dizziness. They may have visual or auditory disturbances such as blurred vision or tinnitus. They may become disorientated and confused. Shivering, twitching and tremors may occur and as CNS levels increase grand mal convulsions and coma may develop.

Cardiac dysrhythmias occur and may culminate in ventricular fibrillation.

What factors can pre-dispose the patient to local anaesthetic toxicity?

Many factors can pre-dispose to toxicity and these should always be considered.

- The vascularity of the area of injection should be considered. More vascular areas will result in a higher absorption of drug into the circulation so higher risk of toxicity. Blocks such as intercostals, paracervical, caudals and epidurals are higher risk.
- The presence of other tissues such as adipose tissue that may bind the local anaesthetic will reduce the risk of systemic absorption.
- The drug used and their doses have obvious implications on the likelihood of toxicity. It is shown that the peak level and rate of rise are important factors in causing toxicity, so

not only the total dose administered but the more concentrated solutions have a higher rate of risk and higher peak levels than a more dilute solution containing the same total dose.

- The concurrent use of vasoconstrictors can reduce the systemic absorption and maximum blood concentrations and therefore the risks of toxicity.
- Acidosis and hypoxia causing a low pH can increase the chance of toxicity as the protein binding decreases in such situations.

How would you manage local anaesthetic toxicity?

I would stop the injection of local anaesthetic immediately and call for help. The initial management of local anaesthetic toxicity would be the standard approach of Airway, Breathing and Circulatory management appropriate to the state of the patient.

Specific management of seizures with benzodiazepines, thiopental or propofol would be undertaken as necessary. Continuous ECG assessment would be undertaken, and management of cardiac dysrhythmias includes anti-arrhythmic drugs as appropriate, amiodarone is the drug of choice unless the patient is in ventricular fibrillation, when a direct current (DC) shock in accordance with Advanced Life Support (ALS) protocol should be used.

In the case of cardiac arrest due to local anaesthetic toxicity ALS guidelines should be followed and 20% intra-lipid administered promptly in accordance with the AAGBI Local Anaesthetic Toxicity Guidelines.

A 1.5 ml/kg of 20% intra-lipid should be given as an immediate bolus under these circumstances. This should be followed by 0.25 ml/kg/min for 20 minutes if there is no return of spontaneous output. The initial bolus can be repeated twice at further 5-minute intervals, followed after another 5 minutes of 0.5 ml/kg/min over 10 minutes until return of spontaneous circulation is achieved. CPR must be continued throughout, and it should be remembered that if bupivacaine was the agent used then resuscitation might be prolonged.

What is EMLA?

EMLA stands for eutectic mixture of local anaesthetic. A eutectic mixture is when two compounds mix to produce a substance that behaves with a single set of characteristics. EMLA contains crystalline bases of 2.5% lidocaine and 2.5% prilocaine in a white oil:water emulsion. It is presented as an emulsion containing 5 or 30 grams and applied to skin under a clear plastic dressing for at least 60 minutes. It is used to anaesthetise skin prior to cannulating, usually in paediatric practice, and prior to harvesting skin grafts. EMLA should be avoided in methaemoglobinaemia or patients taking drugs that can induce methaemoglobinaemia such as sulphonamides or phenytoin. One of the metabolites of prilocaine is o-toluidine, which can cause methaemoglobinaemia. It should not be applied to mucous membranes because of rapid systemic absorption. Care is required with its use in patients taking class 1 anti-arrhythmic drugs as toxic effects can be additive and synergistic.

Chapter

2.6

Analgesic agents

2.6.1. Analgesic agents – Dana L Kelly

What is the difference between an opiate and an opioid?

This is a common question so make sure you can give a clear definition of an opiate and an opioid.

The term "opiate" refers to all naturally occurring substances that have morphine like properties. This is different to an "opioid" which is a much more general term that includes synthetic substances that have an affinity for opioid receptors.

What is the classification, action and distribution of each type of opioid receptor?

Opioid receptors are G-protein coupled receptors that are located throughout the central nervous system. They are present in high concentrations in the nuclei of the tractus solitarius, the peri-aqueductal grey area, the cerebral cortex and the thalamus. They are also located within the spinal cord, the gastrointestinal tract and have been found on peripheral afferent nerve terminals and many other organs.

The classification of opioid receptors is confused by different terminology. There are three types of receptor that are considered true opioid receptors, traditionally classified as μ-, κ- and δ-receptors. The receptors were named using the first letter of the first ligand that was found to bind to them, for example morphine was the first chemical shown to bind to μ-receptors. A number of different subtypes of each receptor exist: two μ, three κ and two δ.

These receptors have been reclassified recently into OP1 (δ), OP2 (κ) and OP3 (μ). In addition, a new opioid receptor has been identified, known as nociceptin receptor or ORL 1 receptor.

The International Union of Pharmacology subcommittee has now recommended that appropriate terminology for the three classical receptors, the μ-, δ- and κ-receptors, and the non-classical (nociceptin) receptor, should be MOP, DOP, KOP and NOP, respectively.

Dr Podcast Scripts for the Primary FRCA, ed. Rebecca A. Leslie, Emily K. Johnson and Alexander P. L. Goodwin.   Published by Cambridge University Press. © R. A. Leslie, E. K. Johnson and A. P. L. Goodwin 2011.

The sigma receptor, previously thought to be an opioid receptor, is no longer classified as such, because it does not meet all the necessary criteria, for example naloxone does not reverse the effects of its stimulation.

The actions and distributions of the "classical" opioid receptors are as follows:

The μ-receptor activation causes analgesia, miosis and euphoria, which are predominantly μ1-subtype-mediated effects. It also causes respiratory depression, bradycardia and inhibition of gut motility, which are predominantly μ2-subtype-mediated effects. The μ-receptors are responsible for "supra-spinal analgesia" so therefore act at brain level. Stimulation of μ-receptors also causes physical dependence. The prototype agonist for μ1- and μ2-receptors is morphine.

The δ-receptor activation results in analgesia and respiratory depression. Analgesia is produced at spinal level. Their precise role is unclear. The prototype agonists are enkephalins.

The κ-receptor activation results in sedation, miosis, respiratory depression, inhibition of ADH release and analgesia, which is again at spinal level. Stimulation also causes physical dependence, though different to that caused by μ-receptor activation. The prototype agonist is ketocyclazacine.

How do opioids work at a molecular level?

Opioid receptors are essentially presynaptic and are coupled with inhibitory G-proteins. Their activation has a number of actions including closing of voltage sensitive calcium channels, stimulation of potassium efflux leading to hyperpolarisation of the cell membrane and reduced cyclic adenosine monophosphate production. Overall, the effect is a reduction in neuronal cell excitability that results in reduced transmission of nociceptive impulses.

What are the routes of administration available for opioids?

Opioids can be administered intra-venously, intra-muscularly, orally, via the epidural or intra-thecal route, or transdermally.

What are the pharmacodynamic effects of opioids?

Remember, whenever describing the effects of any drug make sure you classify your answer. This question is best answered by looking at individual body systems in turn.

There are many effects of opioids on numerous body systems.

Effects on the central nervous system include analgesia, sedation, euphoria and dysphoria, hallucinations, tolerance and dependence. Opioids are most effective in relieving dull, continuous and poorly localised pain arising from viscera. They are typically less effective against superficial and sharp pain. Neuropathic pain can be very resistant, but opioids may reduce pain intensity. Tolerance is the decrease in effect seen despite maintaining a given concentration of a drug. The mechanism is not fully understood but could involve down-regulation of opioid receptors or decreased production of endogenous opioids. Dependence exists when the sudden withdrawn of an opioid, after repeated use over a prolonged period, results in various physical and psychological signs. These signs include restlessness, irritability, sweating, muscle cramps, vomiting and diarrhoea.

In terms of cardiovascular effects, mild bradycardia is common as a result of decreased sympathetic drive and a direct effect on the sino-atrial (SA) node. Peripheral vasodilatation caused by histamine release and reduced sympathetic drive may result in a slight fall in blood pressure that may be significant in hypovolaemic patients.

Opioids also affect the respiratory system. Respiratory depression is mediated via μ-receptors at the respiratory centres in the brainstem. Respiratory rate falls more than the tidal volume and the sensitivity of the brainstem to carbon dioxide is reduced. The brainstem response to hypoxia is less affected, but notably if hypoxic stimulus is removed by supplemental oxygen, there may be augmentation of respiratory depression. Opioids also have an anti-tussive action, i.e. act to suppress cough. Large doses of opioids, particularly remifentanil, may occasionally produce generalised muscle rigidity especially of thoracic wall, and can interfere with ventilation.

Direct stimulation of the chemoreceptor trigger zone causes nausea and vomiting.

Smooth muscle tone is increased by opioids, but motility is decreased resulting in delayed absorption, increased pressure in the biliary system (which may result in spasm of the sphincter of Oddi) and constipation.

Endocrine effects include inhibition of release of ACTH, prolactin and gonadotrophic hormone and increased secretion of ADH.

Stimulation of μ- and κ-receptors in the Edinger–Westphal nucleus of the occulomotor nerve results in constriction of the pupils (meiosis).

Some opioids, especially morphine, cause histamine release from mast cells resulting in urticaria, itching, bronchospasm and hypotension. Itching occurs most often after intrathecal opioids and is more pronounced on the face, nose and torso. The mechanism is centrally mediated and may be reversed by naloxone.

Why do fentanyl, morphine and alfentanil have such different onset times and duration of actions?

This is a commonly asked question so make sure you prepare an answer before the exam. If you cannot remember the specific figures just clearly state the principles involved.

The terminal half-life of alfentanil (100 min) is half that of fentanyl (190 min) but the clearance of alfentanil is less (6 ml/kg/min as opposed to 13 ml/kg/min). The shorter terminal half-life of alfentanil is due to the smaller volume of distribution of alfentanil compared to fentanyl (0.53 L/kg as opposed to 4.0 L/kg). This is because fentanyl is highly lipid soluble and is extensively taken up by fat and muscle.

This redistribution also explains why fentanyl has a shorter duration of action when compared to morphine despite a slower clearance (morphine has a clearance of 16 ml/kg/min and similar terminal half-life. The high lipid solubility of fentanyl (when compared to morphine) also means it therefore crosses the blood–brain barrier more quickly, and therefore exerts a more rapid onset of action.

Alfentanil is poorly lipid soluble and therefore has a much smaller initial volume of distribution. Despite this, it has a rapid onset of action as it is a weak base (pKa 6.5) and therefore at body pH the unbound drug is nearly 90% unionised. As it is the unionised molecules that can cross the blood–brain barrier, it therefore has rapid effect centrally.

How is morphine metabolised and excreted?

Morphine is conjugated in the liver to morphine-3-glucuronide (70%), morphine-6-glucuronide (5–10%) and demethylated to normorphine (20–25%). Morphine-6-

glucoronide is an active metabolite, more potent than morphine. It is excreted predominantly in the urine as conjugated metabolites, less than 10% is excreted unchanged.

Tell me about Remifentanil

Remifentanil is a pure μ agonist. It is a synthetic anilino-piperidine opioid with methyl ester linkage. While it shares many of the effects associated with opioids, its metabolism makes it unique. It is mainly used to provide the analgesic component during general anaesthetic, but has a developing role in many other areas of anaesthetics, including analgesia on intensive care and in obstetrics. It is presented as a lyophilised white powder, in 1-mg, 2-mg or 5-mg vials of remifentanil hydrochloride in a glycine buffer. This is reconstituted, forming a clear, colourless solution for injection. Due to the glycine buffer, remifentanil is not licensed for epidural or intra-thecal use. It is used intra-venously, in boluses of 1 μg/kg and may be infused at a rate of 0.0125–1 μg/kg/min. The peak effect of the drug occurs within 1–3 minutes. The offset is rapid and predictable even after prolonged infusion. This is because the context sensitive half-time is independent of the time it has been infused. It can therefore be used to give high-dose opioid analgesia to provide cardiovascular stability during very stimulating surgery without post-operative effects. However it is important to remember that other analgesics must be given post-operatively as the effects of remifentanil will have worn off.

Remifentanil decreases the mean arterial pressure and particularly heart rate by 20%. Myocardial contractility and cardiac output may also decrease. It is a potent respiratory depressant, causing a decrease in both respiratory rate and tidal volume. It also diminishes the ventilatory response to hypoxia and hypercarbia. Chest wall rigidity ("wooden chest" phenomenon) can occur, which appears to be an effect via μ-receptors located on GABA-ergic interneurones, this phenomenon can be relieved by muscle relaxants. Remifentanil does not cause histamine release and therefore does not precipitate bronchospasm. It has centrally mediated vagal activity. It has minimal hypnotic or sedative effects. Remifentanil, like other opioids, decreases gastrointestinal motility, but appears to have a relatively low incidence of nausea and vomiting associated with its use.

Side effects include respiratory depression, bradycardia, nausea and vomiting.

The metabolism of remifentanil is what really distinguishes it from other opioids. It rapidly undergoes ester hydrolysis by non-specific and plasma esterases to a carboxylic acid derivative which is 300- to 1000-fold less potent than remifentanil and is excreted in the urine. The clearance of remifentanil is 40 ml/kg/min and the elimination half-life is 10 minutes.

How does nalbuphine work?

Nalbuphine is a mixed opioid agonist–antagonist, that is it exerts agonist effects at one opioid receptor and antagonistic effects at the other. It is a semi-synthetic phenanthrene derivative, and is presented as a clear, colourless solution for injection containing 10 mg/ml of nalbuphine. It can be administered IV, IM or SC. It is an agonist at κ-receptors and antagonist at μ-receptors. Nalbuphine therefore produces analgesia (a κ effect) whilst antagonising respiratory depression and dependency problems that are associated with the μ receptor. Side effects include sedation, dizziness, vertigo, dry mouth and headache. Importantly, nalbuphine is ineffective in obtunding cardiovascular responses to laryngoscopy. The drug will precipitate withdrawal symptoms in opioid addicts. It is reversed by naloxone.

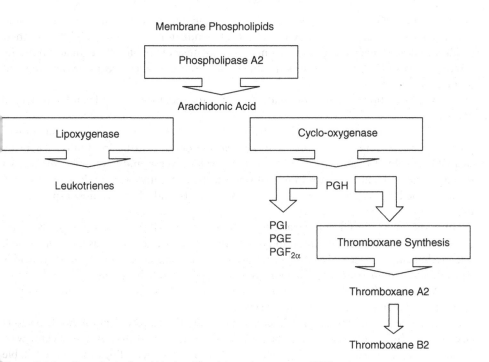

Figure 2.6.1a. Biosynthesis of arachidonic acid and the cyclo-oxygenase (COX) pathway.

What is the mode of action of NSAIDs?

Non-steroidal anti-inflammatory drugs (NSAIDs) inhibit the enzyme cyclo-oxygenase (COX) (see Figure 2.6.1a). They therefore prevent the production of both prostaglandins and thromboxanes from membrane phospholipids. Decreased PGE_2 and PGF_2 synthesis results in anti-inflammatory action, whilst reduced thromboxane synthesis results in decreased platelet aggregation and adhesiveness. The anti-pyretic effects of NSAIDs are due to inhibition of centrally produced prostaglandins. Reduced prostaglandin synthesis in gastric mucosal cells can lead to ulceration.

Lipoxygenase is not inhibited by NSAIDs. When NSAIDS are given and the cyclo-oxygenase pathway is blocked, more arachidonic acid is converted into leukotrienes. This is the likely mechanism behind exacerbation of asthma with NSAID use.

Aspirin produces irreversible inhibition by enzyme acetylation, so synthesis of new cyclo-oxygenase must occur for further production of prostaglandins and thromboxanes. Other NSAIDs produce reversible enzyme inhibition, so when plasma NSAID levels fall, the activity of cyclo-oxygenase resumes.

What is the difference between COX-1 and COX-2 inhibition, and the respective side effects

COX exists as two isoenzymes: COX-1 and COX-2. COX-1 is a constitutive enzyme, whereas COX-2 is induced at sites of inflammation. The existing NSAIDs are not selective.

Inhibition of COX-1 appears to underlie the majority of unwanted effects of NSAIDs, such as gastrointestinal irritation, bleeding and nephrotoxicity. In the stomach, the prostaglandins PGE_2 and PGI_2 inhibit acid secretion and have a gastroprotective action, whereas in the kidney PGE_2 and PGI_2 act as local vasodilators. Therefore, inhibition of their synthesis reduces renal blood flow and may precipitate acute renal failure. In addition, the prolonged use of NSAIDs is associated with risk of chronic renal failure due to development of interstitial nephritis.

COX-2 inhibition appears to provide the anti-inflammatory, analgesic and anti-pyretic effects.

However, this may be a simplistic division as COX-2 is also involved in the production of protective prostaglandins in the presence of *H pylori*–induced gastritis. In addition, it appears that COX-2 inhibitors may increase the risk of cardiac events, and have only been shown to reduce the incidence of gastrointestinal side effects. Currently COX-2 inhibitors are only recommended in those at increased risk of GI side effects, and where low dose aspirin is not used.

In addition to the GI and renal effects discussed, NSAIDs also can trigger NSAID-sensitive asthma. This occurs in up to 20% of asthmatics. Children are usually unaffected. The mechanism is suggested as that by inhibiting cyclo-oxygenase, more arachidonic acid is converted to leukotrienes, which are known to precipitate bronchospasm.

NSAIDs also affect platelet function due to reduced thromboxane A_2 production preventing platelet aggregation and vasoconstriction.

There are several important drug interactions involving NSAIDs. Caution should be exercised when administering with anti-coagulants such as heparin or warfarin, especially warfarin, as it may be displaced from its plasma protein binding sites, leading to an unpredictable increased effect. Serum lithium levels may also be affected.

Up to 15% of patients may have raised serum transaminase levels as a result of NSAID-induced hepatotoxicity.

Compare and contrast the properties and uses of ketorolac and ibuprofen

Ibuprofen is a proprionic acid. It is licensed for adult and paediatric use above 1 year of age. The suggested maximum adult dose is 1.8 g daily. The recommended paediatric dose is 20 mg/kg daily. It has mild anti-pyretic, anti-inflammatory and analgesic effects. It has the lowest incidence of side effects of the commonly used NSAIDs. Ibuprofen has an elimination half-life of 2–3 hours and it is 99% protein bound.

Ketorolac is an acetic acid derivative. It has potent analgesic and anti-pyretic activity, but limited anti-inflammatory action. It shares the side effect profile with other NSAIDs. It is specifically contraindicated in patients on heparin, despite evidence suggesting that there may not be any reaction of clinical significance. Ketorolac has an elimination half-life of 5 hours and it is 99% protein bound.

How does paracetamol work?

Despite having no effect on cyclo-oxygenase in vitro, paracetamol has been classified as an NSAID because of its moderate analgesic and anti-pyretic effects. It is an acetanilide derivative. The mode of action is poorly understood. It has been proposed that its anti-pyretic actions are due to inhibition of prostaglandin synthesis within the central nervous system. It acts peripherally by blocking impulse generation within the bradykinin-sensitive chemoreceptors responsible for the generation of afferent nociceptive impulses.

What is the mechanism of paracetamol toxicity?

Paracetamol is metabolised by the liver to mainly glucuronide conjugates, but also to sulphate and cysteine conjugates. These are actively excreted in the urine, with only a small fraction being excreted unchanged. N-acetyl-p-amino-benzoquinone imine is a highly toxic metabolite of paracetamol. It is normally produced in very small quantities and is rapidly conjugated by hepatic glutathione, which renders it harmless.

Following a toxic dose, the hepatic conjugation pathways become saturated. Glutathione supply becomes depleted and N-acetyl-p-amino-benzoquinoneimine accumulates. It forms covalent bonds with sulphydryl groups on hepatocytes, resulting in centrilobar necrosis. N-acetylcysteine and methionine act as alternative supplies of glutathione and can protect against paracetamol-related hepatotoxicity if administered within 10–12 hours of ingestion. N-acetylcysteine is hydrolysed to cysteine, which is a glutathione precursor, whilst methionine enhances glutathione synthesis.

Chapter

Drugs acting on the central nervous system

2.7.1. Anti-convulsants – Rebecca A Leslie

What are the mechanisms of action of the commonly used anti-convulsants?

This is a tough question. If you get stuck think about the anti-convulsants you know. For example you know that benzodiazepines act on the GABA receptor, and it makes sense that sodium valproate acts on sodium channels.

Epileptic seizures occur as a result of repetitive neuronal discharges of neurones in the central nervous system.

Broadly speaking anti-convulsant drugs act by two mechanisms to prevent these neuronal discharges, they either act on sodium channels or by increasing the activation of GABA receptors.

Anti-convulsants that affect sodium channels act by:

- Blocking the inactive fast sodium channels (phenytoin)
- Stabilising the pre-synaptic sodium channels (lamotrigine).

Phenytoin is an example of a drug that blocks inactive fast sodium channels. It is the fast sodium channels that are responsible for depolarisation during the propagation of an action potential. Therefore by blocking these channels phenytoin prevents further generation of action potentials which are central to seizure activity. Lamotrigine, on the other hand, stabilises the pre-synaptic sodium channels thus preventing the release of excitatory neurotransmitters.

Drugs that affect GABA can be further sub-classified into three types:

- Drugs which facilitate GABA (benzodiapines/barbiturates)
- Drugs which are GABA agonists
- Drugs which inhibit GABA transaminase (sodium valproate/vigabatrin).

The benzodiazepines and barbiturates both facilitate the effects of GABA by opening of the chloride channel in the GABA receptor. This allows chloride ions to flow down their concentration gradient into the cell, making it hyperpolarised and therefore much less excitable.

Sodium valproate and vigabatrin both act to prevent the breakdown of GABA by inhibiting GABA transaminase, the enzyme that normal catalyses the breakdown of GABA.

What do you know about phenytoin?

You must have a good, logical format that you can apply to any drug that will help you structure your answer.

Phenytoin is an anti-convulsant which has been used for many years in the treatment of grand mal seizures, partial seizures, status epilepticus, and trigeminal neuralgia. Phenytoin also has type Ib anti-arrhythmic properties, and is used especially for digoxin-induced arrhythmias.

The site of action of phenytoin is the fast sodium channels which are responsible for depolarisation of an action potential. Because it binds to sodium channels when they are in the refractory period after opening, it is most effective at blocking cells that are firing at a high frequency. This allows the action of phenytoin to discriminate between epileptic and physiological activity.

Phenytoin can be given orally or by intra-venous administration, but must not be given by intra-muscular injection. It has a narrow therapeutic window so levels must be carefully monitored.

Idiosyncratic side effects include hirsutism, gum hyperplasia, acne, coarsening of facial features, peripheral neuropathy and megaloblastic anaemia. At high doses phenytoin will cause ataxia, nystagmus, parasthesia and slurred speech. Phenytoin also has teratogenic effects such as craniofacial abnormalities, growth and mental retardation and limb and cardiac defects.

There is significant risk of drug interactions with the use of phenytoin, because it induces the hepatic oxidase enzymes that are responsible for the metabolism of warfarin, benzodiazepines and the oral contraceptive pill. Drugs such as metronidazole, chloramphenicol and isonazid inhibit the metabolism of phenytoin.

The oral bioavailability of phenytoin is approximately 90% and it is 90% protein bound. It is metabolised in the liver and inactive metabolites are excreted in the urine. It undergoes saturation kinetics at a dose just above the therapeutic range, therefore it normally follows first-order kinetics but at high doses it follows zero-order kinetics, due to saturation of the enzyme systems.

Tell me about sodium valproate

Sodium valproate is an anti-convulsant which is used for petit mal seizures, myoclonic epilepsy and for the management of chronic pain, especially trigeminal neuralgia.

Sodium valproate stabilises inactive fast sodium channels in a similar manner to phenytoin but it also stimulates central GABA inhibitory pathways by inhibiting GABA transaminase.

Sodium valproate is normally well tolerated but can cause nausea and gastric irritation, thrombocytopenia, transient hair loss and neural tube defects.

Sodium valproate is well absorbed orally, and approximately 90% is protein bound. It is metabolised in the liver and excreted renally.

What are the effects of anti-convulsants in pregnancy?

Most anti-convulsants carry a risk of neural tube defects, teratogenicity and coagulation disorders of the newborn. However the greatest risk to the mother and the baby is if the convulsions occur. The mother must undergo counselling, antenatal screening, folate supplements and pre-delivery vitamin K should be considered.

Lamotrigine is one of the newer anti-convulsants that is considered safer in pregnancy.

How would you manage a patient with status epilepticus?

Start by giving a brief definition of status epilepticus.

Status epilepticus is a continuous or rapidly repeating convulsion which has persisted for longer than 30 minutes without the patient regaining consciousness.

General management of status epilepticus consists of rapid assessment of the airway, breathing and circulation. Oxygen should be given and IV access gained. Tracheal intubation may become necessary. Measurement of blood pressure, pulse, oxygen saturation and temperature should be carried out where possible.

Ten milligrams of IV diazepam should be given as first line treatment. This dose can be repeated after 15 minutes if the seizure has not terminated. In addition, phenytoin at a dose of 15 mg/kg can be given to try to terminate the seizure.

If the patient remains resistant to these measures then they will require transfer to a specialist unit with EEG monitoring and given anaesthesia with thiopentone or propofol.

Gabapentin was initially introduced as an anti-convulsant, but what is it most commonly used for now?

Gabapentin is used extensively in the management of chronic neuropathic pain. It is also used in the management of trigeminal neuralgia and post-herpetic neuralgia.

It is an amino acid which is a structural analogue of GABA. Although it is structurally related to GABA it does not interact with GABA receptors, instead it is thought to bind to and modulate voltage-sensitive calcium channels. The mechanism of action of gabapentin is not completely understood. It is thought that it may also increase the synthesis of GABA in the brain, inhibit the excitatory neurotransmitter glutamate, increase serotonin levels and inhibit voltage-dependent sodium channels.

What considerations do you have to take when anaesthetising an epileptic patient?

Classify your answer into the pre-operative, intra-operative and post-operative considerations that you would make.

In the pre-operative period in addition to the normal pre-operative assessment, a careful history of the nature, timing and frequency of seizures should be recorded. A thorough drug history should be taken with the timings of anti-convulsants recorded. The anaesthetist must ensure that the patient continues to take all their anti-convulsant treatment right up until the time of surgery.

If possible regional anaesthetic techniques should be considered to allow early oral intake post-operatively.

In the intra-operative period caution should be taken not to hyperventilate the patient as hypocapnia will lower the seizure threshold.

Conveniently, all currently used anaesthetic agents are anti-convulsant at therapeutic doses. Thiopentone is an especially powerful anti-convulsant and should be considered for induction of anaesthesia.

When choosing a muscle relaxant, you should use a benzylquinolinium such as atracurium, as the common anti-convulsants such as phenytoin, carbamazepine and the barbiturates are hepatic enzyme inducers which will lead to rapid metabolism of the aminosteroidal muscle relaxants such as vecuronium and rocuronium.

Anti-emetics that cause dystonias such as prochlorperazine, metochlopramide and droperidol should be avoided. Ondansetron and cyclizine are safe to use.

In the post-operative period oral intake should be re-instituted early to avoid missing the anti-convulsant doses. If oral or nasogastric therapy is not possible parenteral anti-convulsant therapy should be started.

What do you know about the use of propofol in epileptic patients?

Although propofol is well known to be associated with abnormal movements on both induction and emergence of anaesthesia, EEG studies have failed to show epileptiform activity during these episodes. It is thought that epileptics are prone to seizures during rapid emergence from propofol anaesthesia. However it has also been reported that propofol is effective in status epilepticus in the intensive care setting.

In general, caution is advised in administering propofol to patients with poorly controlled epilepsy and induction with thiopentone is recommended. If propofol has to be used, the coadministration with a benzodiazepine may reduce its potential to produce abnormal movements and reduce the likelihood of post-operative seizures.

2.7.2. Benzodiazepines – Dana L Kelly

What are benzodiazepines?

Don't over complicate this! Keep it short—you will soon be guided towards a specific area of questioning.

The benzodiazepines are a class of psychoactive drugs with varying hypnotic, sedative, anxiolytic, anti-convulsant, muscle relaxant and amnesic properties.

Classify the benzodiazepines, giving examples

Most simply done based on their pharmacokinetic parameters.

Benzodiazepines are commonly divided into three groups by their half-lives:

- Short-acting compounds have a half-life of less than 12 hours, for example midazolam.
- Intermediate-acting compounds have a half-life of 12–24 hours, for example lorazepam.
- Long-acting compounds have a half-life greater than 24 hours, for example diazepam.

Describe the various effects of benzodiazepines

The main actions of the benzodiazepines include hypnosis, sedation, anxiolysis, anterograde amnesia, anti-convulsant activity and muscle relaxation. Benzodiazepines reduce the MAC of co-administered anaesthetic agents. Other effects of the benzodiazepines include a varying degree of cardiorespiratory depression, particularly impairing the ventilatory response to hypercapnia.

Describe the mechanism of action of benzodiazepines

Benzodiazepines are thought to act via specific benzodiazepine receptors found throughout the central nervous system, but especially concentrated in the cortex and midbrain. Benzodiazepine receptors are closely linked with GABA receptors and appear to facilitate the activity of the latter. Activated GABA receptors open chloride ion channels, which either hyperpolarise or short circuit the synaptic membrane.

Describe the subtypes of GABA receptors and the mechanisms associated with them

GABA is the main inhibitory neurotransmitter within the CNS. It acts via two different receptor subtypes, GABAA and GABAB receptors.

The GABAA receptor is a ligand-gated chloride ion channel. It consists of five subunits (2α, β, δ, γ) arranged to form a central ion channel. GABA binds to and activates GABAA receptors, increasing the frequency of opening of the associated chloride ion channel and hyperpolarising the membrane. Chloride ion conductance is potentiated by binding of benzodiazepines to the α-subunit of the activated receptor complex. This is because the benzodiazepine locks the GABAA receptor into a conformation where the neurotransmitter GABA has much higher affinity for the GABA-A receptor. GABAA receptors are mainly located post-synaptically and are widely distributed throughout the CNS.

The GABAA receptor can be further sub-classified depending on the type of α-subunit it contains. Two different receptor subtypes have been identified, and the specific α-subunits these receptors contain determine the predominant benzodiazepine pharmacology; anxiolytic or sedative. BZ_1 receptor subtypes are found in the spinal cord and cerebellum, and are responsible for anxiolysis. BZ_2 receptor subtypes are found in the spinal cord, hippocampus and cerebral cortex, and are responsible for sedative and anti-convulsant activity.

The GABAB receptor is metabotrophic (i.e., it acts via a G-protein and second messenger system). When stimulated it increases potassium conductance, and thereby acts to hyperpolarise the neuronal membrane. GABAB receptors are located pre- and post-synaptically. Baclofen acts via GABAB receptors.

How are the benzodiazepines metabolised?

Diazepam is metabolised in the liver by oxidation to desmethyldiazepam, oxazepam and temazepam, all of which are active. Midazolam is metabolised by hydroxylation to the active compound 1α hydroxymidazolam, which is conjugated with glucuronic acid prior to excretion (see Figure 2.7.2.) Less than 5% is metabolised to oxazepam. Oxazepam and lorazepam are conjugated with glucuronic acid to produce inactive metabolites that are excreted renally.

What are the advantages of midazolam?

Midazolam is presented as a clear solution at pH 3.5. It is unique amongst the benzodiazepine group in that its structure is dependent on the surrounding pH. At pH 3.5 its ring structure is

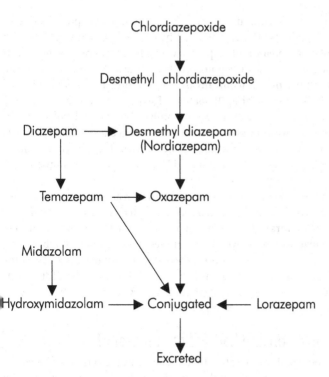

Chlordiazepoxide

Desmethyl chlordiazepoxide

Diazepam ⟶ Desmethyl diazepam
(Nordiazepam)

Temazepam ⟶ Oxazepam

Midazolam

Hydroxymidazolam ⟶ Conjugated ⟵ Lorazepam

Excreted

Figure 2.7.2. Metabolic inter-relationships of the benzodiazepine family. Reproduced with permission from Smith, T., Pinnock, C. and Lin, T. 2009. *Fundamentals of Anaesthesia.* Cambridge: Cambridge University Press. © Cambridge University Press 2009.

open resulting in an ionised molecule, which is therefore water-soluble. In this form it causes less pain on injection. However, when the surrounding pH is greater than 4, the ring structure closes, it is no longer ionised, and therefore becomes lipid soluble. The pK_a of midazolam is 6.5; therefore, at physiological pH it is 90% unionised, and able to cross lipid membranes.

Other advantages include the fact it is available in a wide range of preparations including orally (bioavailability 40%), intra-nasally, intra-muscularly or intra-venously. Also compared to other benzodiazepines, it has a short elimination half-life (1–4 hours), and a large clearance (approximately 6–10 ml/kg/min), making it more suitable for infusion. Midazolam, in combination with fentanyl, has been shown to reduce the pressor response to intubation to a greater extent than thiopentone with fentanyl. The use of midazolam as a pre-medication may decrease MAC requirements by 15%.

What are the principles of treating benzodiazepine poisoning, and can you name a specific antidote for benzodiazepine overdoes?

Don't rush into complex management—with a question like this always start simply with recognition of the problem, involving a senior, and basic resuscitation, before mentioning specific antidotes and treatments.

The principles of managing a benzodiazepine overdose involve recognition, assessment, resuscitation and treatment, including specific antidotes as appropriate.

Benzodiazepine overdose should be recognised as an anaesthetic emergency. I would administer 100% oxygen and call for senior help. My management strategy would include a thorough but rapid initial assessment, and commencement of resuscitation, using an A, B, C, D, E approach. The most important aspect of the management of benzodiazepine overdoses is good supportive care. ECG, non-invasive blood pressure and pulse oximetry monitoring are required for all patients. The airway must be controlled in any patient with significantly decreased level of consciousness or respiratory insufficiency. Endotracheal intubation and ventilation may be required. Intra-venous access is always required. In addition, significant cardiovascular instability may warrant invasive blood pressure monitoring and central venous access. In addition to stabilizing the patient, I would attempt to identify the likely substance involved, particularly details of specific amounts administered and any other likely co-administered substances. I would also like to obtain as much background history as possible, including information on pre-existing medical conditions and regular medications. I would particularly be interested in any details that would lead to suspicion of a proconvulsant state.

As with any overdose, an attempt to minimise toxic effects is warranted. Agents that have been orally ingested may be absorbed by activated charcoal. Activated charcoal is beneficial if it can be administered within 2–4 hours of ingestion, and if the risk of aspiration is minimal.

Specific management in benzodiazepine overdose includes consideration of a benzodiazepine antagonist such as flumazenil. This is a competitive antagonist of the GABA receptor and therefore is a specific antidote for benzodiazepine overdoses; however, use of flumazenil for benzodiazepine overdoses is controversial. Significant adverse effects, such as seizures and acute benzodiazepine withdrawal, have been reported.

What is the mechanism of action and half-life of flumazenil?

Flumazenil is an imidazobenzodiazepine derivative that antagonises the actions of benzodiazepines on the central nervous system. Flumazenil competitively inhibits the activity at the benzodiazepine recognition site on the GABA/benzodiazepine receptor complex.

Generally, doses of approximately 0.1 mg to 0.2 mg produce partial antagonism, whereas higher doses of 0.4 to 1 mg usually produce complete antagonism in patients who have received the usual sedating doses of benzodiazepines. The onset of reversal is usually evident within 1 to 2 minutes after the injection is completed. Eighty percent response will be reached within 3 minutes, with the peak effect occurring at 6 to 10 minutes. The duration and degree of reversal are related to the plasma concentration of the sedating benzodiazepine as well as the dose of flumazenil given.

Flumazenil should be used with caution in patients suspected of taking proconvulsant drugs, for example, tricyclic anti-depressants, mixed overdoses, and patients with a history of epilepsy. This is because it also has inverse agonist activity and may precipitate seizures in susceptible individuals.

Flumazenil is extensively distributed in the extra-vascular space with an initial distribution half-life of 4 to 11 minutes and a terminal half-life of 40 to 80 minutes. Importantly, it has a relatively short half-life compared to the benzodiazepines, meaning that further doses or an infusion may be required. Flumazenil is 50% protein bound and undergoes significant hepatic metabolism to inactive compounds that are renally excreted.

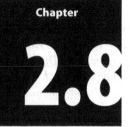

Drugs acting on the cardiovascular system

Chapter

2.8

2.8.1. Anti-hypertensive agents – Caroline V Sampson

Can you classify anti-hypertensive drugs?

These can easily be divided into centrally acting, those acting on the heart and vasculature and those acting on the kidneys. There is some overlap – for example the calcium antagonists act mainly on the vasculature but some also have negative inotropic effects.

Centrally acting anti-hypertensives include clonidine, methyldopa and reserpine. The main anti-hypertensives acting on the heart are the β-blockers. Most of the anti-hypertensives in use act on the vasculature and include α-blockers, calcium channel antagonists, angiotensin-converting enzyme (or ACE) inhibitors, angiotensin 2 receptor antagonists, nitrates such as glyceryl trinitrate and sodium nitroprusside (SNP), potassium channel activators such as diazoxide and monoxidil and hydralazine which is a direct acting arterial vasodilator. Finally there are anti-hypertensives that act on the kidneys such as the diuretics and the direct renin inhibitors.

What is hypotensive anaesthesia and what agents are commonly used?

Hypotensive anaesthesia is defined as deliberately induced hypotension during anaesthesia to minimise blood loss. Hale Enderby is the anaesthetist credited with introducing and publicising the technique of hypotensive anaesthesia.

This technique is often employed during surgery where any bleeding within the surgical field will restrict vision such as in middle ear surgery in ear–nose–throat or neurosurgery.

There are many methods employed to induce hypotension. Patients are usually positioned in a head up tilt and hypotension may be induced merely by increasing the concentration of volatile anaesthetic agent, or by using opiates, especially the short-acting alfentanil or remifentanil. If these simple measures fail, intra-venous agents can be used to induce hypotension. These should be agents with a quick onset and offset of action. Agents commonly used include esmolol, which is a β-blocker, labetalol, which is a combined α- and β-blocker or the nitrates such as glyceryl trinitrate and sodium nitroprusside.

What defines hypotension depends upon the patients starting blood pressure, but systolic blood pressures around 80 could be used in previously normotensive patients. This technique must be used by caution in those with vascular insufficiency, for example in the elderly, as a drop in systemic pressure could cause cerebral insufficiency.

Dr Podcast Scripts for the Primary FRCA, ed. Rebecca A. Leslie, Emily K. Johnson and Alexander P. L. Goodwin.   Published by Cambridge University Press. © R. A. Leslie, E. K. Johnson and A. P. L. Goodwin 2011.

What do you know about β-blockers?

A mnemonic for describing any single drug is "Cup a Dorset Dame", which stands for Chemical, Uses, Presentation, Actions, Dose, Onset, Route (of administration), Side effects, Everything else and Toxic effects, with the Dame standing for the pharmacokinetic parameters of Distribution, Absorption, Metabolism and Elimination. There are many such mnemonics around, it doesn't matter which you use as long as you have a system for describing drugs. This mnemonic can be adjusted slightly for groups of drugs – you will not need to describe the presentation or dose or pharmacokinetics of all drugs in the class so miss these out, but add in any important subdivisions or classifications within the drug group.

The β-blockers have many different uses including the treatment of angina, hypertension, congestive cardiac failure, arrhythmias, hyperthyroidism, glaucoma and certain anxiety disorders. They are also used in migraine prophylaxis and in secondary prevention following myocardial infarction. NICE guidelines published in 2006 state that β-blockers should not be used as the first line agents in the treatment of hypertension and should only be used when several agents are required.

In anaesthetic practice β-blockers can be used to attenuate the hypertensive response to laryngoscopy and intubation or in hypotensive anaesthesia. They may also be used to treat peri-operative hypertension or arrhythmias.

The β-blockers are antagonists at β-adrenergic receptors. They can be subdivided into non-selective β-blockers which affect both β1- and β2-receptors, for example timolol and sotalol, and selective β-blockers which affect mainly β1-receptors such as atenolol and metoprolol. Some β-blockers such as pindolol and acebutolol have intrinsic sympathomimetic activity and some act as membrane stabilisers such as sotalol. Labetalol and carvedilol have α- and β-blocking properties.

β-blockers cause negative inotropy and chronotropy which reduces myocardial work and blood pressure.

β-blockers are commonly administered orally but some can be administered intravenously such as atenolol, labetalol and esmolol.

There are many side effects reported with β-blockers. In the cardiovascular system they produce bradycardia and the negative inotropic effect may worsen cardiac failure. They can worsen peripheral vascular disease and many patients complain of cold extremities. They cause bronchospasm and should be avoided in asthmatic patients. The β-blockers, especially those with higher lipid solubility can cause tiredness, nightmares and sleep disturbance. Metabolically, β-blockers can reduce glycogenolysis and insulin release and blunt the hypoglycaemic response so should be used with caution in diabetics.

β-blockers should never be used with calcium antagonists that have negative inotropic effects such as verapamil and diltiazem, as this can cause profound hypotension, bradycardia and conduction defects.

Which anti-hypertensives are commonly used to treat hypertensive emergencies?

Hypertensive emergencies are usually managed in a high dependency area with continual invasive blood pressure monitoring. Short-acting intra-venous anti-hypertensives are used, commonly glyceryl trinitrate, SNP, labetalol or hydralazine. Agents used in the past include phentolamine, β-blockers, diazoxide and clonidine. Nifedipine and ACE inhibitors are not recommended.

Tell me about sodium nitroprusside

SNP is an inorganic complex. It is used to treat hypertensive emergencies, for example hypertension associated with a dissecting thoracic aneurysm, and in hypotensive anaesthesia.

It is presented as a red–brown powder in a brown glass ampoule and should be diluted in 5% dextrose.

Its actions on the cardiovascular system include widespread vaso- and veno-dilatation resulting in reduced blood pressure, reduced left ventricular end-diastolic pressure and reduced myocardial oxygen demand. There is usually a compensatory tachycardia but cardiac contractility is unaffected. In the central nervous system SNP causes cerebral vasodilatation, which increases intra-cranial pressure. In the respiratory system hypoxic pulmonary vasoconstriction is impaired, which can cause a fall in arterial oxygen tension. Finally, SNP causes a reduction in GI motility.

Dose ranges are 0.1 to 8 μg/kg/min. Higher concentrations have been used but with an increased risk of cyanide toxicity.

The onset is very rapid, within seconds, and SNP must be administered intra-venously.

There are several problems with SNP. It is unstable in solution and must be protected from light so special opaque syringes and giving sets are necessary. The patients will often demonstrate a compensatory tachycardia that could lead to myocardial ischaemia in susceptible individuals. There is often a rebound hypertension on stopping SNP. SNP can raise intra-cranial pressure and worsen VQ mismatching due to its effects on the central nervous and respiratory systems. Finally there is the possibility of cyanide poisoning which is greatly increased at higher dose infusions. SNP is metabolised to produce cyanide ions, which are normally metabolised in the liver but if the metabolic pathway is overwhelmed cyanide ions can accumulate, potentially causing cyanide toxicity. SNP has a small volume of distribution (0.2 L/kg), has a very short half-life and is eliminated at a rate of 1 μg/kg/min.

You mentioned cyanide toxicity, how might this manifest and how is it treated?

Cyanide toxicity presents with non-specific features of dizziness, headache or confusion. Patients may be tachypnoeic or apnoeic. Arterial blood gases will show a decreased aterio-venous oxygen difference and a metabolic acidosis with raised lactate.

The initial management is along the ABC resuscitation lines, with supplemental oxygen. Chelating agents such as dicobalt edetate combine with cyanide to form non-harmful inert compounds. Sodium nitrite could be given, which converts haemoglobin to methaemoglobin which then binds with cyanide to form cyanmethaemoglobin. Finally sodium thiosulphate can be given which converts cyanide to thiocyanate, which is water soluble and therefore excreted in the urine.

What is a diuretic?

A diuretic is any agent that promotes diuresis, which is the increased rate of urine production by the kidney.

Can you classify diuretics and briefly describe how each class works?

Diuretics are usually classified by their site of action. I find it easiest to go through the nephron from Bowman's capsule to collecting duct – that way you shouldn't forget any!

Firstly there are osmotic diuretics such as mannitol, urea and glucose. They mainly act on the proximal convoluted tubule and are freely filterable, non-reabsorbable osmotic agents that reduce the reabsorption of sodium and water.

Carbonic anhydrase inhibitors such as acetazolamide inhibit the enzyme carbonic anhydrase in the luminal membrane of the proximal tubule, which reduces proximal bicarbonate reabsorption and causes a weak diuretic effect.

Loop diuretics such as frusemide and bumetanide inhibit the sodium/potassium/2 chloride$^-$ co-transport system in the thick ascending limb of the loop of Henle.

Thiazide diuretics such as bendroflumethiazide and chlorothiazide inhibit the sodium/chloride co-transporter in the early distal convoluted tubule.

The potassium sparing diuretics act on the distal part of the distal convoluted tubule and the collecting tubules. They are subdivided into spironolactone, which is an aldosterone antagonist, and drugs such as amiloride and triamterene, which inhibit the sodium/potassium pump by reducing Na^+ entry across the luminal membrane.

Other substances can also cause diuresis. These include the xanthines, such as caffeine and aminophylline which reduce sodium excretion, dopamine which increases renal blood flow and reduces sodium reabsorption, water and ethanol which inhibit vasopressin secretion and demeclocycline, which blocks the action of vasopressin on the distal convoluted tubule and collecting ducts.

What are the main indications for using a diuretic?

Diuretics are used in the management of hypertension. Thiazide diuretics are recommended as first line in elderly patients with newly diagnosed hypertension. They are also used in the acute and chronic management of congestive cardiac failure. Frusemide, usually as an intra-venous bolus, is used to treat acute pulmonary oedema. The rapid symptomatic relief is mainly due to its venodilatatory effects.

Diuretics are used in the management of chronic renal failure and also in acute renal failure associated with fluid overload, often as a bridging measure prior to dialysis. Diuretics such as mannitol can be used to reduce intra-cranial pressure and have been used to try to prevent acute renal failure. Spironolactone in particular is also used to treat Conn's syndrome and ascites associated with liver disease. Acetazolamide is used in the treatment of glaucoma, altitude sickness and occasionally in the management of metabolic alkalosis. Thiazide diuretics can be used to prevent the formation of calcium containing renal calculi as they lower urinary calcium excretion.

What are the problems associated with thiazide diuretics?

Thiazide diuretics are a commonly used class of drug but they can cause many electrolyte disturbances. These include hypokalaemia, hyponatraemia, hyperuricaemia, hypomagnesaemia, hypochloraemic alkalosis, hyperglycaemia and hypercholesterolaemia. They should therefore be used with caution in patients with diabetes or gout. Other side effects include exacerbation of renal and hepatic impairment and impotence. Rarely they can cause rashes or thrombocytopenia. Long-term use of thiazide diuretics has been linked

Table 2.8.2a. Vaughan–Williams classification of anti-arrhythmic drugs

Class	Action	Examples
I	Block sodium channels	
Ia	Prolong refractory period of action potential	Quinidine
		Procainamide
Ib	Shorten refractory period of action potential	Lidocaine
		Phenytoin
Ic	No effect on refractory period of action potential	Flecainide
II	β-blockers	Propranolol
		Atenolol
		Esmolol
		Sotalol
III	Block potassium channels	Amiodarone
		Bretylium
		Sotalol
IV	Calcium antagonists	Verapamil
		Diltiazem

to increased levels of homocysteine in the blood, which is a risk factor for developing atherosclerosis.

What would you check pre-operatively if a patient is taking diuretics?

You should check that they are euvolaemic and not dehydrated, especially if they have been nil by mouth for an extended period of time. Urea and electrolytes are important as diuretics can cause hypo- or hyperkalaemia. You would need to assess why they are taking diuretics and whether this condition (for example congestive cardiac failure) could be further optimised prior to surgery.

2.8.2. Anti-arrhythmics – Emily K Johnson

How are anti-arrhythmic drugs classified?

Anti-arrhythmic drugs can be classified in two ways. There is the Vaughan–Williams system of classification or they can be classified according to their clinical uses.

Tell me about the Vaughan–Williams classification and give examples

To answer a question about anti-arrhythmics it is helpful to draw the action potentials for cardiac muscle and pacemaker cells, see Figure 1.2.3d.

It is essential you have a thorough understanding of these action potentials before you can describe the mechanism of action of anti-arrhythmic drugs. You must be able to draw the action potentials quickly and clearly. Please refer to the Action Potentials podcast for more details.

The Vaughan–Williams classification is based on the mechanism of action of anti-arrhythmic drugs (Table 2.8.2a). Anti-arrhythmic drugs are classified into classes Ia, Ib, Ic, II, III and IV.

Class I contains drugs that act like local anaesthetics, blocking sodium channels. These drugs affect non-nodal areas of the heart that are characterised by fast depolarisation. They also affect phase 4 of the action potential of pacemaker cells, reducing the rate of spontaneous depolarisation and so reducing the spontaneous automaticity. Class I is subdivided into class Ia which includes drugs that prolong the refractory period of cardiac muscle such as quinidine and procainamide. Class Ib includes drugs that shorten the refractory period of cardiac muscle such as lidocaine and phenytoin. Class Ic includes drugs that have no effect on the refractory period of cardiac muscle and includes flecainide.

Class II includes β-blockers such as propranolol, atenolol, esmolol and sotalol. These drugs block the effects of catecholamines on the cardiac β1-adrenoceptors. It is phase 4 of the action potential that is shortened by adrenaline and noradrenaline so by blocking this action β-blockers increase the duration of this phase and slow the heart rate. They also reduce the force of contraction.

Class III contains drugs that block potassium channels therefore prolonging repolarisation and so prolonging the action potential and increasing the refractory period. This class includes amiodarone, bretylium and sotalol.

Class IV are calcium antagonists such as verapamil and diltiazem. They block the L-type calcium channels, therefore slowing the calcium influx and reducing the automaticity and rate of conduction of the heart.

What are the limitations of the Vaughan–Williams classification?

There are several limitations to the Vaughan–Williams classification of anti-arrhythmic drugs resulting in it being less of a clinically useful classification system.

There are some drugs, now in regular use, that don't come into the Vaughan–Williams classification, often because this classification system excludes some potential sites of action. For example, digoxin and adenosine find no place in this system.

There are also drugs that fall into the same category that are not necessarily clinically similar. There are drugs which have multiple actions such as sotalol which falls into category I, II and III. It is not clear which of its actions are responsible for the anti-arrhythmic effects, therefore it is difficult to accurately classify such drugs.

In addition to these points the Vaughan–Williams classification does not allow for the fact that drug may acts differently on healthy and diseased heart tissue.

Tell me more about the classification of anti-arrhythmics according to their clinical uses and give some examples

Anti-arrhythmics can be classified into those which are effective in supra-ventricular arrhythmias such as adenosine, those effective in ventricular arrhythmias such as lignocaine and those effective in both types of arrhythmia such as amiodarone.

Give more information about the drugs that may be used for supra-ventricular arrhythmias

Drugs used for supra-ventricular arrhythmias can be divided into those used for tachyarrhythmias and those used for bradyarrhythmias. The drugs used for supra-ventricular tachycardias can be further divided into those used for SVTs and those used for fast atrial fibrillation.

In cases of SVT adenosine or verapamil can be used. For fast atrial fibrillation (AF) digoxin or amiodarone may be used. For bradyarrhythmias atropine or glycopyrronium may be used.

Tell me about adenosine

Whenever you are asked to describe a drug you must have a structure you use to help you start your answer in a logical, well-presented way, and to help prevent you forgetting information you can give. If you learn a structure you will be surprised how much you can say about a drug you feel you know relatively little about!

The structure used here is to classify, describe presentation, routes of administration and dose, then uses and mechanism of action, followed by side effects, interactions and kinetics.

Adenosine is a natural purine nucleoside. It is presented as a colourless solution in vials and stored at room temperature. It is given in doses of 3, 6 and 12 mg at 1–2 minute intervals until an effect is observed. It is used to terminate SVT or identify the underlying rhythm by transiently slowing the rate. It acts on A1 adenosine receptors found in the SA and AV nodes. These open potassium channels that are also sensitive to acetylcholine binding to muscarinic receptors. The opening of these channels hyperpolarises the myocardium and voltage-sensitive calcium channels open less frequently. The effect is to reduce the rate of firing of the SA node and slow conduction through the AV node.

The side effects of adenosine include flushing, bronchospasm, chest pain and dyspnoea. It is contraindicated in asthmatics, sick sinus syndrome and second- and third-degree AV block. The half-life of adenosine is 8–10 seconds due to rapid de-amination and uptake by red blood cells, so it has a short duration of action.

Tell me about verapamil

Verapamil is a calcium channel antagonist. It is presented as tablets from 40 to 240 mg or solution for injection containing 2.5 mg/ml. It is given in divided doses up to 480 mg daily or as injection of 5–10 mg over 30 seconds. It is used to treat SVT and AF or flutter and can also be used in the treatment of hypertension and as angina prophylaxis. It acts by preventing calcium influx through the voltage-gated L-type calcium channels in the SA and AV nodes, and it reduces calcium influx during the plateau phase of the cardiac action potential. This reduces automaticity and reduces rate of conduction. It also causes coronary artery dilatation. Side effects of verapamil include dizziness, flushing, nausea and second- or third-degree heart block with oral administration. IV administration can precipitate LV failure, or in patients with WPW syndrome it can precipitate VT or VF. It can cause bradycardia in combination with other agents that slow AV conduction and it may increase serum digoxin levels. It can be potentiated by grapefruit juice. Verapamil is completely absorbed, but has high first-pass metabolism and oral bioavailability of 25%. It is 90% protein bound, metabolised in the liver and excreted by the kidneys. Its elimination half-life is 3–7 hours but the liver enzymes become saturated so increased dose intervals are necessary in hepatic impairment.

What drugs can be used to treat atrial fibrillation?

Define and classify

Atrial fibrillation is uncoordinated atrial activity with a ventricular rate dependent on the AV node transmission.

It is classified according to time of onset and may be fast or rate controlled. Onset of fast AF within 48 hours or less would generally be treated with a DC cardioversion or flecainide. If onset is greater than 48 hours drug treatment options include digoxin, β-blockers, amiodarone or verapamil.

What are the clinical uses of digoxin?

If you are asked any specific question about an individual drug, stick to your structure for answering. This will aid your thought process and the examiner will get the impression you know a lot about the drug and may move on. If, for example, in answer to this question you simply listed the uses of digoxin, the examiner would ask more questions that may lead you into difficulty. The examiner can always interrupt you and ask for more specific information.

Digoxin is a cardiac glycoside extracted from the leaves of *Digitalis lanata*, the foxglove. It is available as tablets or solution for intra-venous injection. It has a loading dose of 1 to 1.5 mg in divided doses over 24 hours and a maintenance dose of 125 to 500 μg daily in divided doses. The therapeutic range is 1–2 μg/L. The uses of digoxin are in the treatment of, or rarely the prevention of atrial fibrillation and flutter and in heart failure.

It has direct and indirect actions. Its direct action is mediated by binding to the Na-K–ATPase in the cell membrane. This causes increased intra-cellular sodium and decreased intra-cellular potassium concentrations. The increased intra-cellular sodium leads to an increase of the exchange with extra-cellular calcium therefore increasing the availability of intra-cellular calcium, producing positively inotropic effects. Decreased intra-cellular potassium concentrations reduce the automaticity and slow AV conduction. The indirect action is via enhancing the release of acetylcholine at cardiac muscarinic receptors, further prolonging the refractory period in the AV node and bundle of His. The reduced rate of contraction allows better coronary blood flow and more time for ventricular filling and so an increased cardiac output.

Side effects of digoxin are common as it has a narrow therapeutic range, which can therefore easily be exceeded. They can be divided into cardiac, gastrointestinal, neurological and other side effects. The cardiac side effects include arrhythmias and conduction defects, most commonly junctional bradycardia, bigemini and second- or third-degree heart block. These effects can be precipitated by hypokalaemia, hypercalcaemia or altered pH. Gastrointestinal side effects include anorexia, nausea and vomiting, diarrhoea and abdominal pain. Neurological side effects include headache, drowsiness and confusion, visual disturbances, impaired colour vision, muscular weakness and coma. Other side effects are gynaecomastia and rashes. Digoxin levels can be influenced by some other drugs. The plasma levels are increased by amiodarone, erythromycin and captopril and decreased by antacids, phenytoin and metoclopramide.

Digoxin is unpredictably absorbed from the gut and has an oral bioavailability of greater than 70%. It is approximately 25% protein bound in the plasma. It is secreted largely unchanged by filtration in the glomerulus and active tubular secretion, so its elimination is reduced in renal impairment. Its elimination half-life if around 35 hours.

What are the symptoms and signs of digoxin toxicity?

Digoxin toxicity is generally seen with plasma levels above 2.5 μg/L. Serious toxicity occurs with levels above 10 μg/L. The symptoms are nausea, vomiting, diarrhoea, headache, malaise and confusion. Impaired colour vision is an early symptom. Signs include any cardiac arrhythmia and ECG findings of a prolonged PR interval, heart block, T-wave inversion and ST segment depression in a reverse tick pattern. These findings may occur in toxicity but are not necessarily indicators of toxicity.

How would you treat digoxin toxicity?

In a patient with suspected digoxin toxicity I would follow the ABC approach to treatment, administering oxygen and requesting senior assistance if required. Electrolytes should be checked and any hyperkalaemia, which may be a feature, should be corrected. Likewise hypokalaemia may exacerbate the toxicity so should be corrected. Atropine or pacing may be required for bradyarrhythmias. Ventricular arrhythmias should be treated with lidocaine or phenytoin.

Levels greater than 20 μg/L should be treated with digoxin-specific anti-body fragments. These IgG fragments bind digoxin with greater affinity than its receptor therefore terminate its action. The complex of anti-body fragment and digoxin is removed by the kidney. The anti-body fragments carry the risk of anaphylaxis on re-exposure.

How does amiodarone work?

Again, however the question on a particular drug is asked, stick to your structure and you will answer it picking up bonus points on the way!

Amiodarone is a benzofuran derivative and a class III anti-arrhythmic agent. It is presented as tablets or as a solution for mixture with 5% dextrose prior to injection. It is administered as a loading dose of 5 mg/kg over 1 hour followed by 15 mg/kg over 24 hours. The starting oral dose is 200 mg three times daily, then reduced slowly to 200 mg once daily.

It is used for the treatment of SVTs, VTs and WPW syndrome. It acts by blocking potassium channels therefore slowing the rate of repolarisation and increasing the duration of the action potential and the refractory period.

You may be asked to draw the normal action potential and show the differences amiodarone will make.

What are the side effects of amiodarone?

Amiodarone has numerous side effects, some of which can be severe and have led to the reduced use of long-term amiodarone treatment.

The side effects can be divided into systems:

- Cardiac side effects include bradycardia and hypotension if rapidly administered. It can prolong the QT interval.
- Pulmonary side effects include a 10% incidence of developing pneumonitis, fibrosis or pleuritis.
- Hepatic side effects include cirrhosis, jaundice, and hepatitis so LFTs should be monitored in long-term treatment.
- Eye side effects are corneal microdeposits, which are reversible.
- The thyroid can be affected and there is a 0.9% incidence of hyperthyroidism and 6% incidence of hypothyroidism, which is also reversible.

- Neurological side effects include a peripheral neuropathy or a myopathy.
- Dermatological side effects are photosensitivity and a slate grey skin colour.

Amiodarone has numerous interactions with other drugs as it is a potent inhibitor of the cytochrome P450 enzyme system. It also affects other highly protein bound drugs such as phenytoin, digoxin and warfarin as it displaces them increasing their actions. It should be used cautiously with other drugs slowing AV conduction such as β-blockers, and avoided in those increasing the QT interval such as TCAs.

2.8.3. Inotropes – Caroline V Sampson

This podcast complements the podcast on the "Autonomic nervous system and adrenoceptors".

What is an inotrope?

An inotrope alters the force of contraction of cardiac muscle without changing pre-load or after-load. Positive inotropes increase cardiac contractility whilst negative inotropes decrease cardiac contractility.

Can you name some positively inotropic drugs?

It is really important to have a classification here. Don't just launch straight in with nora-drenaline or adrenaline as although few of the inotropes are actually used in clinical practice you need to demonstrate you are aware of the rarer or newer classes of drug.

Class I inotropes increase intra-cellular calcium and can be subdivided into calcium ions, drugs that increase cardiac cAMP such as adrenoceptor agonists, phosphodiesterase inhibitors and glucagon and finally drugs affecting the Na–K–ATPase pump such as digoxin.

Class II inotropes increase the sensitivity of actomyosin to calcium and include levosimendan.

Class III inotropes act via metabolic or endocrinological pathways and include tri-iodothyronine or T3.

The most commonly used positive inotropic agents belong to Class I and are adreno-receptor agonists. These can be naturally occurring such as adrenaline, noradrenaline and dopamine or synthetic such as dopexamine, dobutamine, isoprenaline and salbutamol.

Can you explain how digoxin acts as an inotrope?

This is controversial as it is questionable whether digoxin acts as an inotrope at all. However always explain the mechanism before arguing the toss!

Digoxin is mainly used as rate control in atrial fibrillation and atrial flutter, but has also been used for many years in heart failure, especially if this is resistant to other treatments. Digoxin inhibits the Na^+/K^+ pump on the sarcolemmal membrane, which causes an increase in intra-cellular Na^+. Na is normally pumped into the cell by a $Na^+/Ca2^+$ exchange pump that relies on the high Na^+ gradient from outside to inside the cell. Increasing the concentration of Na^+ in the cell decreases this concentration gradient therefore less Na^+ is pumped into the cell and consequently less $Ca2^+$ is pumped out in return, therefore increasing the concentration of $Ca2^+$ in the cell. An increase in intra-cellular $Ca2^+$ causes the positive inotropic effect. Any positive inotropic effect is somewhat offset by digoxin's other effect, which is to activate the parasympathetic nervous system. Some might argue that digoxin only acts as an inotrope in a minority of patients.

When do you give calcium and why is it important in cardiac contractility?

Calcium is given to correct hypocalcaemia, especially when the ionised calcium is low. It is also used to antagonise the effects of hyperkalaemia and hypermagnesaemia.

Ionised calcium is vital in normal myocyte contraction. Calcium enters through voltage-gated Ca channels in the sarcolemma in response to depolarisation. This increase in cytoplasmic Ca^{2+} causes more Ca^{2+} to be released from the sarcoplasmic reticulum. In resting cardiac myocytes tropomyosin overlays the myosin binding site on actin preventing cross-linkage between these two and therefore contraction. If Ca^{2+} is available, it binds to troponin C which causes a conformational change in the tropomyosin complex, allowing the myosin heads access to the binding sites on actin and therefore muscle contraction.

Two different intra-venous preparations are available, calcium gluconate 10% and calcium chloride 10%. Although calcium gluconate is classically used to antagonise the effects of hyperkalaemia, it contains less elemental calcium – approximately 9 mg in 10 ml compared to 27 mg in 10 ml 10% calcium chloride.

Where do you use adrenaline in your practice and at what dose?

This is being asked in a set of questions on inotropes so it would be easy to get stuck just on this as an answer – but always think laterally, there are many areas in your practice where you use adrenaline. Don't forget its use as an addition to local anaesthetics.

Adrenaline is used in cardiac arrest situations at a dose of 1 mg every 2–3 minutes or a dose of 10 µg/kg in paediatric arrests. It is also used in cases of anaphylaxis at incremental doses of 100 µg intra-venously or 0.3–0.5 mg intra-muscularly. Adrenaline infusions are used as an inotrope in critical care in the dose range 0.01 µg/kg/min up to 0.3 µg/kg/min and higher. Nebulised adrenaline at a dose of 1 mg in 2 ml of normal saline can be used for severe asthma attacks and to reduce airway oedema where there is upper airway obstruction. Finally adrenaline is added to local anaesthetic solutions usually in a dose of 1 in 200 000. This serves several useful functions, including prolonging the action of the local anaesthetic, decreasing bleeding at the site of infiltration and acting as a marker for intra-venous injection. Adrenaline also reduces systemic uptake and increases the safe concentration of lidocaine from 3 mg/kg to 7 mg/kg but does not alter the safe concentration of bupivicaine.

What is the mechanism of action of adrenaline?

This is asking about adrenoceptors, so could come up in physiology or a pharmacology structured oral examination.

Adrenaline is a naturally occurring catecholamine. It is secreted into the bloodstream by the adrenal medulla in response to sympathetic stimulation. It stimulates α1-, β1- and β2-adrenoreceptors. Adrenoreceptors are G-protein coupled receptors that when activated result in an increase in calcium influx into cells. α-adrenoreceptors are linked to a Gq-proteins, which stimulates phospholipase C to produce second messengers inositoltriphosphate (ITP) and diacylglycerol. β-adrenoreceptors are linked to Gs-protein, which stimulates adenylate cyclase to produce cyclic AMP as the second messenger from ATP. cAMP goes on to activate protein kinase A.

Low dose adrenaline infusions of 0.01–0.02 µg/kg/min mainly stimulate β2 adrenoreceptors. This leads to smooth muscle relaxation in the bronchi, uterus and gastrointestinal tract, dilatation of skeletal muscle arteries and an increase in glycogenolysis. Mid-range infusions of 0.03–0.2 µg/kg/min stimulate mainly β1-adrenoreceptors. This results in inotropy and chronotropy, with an increased contractility and automaticity in sino-atrial node, atrial, atrio-ventricular node and ventricular muscle cells as well as increased renin release and an increase in lipolysis in adipose tissue. High dose infusions of 0.2 to 0.3 µg/kg/min stimulate mainly α receptors. These cause generalised vaso- and venoconstriction, increasing systemic vascular resistance and, therefore, pre-load and after-load.

What are the side effects of adrenaline?

- Cardiovascular – in common with all inotropes adrenaline increases myocardial oxygen demand, which could lead to myocardial ischaemia in susceptible patients. Adrenaline causes tachycardia and may cause ventricular arrhythmias. This was a particular problem during halothane anaesthesia. Adrenaline infusions can cause down-regulation of β-adrenoreceptors if used for longer than 24 hours and therefore the patient may demonstrate tachyphylaxis.
- Gastrointestinal – especially at high doses adrenaline can cause splanchnic vasoconstriction, which can lead to ischaemia and has been linked to bacterial translocation.
- Metabolic – adrenaline increases glycogenolysis, gluconeogenesis and lipolysis. This causes hyperglycaemia and all patients will require an insulin sliding scale. There is also an increase in lactic acidosis.

Can you compare and contrast adrenaline with noradrenaline?

It is really important to have a structure here. The examiner may want you to write a table – in which case they would probably ask you to construct a table comparing the two. If not, you need to construct a table in your head.

Both adrenaline and noradrenaline are naturally occurring catecholamines secreted by the adrenal medulla in response to sympathetic stimulation. Adrenaline is secreted in much greater amounts by the adrenal glands. Noradrenaline functions as the neurotransmitter at synapses in the sympathetic nervous system.

Noradrenaline is a vasopressor used in critical care to maintain or increase mean arterial pressure in vasodilated states. It is particularly suited to patients in septic shock. Adrenaline has many uses including in adult and paediatric arrests, in anaphylaxis, nebulised in severe asthma or cases of upper airway obstruction secondary to oedema, as an inotrope and as a local anaesthetic additive.

Both are presented as a clear colourless solution in glass vials. Adrenaline comes in concentrations of 1 in 1000 and 1 in 10,000, mini-jets contain 10 ml of 1 in 10,000. Noradrenaline comes as 4 mg which is usually diluted with 50 ml 5% dextrose to give a concentration of 80 µg/ml.

Both act on adrenoreceptors in the body. Adrenaline, at low dose, stimulates β-adrenoreceptors causing bronchodilatation, glycogenolysis, inotropy and chronotropy and at high doses stimulate mainly α adrenoreceptors, causing widespread vaso- and venoconstriction. Noradrenaline has mainly α adrenoreceptor action with some β1-agonist effects.

The dose range used in noradrenaline is an infusion of 0.01 to 0.4 µg/kg/min. Adrenaline is used at different doses depending on the clinical circumstances. The dose in adult arrest is 1 mg, with 10 µg/kg in paediatric arrests. In anaphylaxis 0.5 mg IM or increments of 100 µg IV are given. Infusions of 0.01 to 0.3 µg/kg/min are used in critical care and adrenaline is usually added to local anaesthetic solutions in a concentration of 1 in 200 000.

Both have a quick onset and offset with a plasma half-life of 2 minutes.

Noradrenaline must be administered intra-venously through a central line. Adrenaline can be administered IV, IM, SC or via a nebuliser and can be administered peripherally, but infusions should be given through a central line. Cardiovascular effects include an increased myocardial oxygen demand with both drugs that can lead to cardiac ischaemia. Adrenaline can cause a tachycardia and ventricular arrhythmias whilst noradrenaline typically causes a bradycardia. Systolic blood pressures are increased with both agents. If adrenaline infusions are continued for over 24 hours a down-regulation of β receptors can occur.

Adrenaline is a potent bronchodilator whilst noradrenaline has no effect on airway calibre. Both agents cause pulmonary vasoconstriction.

Both noradrenaline and adrenaline at high doses can cause splanchnic vasoconstriction. Adrenaline increases renal blood flow whereas noradrenaline reduces renal blood flow but renal perfusion may be actually improved with noradrenaline due to the increase in blood pressure.

Adrenaline has greater metabolic effects causing an increase in basal metabolic rate, glycogenolysis, gluconeogenesis and lipolysis. This results in hyperglycaemia and lactic acidosis.

Both agents have a similar metabolism, by catechol O-methyl transferase in the liver and monoamine oxidase in adrenergic neurones to inactive metabolites that are excreted in the urine.

Chapter

Drugs acting on the gastrointestinal tract

2.9.1. Drugs acting on the GI tract – Rebecca A Leslie

Classify drugs acting on the GI tract

Drugs that act on the GI tract can be broadly classified into four main categories.

- Antacids
- Drugs that affects gastric acid secretion
- Drugs which affect gastric motility
- Drugs that act as mucosal protectors.

Drugs that affect gastric acid secretion can be further sub-classified depending on their mechanism of action, such as H2 receptor antagonists, proton pump inhibitors and prostaglandin analogues.

Tell me about antacids

Antacids are used to relieve the symptoms of dyspepsia and gastro-oesophageal reflux by neutralising the gastric acidity.

There are several different types of antacids:

- Magnesium-containing antacids
- Aluminium-containing antacids
- Sodium citrate.

Aluminium- and magnesium-containing antacids are useful because neither of them are absorbed from the gut, and as they are relatively insoluble in water they have a long duration of action. However aluminium-containing antacids can produce constipation whilst magnesium-containing antacids can cause diarrhoea.

Sodium citrate has a very short duration of action so must be given less than 10 minutes before the start of surgery. It is however commonly used to neutralise gastric acidity prior to an emergency caesarean section.

Dr Podcast Scripts for the Primary FRCA, ed. Rebecca A. Leslie, Emily K. Johnson and Alexander P. L. Goodwin.   Published by Cambridge University Press. © R. A. Leslie, E. K. Johnson and A. P. L. Goodwin 2011.

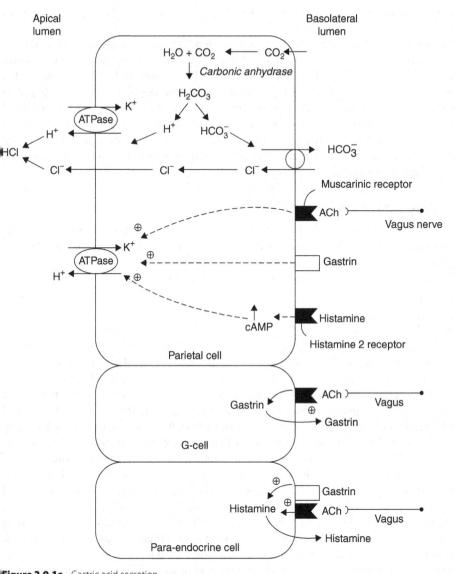

Figure 2.9.1a. Gastric acid secretion.

Tell me how gastric acid is produced

This question will be much easier to answer if you draw a simple diagram of a parietal cell, marking on the basolateral and the apical membranes. Remember the basolateral membrane is the membrane that is in contact with the systemic blood supply and the apical membrane is the membrane that is in direct contact with the stomach lumen. You should also include on your diagram muscarinic, histamine and gastrin receptors, which are present on the basolateral membrane. See Figure 2.9.1a.

Gastric acid is secreted by the parietal cells of the stomach. It is estimated that 2 litres of acid can be produced by the parietal cells per day, and the hydrogen ion concentration is approximately one million times higher than in the blood with a pH of between 1 and 3.5.

Carbon dioxide diffuses into the cell, from the blood, through the basolateral membrane. The carbon dioxide combines with water under the action of carbonic anhydrase to produce carbonic acid. The carbonic acid then dissociates into bicarbonate and hydrogen ions. At the apical membrane these intra-cellular hydrogen ions are exchanged for extracellular potassium ions in a process that requires energy produced from ATP. This exchange is achieved using a hydrogen/potassium ATPase protein, often called the proton pump. At the basolateral membrane the bicarbonate ions are rapidly exchanged for chloride ions. These chloride ions then leak down their concentration gradient into the gastric lumen, where they combine with hydrogen ions to produce hydrochloric acid.

What causes gastric acid secretion?

Try and keep your answer simple. Work through the three different phases of gastric acid secretion in a logical manner. The three main stimulators for gastric acid that you must mention are acetylcholine, histamine and gastrin.

These are three different phases of gastric acid secretion:

- The cephalic phase
- The gastric phase
- The intestinal phase.

The cephalic phase occurs due to the sight, smell, taste and mastication of food. At this stage there is no food in the stomach and the gastric acid secretion is brought about by the vagus nerve, which releases acetylcholine, which acts on muscarinic receptors on the basolateral membrane and through second messenger systems stimulates gastric acid secretion. Vagal stimulation also causes the release of gastrin from G-cells in the antrum of the stomach. Gastrin is released into the bloodstream and when it reaches the parietal cells it too stimulates gastric acid secretion. In addition both vagal activity and gastrin stimulate the release of histamine from mast cells, which acts on histamine receptors on the basolateral membrane of the parietal cell and, through the use of second messenger systems, stimulate gastric acid secretion.

During the gastric phase, food directly stimulates the parietal cells to secrete acid. Whole proteins do not affect the secretion of gastric acid, it is only their breakdown products such as peptides and amino acids that stimulate gastric acid secretion.

In addition mechanoreceptors in the gastric wall are stretched due to the distension of the stomach when food enters. This stimulates the vagus nerve, and again causes the release of acetylcholine, which stimulates the release of gastrin and histamine. In turn acid is secreted into the gastric lumen.

A low pH will inhibit gastric acid secretion, so when there has been no food in the stomach for a long period of time the parietal cells will stop producing acid. In contrast when food enters the stomach, and as a result the pH rises, more gastric acid will be produced.

In the intestinal phase, the duodenum becomes distended as chyme passes from the stomach into the small intestine. This stimulates a number of reflexes that inhibit gastric acid secretion. Several hormones are responsible for these reflexes. Secretin is released in response to fatty acids and a low pH in the duodenum and enters the bloodstream. When secretin reaches the stomach it inhibits the release of gastrin. The presence of fatty acids in the duodenum also stimulates the release of two polypeptides called gastric inhibitory peptide and cholecystokinin, which both inhibit the release of gastrin and acid.

Which drugs do we commonly use to reduce gastric acid secretion?

Remember to listen to the question. They are specifically asking about drugs which reduce gastric acid secretion, don't start talking about antacids which neutralise gastric acid.

We commonly use histamine-2 (H2) antagonists such as ranitidine, and proton-pump inhibitors such as omeprazole, lansoprazole and pantoprazole.

As we have already mentioned, acetylcholine and gastrin indirectly stimulate gastric acid secretion by releasing histamine from adjacent paraendocrine cells. The histamine binds to H2 receptors on the basolateral membrane of the parietal cells and stimulate gastric acid secretion through the use of the second messenger cylic AMP. H2 receptor antagonists prevent histamine from stimulating the release of gastric acid by antagonising the histamine receptor on the basolateral membranes of gastric parietal cells.

Proton-pump inhibitors reversibly block the hydrogen/potassium ATPase pump and therefore block the final common pathway of gastric acid secretion and can produce complete achlorhydria.

What are the unwanted side effects of cimetidine?

Cimetidine is no longer used very often as there are more potent H2 antagonists with less side effects. However you will still be expected to know the side effects. Remember when you are discussing side effects of drugs try to go through with a systematic approach, starting with the most important side effects.

Cimetidine inhibits hepatic cytochrome P450 and as a result will slow down the metabolism of many commonly used drugs that rely on this enzyme system for their metabolism. Examples of drugs whose actions may become prolonged when used in conjunction with cimetidine include warfarin, phenytoin, lignocaine, propranolol, diazepam and aminophylline.

Endocrine effects of cimetidine include anti-androgenic effects such as gynaecomastia, impotence and reduced sperm count.

Cimetidine also has effects in the central nervous system such as hallucinations, confusion and seizures. However these effects are normally only seen when levels get really high.

If cimetidine is infused rapidly intra-venously then H2 receptors in the heart may blocked causing bradycardia and hypotension.

What is the role of prostaglandins in gastric acid secretion?

Local mediators such as prostaglandin E_2 and prostaglandin I_2 are released when the gastric mucosa is damaged. They stimulate the production of a mucous layer that coats the gastric epithelial cells and protects the cells from further damage or autodigestion. The prostaglandins also stimulate the production of bicarbonate which helps to neutralise the acidity of the gastric lumen.

Do we use any prostaglandin analogues?

Yes we use misoprostil in the prevention and treatment of non-steroidal anti-inflammatory–induced ulcers. Because misoprostil is a prostaglandin analogue it stimulates the secretion of productive mucous layer therefore protecting the gastric mucosa.

Which other drugs do we use that protect the gastric mucosa?

We also use a drug called sucralfate that forms a viscous barrier over the stomach lumen. It adheres preferentially to ulcerated regions via ionic binding so protects against further damage. It is consequently used in the treatment of peptic ulcer disease and for the prevention of stress ulceration in the critically ill.

What do you mean by prokinetic drugs?

Prokinetic drugs are drugs which stimulate gastric motility by increasing the contraction of the stomach wall and enhancing the emptying of the stomach into the small intestine.

Why do anaesthetists use prokinetic drugs?

Anaesthetics use pro-kinetic drugs to speed up gastric motility and to reduce the risk of gastric aspiration. They are used in patients who are at risk of aspiration due to gastric stasis, often as a result of autonomic neuropathy in patients with diabetes mellitus, or in patients who have a hiatus hernia.

Metoclopramide is one of the most frequently used prokinetics. It acts as an antagonist of peripheral dopaminergic receptors and selectively stimulates gastric muscarinic receptors. An unwanted side effect of metoclopramide in the young and the elderly are extra-pyramidal effects, such as akinesia and occulogyric crisis.

In the intensive care setting the anti-biotic erythromycin is also commonly used as a pro-kinetic. Erthromycin is an agonist of the motilin receptor. Motilin is a powerful prokinetic that acts on the motilin receptor in the gastric mucosa, which acts via a G-protein to produce gastric motility.

2.9.2. Anti-emetics – Emily K Johnson

Can you explain what happens when someone vomits and how it is controlled?

Vomiting is retching followed by the expulsion of gastric contents. The abdominal muscles contract and relax during retching, followed by sustained contraction of abdominal muscle and coordination of intercostal muscles and muscles of the pharynx and larynx during expulsion. A large autonomic involvement causes pallor, salivation, hypotension and sweating. This process is controlled by efferent neurones in the medulla oblongata in an undefined area known as the vomiting centre.

The control of vomiting is easier to describe if you sketch a diagram of all the relevant areas. Practice doing this as this question is a popular one (Figure 2.9.2a).

The vomiting centre is stimulated to produce this response by a number of different afferents. These include vagal and some sympathetic afferents from the GI tract, which can induce

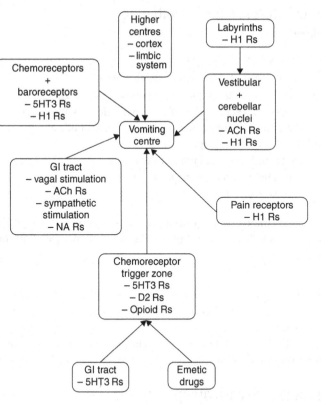

Figure 2.9.2a. The control of vomiting.

vomiting if the upper GI tract is distended or irritated. These signals are received in the area postrema and the nucleus tractus solitarius in the medulla. 5HT3 receptors are present in the GI tract and if 5-hydroxytryptamine is released from enterochromaffin cells it interacts with the 5HT3 receptors, which cause stimulation of the vagal afferent nerves, and can therefore induce vomiting. Substance P from gastric mucosa may act indirectly on 5HT3 receptors to produce the same effect.

As well as stimulus from the GI tract, central stimulus can result in vomiting. The chemoreceptor trigger zone plays a large role. It is in the area postrema on the caudal floor of the fourth ventricle and functionally outside the blood–brain barrier. There are high concentrations of 5HT3, dopamine D2 and opioid receptors in this area of the brain. When stimulated, the chemoreceptor trigger zone sends messages to the vomiting centre to initiate vomiting.

Motion sickness is another cause of vomiting by a different pathway. It involves the vestibular nuclei, where there are cholinergic and histamine H1 receptors. Again, this area, when stimulated sends signals to the vomiting centre where the action of vomiting is initiated.

Higher centres such as the limbic system can also have an effect on the vomiting centre but the mechanisms are unclear.

In summary, vomiting is coordinated by the vomiting centre and there are several different afferent inputs. These are the chemoreceptor trigger zone, the vestibular system, higher centres and vagal stimuli from the GI tract.

Summarise the different receptors involved in initiating vomiting and their locations

The receptors involved in the initiation of vomiting are:

- Dopamine D2 receptors – present in the chemoreceptor trigger zone
- 5HT3 receptors – present in the upper GI tract and the chemoreceptor trigger zone
- Muscarinic acetylcholine receptors – present in the parasympathetic nervous system (initiates vomiting due to distension of the upper GI tract), also acetylcholine is important in transmission from the vestibular apparatus
- Histamine H1 receptors – present in the vestibular apparatus
- Opioid receptors – present in the chemoreceptor trigger zone
- Noradrenergic receptors – may also play a role

These receptors are those targeted in the treatment of nausea and vomiting but it is likely that the actual mechanisms are not this clear cut, and the precise site and nature of all the receptors involved are not known.

Can you classify anti-emetics?

Anti-emetics are drugs given to treat nausea and vomiting and they can be classified according to the receptor types at which they act.

There are dopamine antagonists, 5HT3 antagonists, anti-cholinergics, anti-histamines and a miscellaneous group with unknown action.

Tell me which drugs you know of in each group

Dopamine antagonists include the phenothiazines, which are mainly used as anti-psychotics and have a minor role in the treatment of nausea and vomiting. They are divided into three groups, propylamines such as chlorpromazine, piperidines such as thioridazine and piperazine such as prochlorperazine. Another group of drugs, the butyrophenones, are also dopamine antagonists. This group includes drugs such as droperidol and domperidone. Metoclopramide is also a dopamine antagonist.

5HT3 receptor antagonists include ondansetron and granisetron.

Anti-cholinergics include atropine, hyoscine and glycopyrolate. Atropine and hyoscine cross the blood–brain barrier and therefore have anti-emetic properties but glycopyrolate doesn't.

Anti-histamines used in the treatment of nausea and vomiting are cyclizine and promethazine.

Tell me more about ondansetron

Use a structure you are familiar with to describe any drug. The structure used in this answer is classify the drug, describe its presentation, routes of administration and dose, then its uses, mechanism of action, side effects, interactions and kinetics.

Ondansetron is a synthetic carbazole. It is presented as a clear colourless solution for injection and can be administered orally, intra-muscularly or intra-venously at a dose of 4 to 8 mg. It is used in the management and prevention of nausea and vomiting, particularly when induced by chemotherapy or radiotherapy. It is a selective 5HT3 receptor antagonist acting centrally and peripherally. It blocks the activation of vagal afferents from the GI tract which appear to be stimulated by 5HT3 receptor activation, occurring when 5-hydroxytryptophan is released in response to emetogenic stimuli.

Ondansetron is a well-tolerated drug and its main side effects are headache, flushing, bradycardia and constipation. Anaphylaxis has been reported. It is rapidly absorbed and has bioavailability of 60%. It is 76% protein bound. It is extensively metabolised in the liver by hydroxylation and glucuronide conjugation to inactive metabolites. It has a half-life of 3 hours, and its dose should be reduced in hepatic impairment.

Tell me more about cyclizine

Cyclizine is a piperazine derivative. It is presented as a clear colourless solution for injection or tablets for oral administration. It is given in doses of 50 mg to adults, and 1 mg/kg for children.

Cyclizine is used in the treatment of nausea and vomiting, particularly due to general anaesthetic or opioid drugs, motion sickness or Meniere's disease.

It is a histamine 1 receptor antagonist and also has some anti-muscarinic actions, which may contribute to its anti-emetic effects.

The side effects of cyclizine are related to its anti-muscarinic effects, they include a tachycardia, drowsiness, dry mouth, blurred vision and increased lower oesophageal sphincter tone. It is well absorbed orally and has high oral bioavailability of 80%. It is metabolised in the liver to norcyclizine. The elimination half-life is around 10 hours.

Tell me more about metoclopramide

Metoclopramide is a benzamide. It is presented as tablets, a syrup or solution for injection and may be administered orally, intra-venously or intra-muscularly at a dose of 10 mg every 8 hours. It is an anti-emetic used in the treatment of nausea and vomiting due to a variety of causes including general anaesthetics and opiates. It is also a prokinetic and is used in the treatment of digestive disorders such as hiatus hernia and reflux oesophagitis. Both of its actions as anti-emetic and prokinetic are useful in the treatment of migraine.

Metoclopramide acts as an anti-emetic by blocking dopamine receptors centrally at the chemoreceptor trigger zone. Its prokinetic actions are mediated by antagonism of peripheral dopaminergic receptors, augmentation of peripheral cholinergic responses and a direct action increasing smooth muscle tone. It also blocks 5HT3 receptors.

The side effects include extra-pyramidal effects including dystonic reactions and neuroleptic malignant syndrome. Cardiovascular side effects including hypotension and tachy- or bradycardias may occur. Prolactin levels increase. Metoclopramide is well absorbed but has variable first-pass metabolism, between 30 and 90%. It is metabolised in the liver and excreted mainly in the urine.

What are the features of the neuroleptic malignant syndrome and how do you treat it?

The neuroleptic malignant syndrome is characterised by hyperthermia, fluctuating conscious level, muscle rigidity and autonomic dysfunction causing pallor, tachycardia, sweating, labile blood pressure and urinary incontinence. It is a potentially fatal side effect of anti-psychotic drugs and metoclopramide. There is no proven effective treatment so the drug must be discontinued but cooling is appropriate and bromocriptine and dantrolene have been used.

What other drugs can be used as anti-emetics that don't fall into any of the categories we have discussed?

Other drugs found to have anti-emetic properties include steroids. Dexamethasone has been used as an anti-emetic in chemotherapy and is currently used in anaesthesia to prevent nausea and vomiting. Its mechanism of action is not clear. Cannabinoids have some anti-emetic activity and nabilone has been used as an anti-emetic for chemotherapy.

The intra-venous induction agent propofol also has anti-emetic properties and has been used in low doses to treat nausea and vomiting. Benzodiazepines have also been used in cancer chemotherapy as anti-emetics and their mode of action as anti-emetics is also not clear.

Which anti-emetics can be used safely in Parkinson's disease?

Parkinson's disease is caused by loss of dopaminergic neurones so any drugs that reduce dopamine levels or block dopamine receptors will worsen the condition. Therefore dopamine antagonists should be avoided, so metoclopramide, droperidrol and prochlorperazine should not be used. Anti-cholinergic drugs that act centrally, atropine and hyoscine, should also be avoided as they can precipitate central anti-cholinergic syndrome.

Domperidone can be used safely as although it is a dopamine antagonist it does not cross the blood–brain barrier. The 5HT3 receptor antagonists and histamine 1 receptor antagonists can be safely used as anti-emetics.

Have you heard about NK1 receptors and their role in nausea and vomiting?

Neurokinin 1 receptors can be found in the GI tract. They are activated by substance P, which is released from gastric mucosa if it becomes damaged. It is thought they may act in association with 5HT3 receptors to trigger vagal afferents and induce vomiting. The NK1 receptor is a potential target for anti-emetic therapy, which is currently being investigated.

2.9.3. Hypoglycaemics – Caroline V Sampson

This section covers the pharmacology of hypoglycaemics but could also appear in the clinical structured oral examination and place more relevance on diabetes and the management of patients with diabetes who are undergoing surgery.

How is diabetes classified?

Diabetes is a metabolic disorder characterised by chronic hyperglycaemia, which occurs as a result of insufficient insulin production or peripheral insulin resistance.

The World Health Organization and American Diabetes Association classify the condition into four different types:

- Type I is characterised by beta cell destruction in the pancreas, usually leading to absolute insulin deficiency. These patients are typically diagnosed at a young age, prone to developing ketoacidosis and must be treated with insulin.

- Type II is characterised by insulin resistance (often accompanied with a relative insulin deficiency). This is by far the most common form of diabetes. Typically, it affects an older group of patients, who are often overweight and may demonstrate other features of "syndrome X".
- Type III describes other specific types, of "secondary diabetes". For example, due to disorders of the exocrine pancreas (e.g., pancreatitis, cystic fibrosis), drug-induced (e.g., steroids, thiazides) or endocrinopathies (e.g., Cushing's, acromegaly).
- Type IV is gestational diabetes mellitus.

This classification describes the pathophysiology of the different types of diabetes and is, therefore, a more accurate way of describing the different diabetic groups than previous classification systems, which were based upon common treatment options (e.g., insulin-dependent diabetes mellitus or non–insulin-dependent diabetes mellitus, especially as it is becoming more common for type 2 diabetics to be treated with insulin).

In addition to diabetes itself, two separate conditions, known as impaired glucose tolerance and impaired fasting glucose, are recognised.

How is diabetes diagnosed?

This question involves learning some numbers. In the UK we refer to glucose measurements in mmol/L, which unfortunately means lots of decimal points because the definitions were originally set in mg/dl as used in the United States.

Also, don't be caught out by the difference in serum glucose and plasma glucose values. They are different, and all definitions below use plasma glucose values.

Diagnosis of diabetes is both clinical and biochemical.

Symptoms of hyperglycaemia include polyuria, polydipsia and weight loss.

Biochemical measurement of plasma or serum glucose concentrations can be random, fasting (for at least 8 hours) or part of an oral glucose tolerance test.

1. Random plasma glucose

    - Symptoms of hyperglycaemia (i.e. polyuria, polydipsia and/or weight loss) with a random plasma glucose concentration ≥ 11.1 mmol/L is diagnostic of diabetes.

2. Fasting plasma glucose

    - ≤ 5.6 mmol/L is normal
    - ≥ 7.0 mmol/L is diagnostic of diabetes
    - 5.9–6.9 mmol/L indicates impaired fasting glucose.

3. Oral glucose tolerance test

    - During an oral glucose tolerance test the patient is starved for 8 hours, a fasting baseline plasma glucose level is then checked and the patient given a glucose solution containing 75 g of glucose to drink. A repeat plasma glucose or "post-load glucose" is taken 2 hours later.
    - 2-hour post-load plasma glucose ≤ 7.8 mmol/L is normal.
    - 2-hour post-load plasma glucose ≥ 11.1 mmol/L is diagnostic of diabetes.
    - 2-hour post-load plasma glucose 7.8–11.1 mmol/L indicates impaired glucose tolerance.

What is the clinical relevance of impaired fasting glucose and impaired glucose tolerance?

Impaired fasting glucose and impaired glucose tolerance is thought to be a "pre-diabetic" condition. These patients are at high risk of developing diabetes and are also at risk of hypertension and cardiovascular complications.

Patients with impaired fasting glucose and impaired glucose tolerance should be closely monitored and should receive all the same lifestyle and dietary advice that is offered to diabetics, so that they can reduce their risk of developing diabetes and its complications.

What is insulin?

Insulin is a polypeptide hormone produced by the beta cells of the Islets of Langerhans in the pancreas. Insulin consists of 51 amino acids organised as two chains, A and B, which are joined by two disulphide bridges.

Insulin is formed by the removal of a "c" peptide from "pro-insulin".

What are the actions of insulin?

Insulin is a powerful anabolic hormone. It is secreted when the body is in a "well-fed" state and its actions are therefore related to the breakdown of energy-containing molecules. Insulin increases:

- Glucose uptake by muscle and fat
- Fat and protein synthesis
- Potassium uptake by cells.

Insulin decreases:

- Glycogen breakdown and gluconeogenesis
- Fat and protein breakdown
- Ketone body synthesis by the liver.

What drugs are used to reduce blood sugar in diabetes mellitus?

Drugs used in diabetes can be divided into insulin, which is administered intra-venously or subcutaneously, and the oral hypoglycaemics:

- Sulphonylureas (e.g. gliclazide)
- Biguanides (e.g. metformin)
- Thiazolidinediones (e.g. rosiglitizone)
- Acarbose
- Newer agents including meglitinides (e.g. repaglinide), DPP-4 inhibitors (e.g. sitagliptin) and GLP-1 mimetics (e.g. exenatide).

Tell me about the sulphonylurea group of drugs

Sulphonylureas are oral hypoglycaemic agents used in type 2 diabetes.

They work by enhancing the function of the beta cells of the Islets of Langerhans in the pancreas, making more insulin available to the peripheral tissues. They are also thought to act on the liver, by stimulating the glycolytic pathway and therefore inhibiting glucose production. Long-term sulphonylurea use may also reduce peripheral resistance to insulin.

Examples of commonly used sulphonylureas are gliclazide and glibenclamide. They are known as second-generation agents and have a half-life of 8–12 hours. The most well-known first-generation sulphonylurea is chlorpropramide, which has a much longer half-life of 40 hours.

Sulphonylureas are well absorbed and have oral bioavailabilities of over 80%. They are bound to albumin in the plasma, and are extensively metabolised in the liver to inactive metabolites, which are then excreted in the urine. The only exception to this is chlorpropramide, which is predominantly excreted unchanged in the urine and therefore has a prolonged half-life in renal failure.

Sulphonylureas are generally considered not to cause hypoglycaemic events, however agents with longer half-lives do have a risk of this, particularly in the elderly. This was especially true of chlorpropramide in view of its renal elimination.

How do biguanides work?

Metformin is the only biguanide available in the UK, and it is an oral hypoglycaemic used to treat type 2 diabetes. Biguanides work by decreasing gluconeogenesis and by increasing peripheral insulin utilisation. They act at the level of skeletal muscle by increasing glucose transport across the cell membrane. They are also thought to delay the uptake of glucose from the gut.

Metformin is absorbed slowly and has an oral bioavailability of 60%. It is not plasma-protein bound and is excreted unchanged in the urine. It therefore has a significantly prolonged action in renal failure. It does not cause weight gain and is therefore the agent of choice in treating overweight diabetics.

Biguanides can precipitate severe lactic acidosis, especially if taken in renal impairment, and can also cause hypoglycaemic episodes.

How would you anaesthetise a sick diabetic patient for an amputation of an infected leg?

This clinical question should be approached in the same way as all clinical structured oral examinations, considering carefully pre-, intra- and post-operative issues. The examiner may want you to talk purely about your chosen anaesthetic technique. However it is always worth starting by discussing the importance of pre-operative assessment and optimisation, especially as the condition of the patient will dictate what technique you do eventually decide to use.

I would consider carefully pre-, intra- and post-operative issues relevant to this case, and would want to discuss the management and get help from a senior colleague.

Initially it is important to get a history of the diabetes, how long the patient has had it, how well it is controlled and whether they suffer from any microvascular and macrovascular complications. How often the patient checks their blood sugar, what it normally runs at, and what their HbA1C is, are all helpful pieces of information. It is also useful to know which healthcare professionals manage their diabetes. If it is left to the practice nurse, they are probably easy to control, if they see a diabetologist it is likely to be more complex. If, on the other hand, they don't see anyone, then I would always be suspicious of poor control and of undiagnosed complications.

After taking a full medical and anaesthetic history as for any other case, I would examine the patient, making careful note of their blood pressure, looking for any evidence of cardiovascular or cerebrovascular disease, and assess for both autonomic and sensory neuropathies and evidence of "stiff joint syndrome". I would want to see an ECG and would have a low threshold for requesting an echocardiogram. Important blood tests include full blood count, renal and hepatic function tests and a clotting screen.

In this case the requirement for amputation suggests peripheral vascular disease and also possibly peripheral sensory neuropathy, having allowed the infection to develop to the extent that it has, and it is therefore almost certain that the patient will have cardiovascular disease and that their diabetes is advanced. This needs to be taken into account when determining the most appropriate form of anaesthetic for this patient. He is sick with his infected leg, is likely to have complications and would therefore benefit from the least "aggressive" anaesthetic possible.

After assessing the patient thoroughly it may be necessary to optimise his condition prior to surgery, and the findings of the assessment will guide this.

The next decision is whether to give a regional or general anaesthetic in this case, and this can only be made after a careful and thorough pre-op assessment. Personally I would choose....

At this point you need to say what you personally would do, and why. If you want to do a spinal (assuming there are no contraindications) then this is perfectly acceptable and indeed probably what the majority of anaesthetists would do in this case. If you would want to give a general anaesthetic and you can justify your reasons for doing so then this would also be fine. Either way, you need to consider the safety of the patient during the anaesthetic and therefore talk about intra-operative monitoring and the need for invasive monitoring, appropriate doses of anaesthetic drugs and how you will control the blood glucose during the procedure.

Post-operatively this patient should be managed on a high dependency unit where he can be closely monitored to minimise the risk of further complications developing.

What complications of diabetes have an effect on the administration of anaesthesia?

Diabetes is a multi-system disorder and as a result can affect most organ systems of the body. Complications of diabetes can be classified as macrovascular and microvascular. They arise not only as a result of chronic hyperglycaemia, but also due to poorly controlled hypertension. It is for this reason that good blood pressure control is imperative in the day-to-day management of diabetes.

Macrovascular complications include hypertension, ischaemic heart disease and cerebrovascular disease.

Microvascular complications can be broken down into nephropathy, neuropathy (which can be autonomic and peripheral) and retinopathy. In addition some patients get what is known as "stiff joint syndrome", which can have implications for the anaesthetist.

All of these complications have an effect on the administration of anaesthesia, either by dictating the technique of anaesthetic used or by making it a higher-risk event. Priorities should be on optimising the patient pre-operatively and on minimising the risk of further complications arising during the peri-operative period.

Chapter

2.10

Antibiotics

2.10.1. Antibiotics – Caroline SG Janes

This is a huge topic that whole textbooks have been dedicated to so don't be disheartened by these questions. You will only be expected to know the basics concerning anti-biotic use in intensive care and surgical prophylaxis.

When answering a question about anti-biotic prescribing in a specific condition it is advisable to begin the answer by referring to local anti-biotic guidelines and in complicated cases by stating that you would seek the opinion of a microbiologist. You will, however, still be expected to come up with a sensible suggestion for what could be used.

What is an antibiotic?

Generally speaking an anti-biotic is an agent that is used systemically or topically to treat infection. They act by inhibiting or abolishing the growth of micro-organisms such as fungi, bacteria or protozoa. Such agents include anti-bacterials, anti-fungals and anti-parasitic agents. However, strictly speaking an anti-biotic is a naturally occurring microbial product and we should refer to the above agents as chemotherapeutic agents.

What do you understand by the terms bactericidal and bacteriostatic?

Bactericidal agents kill bacteria directly and bacteriostatic agents prevent them dividing. These classifications are based on the behaviour of bacteria in a laboratory and cannot be directly translated to clinical situations.

How are bacteria classified?

"True bacteria" are best classified using the Gram stain. Gram-positive bacteria possess a thick cell wall containing many layers of peptidoglycan and stain purple. In contrast, Gram-negative bacteria have a relatively thin cell wall consisting of a few layers of peptidoglycan surrounded by a second lipopolysaccharide layer and these stain pink.

Bacteria can be further classified according to their morphology which is either spherical called cocci or rod-shaped called bacilli. Therefore the four main groups of bacteria are Gram-positive cocci, Gram-positive bacilli, Gram-negative cocci and Gram-negative bacilli.

Dr Podcast Scripts for the Primary FRCA, ed. Rebecca A. Leslie, Emily K. Johnson and Alexander P. L. Goodwin.   Published by Cambridge University Press. © R. A. Leslie, E. K. Johnson and A. P. L. Goodwin 2011.

Gram-positive cocci include staphylococci and streptococci, and important Gram-positive bacilli comprise clostridium and bacillus amongst others. Neisseria are the most common Gram-negative cocci and the Gram-negative bacilli include the enterobacteria, campylobacter and pseudomonas.

For other types of bacteria the Gram stain cannot be used as they differ in structure and do not have a peptidoglycan layer in their cell wall. These include filamentous bacteria, spirochaetes, mycoplasma, rickettsiae and chlamydiae. Filamentous bacteria are capable of branching and can produce mycelium, this group includes actinomyces and mycobacteria – the latter shows acid-fastness on Ziehl–Neelsen staining. Spirochaetes differ by being able to multiply by binary fission. Mycoplasma, on the other hand, lack a rigid cell wall and are smaller in size. Rickettsiae and chlamydiae are strict intra-cellular parasites.

What classes of anti-bacterial drugs exist?

At first this question may seem difficult, but just start off simply by explaining the three main ways in which they act and try to remember a couple of examples for each class. You will be expected to know the β-lactam agents well so spend a bit more time learning these.

There are many anti-bacterial agents and they are mostly classified into three main groups according to the site of action. Firstly there are inhibitors of cell wall synthesis which include β-lactam agents and glycopeptides. The second group inhibit bacterial protein synthesis which include tetracyclines, aminoglycosides, chloramphenicol, macrolides, clindamicin and fusidic acid. And thirdly there are inhibitors of nucleic acid synthesis which include sulphonamides, quinolones, metronidazole, nitrofurantoin and rifampicin.

Another method is to divide anti-bacterial agents into those that have β-lactam activity and those that do not. The β-lactam anti-bacterials include penicillins, cephalosporins, carbapenems and monobactams.

What is a β-lactam anti-bacterial?

This is a broad class of anti-bacterials that contains a β-lactam nucleus in its molecular structure. They act by inhibiting the synthesis of the peptidoglycan layer of bacterial cell walls. They do this by irreversibly binding to the active site of penicillin-binding proteins (PBPs). This then prevents the final cross-linking of the peptidoglycan layer, disrupting cell wall synthesis and ultimately triggering the digestion of existing peptidoglycan by autolytic hydrolases.

What anti-bacterial activity do penicillins have?

The penicillin benzylpenicillin has almost unrivalled activity against streptococci, staphylococci, spirochaetes and neisseria, although due to resistance its activity against staphylococci has been reduced. Other important penicillins include the anti-staphylococcal flucloxacillin, amoxycillin/ampicillin which have activity against some enterobacteria and piperacillin which is used in combination with tazobactam to make tazocin. Tazocin has a broad spectrum of activity and is commonly used on intensive care. The biggest problem with penicillin use is increasing bacterial resistance.

Tell me more about the cephalosporins and carbapenems?

Cephalosporins are similar to penicillins, but differ by having a β-lactam ring fused to a dihydrothiazidine ring instead of a thiazolidine ring. They are stable to staphylococcal penicillinase, exhibit a broader spectrum of activity and are less likely to cause hypersensitivity reactions. They are classified into first-, second- and third-generation agents. First-generation agents include cephradine which lacks Gram-negative cover, second-generation agents include cefuroxime which has better Gram-negative cover and is sometimes used for surgical prophylaxis. Third-generation agents include ceftriaxone which is more broad-spectrum and ceftazidime which has activity against pseudomonas. Third-generation agents also penetrate the meninges better, therefore are used to treat suspected meningitis.

Carbapenems have the broadest activity of the β-lactam agents against Gram-positive, Gram-negative and anaerobic bacteria. They include the widely used agents imipenem, ertapenem and meropenem.

How do bacteria become resistant to β-lactam antibiotics?

The effectiveness of these β-lactam antibiotics relies on their ability to reach the PBP intact and their ability to bind to the PBP. There are two modes of resistance. In the first the bacteria confers resistance by producing the enzymes β-lactamase or penicillinase which breaks open the β-lactam ring of the anti-biotic, rendering it ineffective. The genes encoding these enzymes may be present on the bacterial chromosome or may be acquired via plasmid transfer. β-lactamase gene expression may be induced by exposure to β-lactams. The production of a β-lactamase by a bacterium does not necessarily rule out all treatment options with β-lactam antibiotics. In some instances, β-lactam antibiotics may be co-administered with a β-lactamase inhibitor, such as clavulanic acid and tazobactam.

The second mode of β-lactam resistance is due to possession of altered penicillin-binding proteins. β-lactams cannot bind as effectively to these altered PBPs, and, as a result, the β-lactams are less effective at disrupting cell wall synthesis. Notable examples of this mode of resistance include methicillin-resistant *Staphylococcus aureus* (MRSA) and penicillin-resistant *Streptococcus pneumoniae*.

What is MRSA?

MRSA stands for methicillin-resistant *Staphylococcus aureus* – it is a strain of staphylococcus aureus that has developed resistance not only to penicillins but to all β-lactam anti-bacterials. Glycopeptides such as vancomycin which also inhibit cell wall synthesis but are not β-lactams are therefore used to treat MRSA.

What are the adverse effects of β-lactam antibiotics?

Common adverse drug reactions to β-lactam antibiotics include diarrhoea, nausea, rash, urticaria and opportunistic infection, especially fungal. Pain and inflammation at the injection site is also common for parenterally administered β-lactam antibiotics. Other reactions include fever, vomiting, erythema, dermatitis, angioedema and pseudomembranous colitis.

Immunologically mediated adverse reactions to any β-lactam anti-biotic can occur in up to 10% of patients receiving that agent, but only a small fraction are IgE-mediated. Anaphylaxis occurs in approximately 0.01% of patients. There is a 5–10% cross-sensitivity between penicillins, cephalosporins, and carbapenems. The risk of cross-reactivity warrants the contraindication of all β-lactam antibiotics in patients with a history of severe allergic reactions to any β-lactam anti-biotic.

Some drug-specific side effects include convulsions with benzylpenicillin and imipenem, abnormal liver function with ceftazidime and a positive Coomb's test with cefuroxime and imipenem.

Tell me more about the remaining group that inhibits cell wall synthesis – the glycopeptides

Glycopeptides act by inhibiting the glycopeptide synthetase and preventing peptidoglycan formation. They have good activity against Gram-positive organisms and are used increasingly in MRSA infection. They are also important in penicillin-allergic individuals. Vancomycin and teicoplanin are the most commonly used. They have very variable pharmacokinetics and therefore levels need to be checked regularly. Vancomycin is not absorbed intestinally and for this reason has a role in the treatment of *Clostridium difficile* infection where it is administered orally.

Tell me about the anti-bacterials that inhibit protein synthesis

These include tetracyclines, aminoglycosides, macrolides and clindamicin.

Tetracyclines prevent the binding of t-RNA to the ribosome. They have important activity against chlamydiae, rickettsiae and mycoplasma as well as Gram-negative and -positive bacteria. Doxycycline and minocycline are in most common use but their value has been limited by resistance.

Aminoglycosides inhibit the 30S ribosomal RNA unit and have activity against a wide range of Gram-negative enterobacteria and some Gram-positive – namely staphylococci, but they have no anaerobic cover. Aminoglycosides have to be given parenterally, they are excreted renally and have a narrow therapeutic index. Their levels therefore need to be monitored, especially in renal impairment. The most commonly used agent is gentamicin, which has many important side effects – these include ototoxicity, nephrotoxicity and muscle weakness.

Macrolides act by binding to the 50S ribosomal unit thus inhibiting translocation. They have similar activity to penicillins and are often used in people who are penicillin allergic. The main agents are clarithromycin and erythromycin. Macrolides often cause GI upset, especially erythromycin. Importantly erythromycin is an enzyme inhibitor and causes increased levels of alfentanyl and midazolam when co-administered.

Clindamicin is a lincosamide, it is highly active against Gram-positive aerobes and anaerobes. It disrupts the function of the 50S ribosomal sub-unit. Its use has been limited by its association with the development of life-threatening pseudomembranous colitis.

The remaining group of anti-bacterials inhibit nucleic acid synthesis, give me some examples

Anti-bacterials which inhibit nucleic acid synthesis include nitroimidazoles, quinolones and rifamycins.

Nitroimidazoles are synthetic anti-microbials of which the best known is metronidazole. Metronidazole is widely considered the anti-biotic of choice in the treatment of anaerobic infections and is commonly used in surgical prophylaxis and the treatment of GI tract infections. It is also the first line treatment of *C difficile* infection.

The quinolones act by inhibiting the α-subunit of the DNA gyrase enzyme which inactivates the supercoiling of the bacterial DNA resulting in cell death. The main quinolones are ciprofloxacin, norfloxacin, levofloxacin and ofloxacin. They have activity against Gram-positives including legionella, mycoplasma, rickettsiae, Chlamydiae and pseudomonas, although resistance to pseudomonas can be rapidly acquired. Quinolones are often used for urinary tract infections although as with other anti-bacterials their association with *C. difficile* colitis has curtailed their use.

Rifampicin is a rifamycin and is best known for its use in the treatment of tuberculosis and leprosy. It is also used in Legionnaire's disease and is given as prophylaxis in contacts of patients with haemophilus influenza B and meningococcal disease. It is well absorbed by the oral route. Hepatotoxicity is a well-recognised side effect and it is an enzyme inducer thus reducing the effectiveness of oral contraceptives. Patients should always be warned that rifampicin will cause a strong red pigmentation of urine and other bodily secretions. Resistance is a problem and the drug is usually given in combination with other agents.

Chapter

Anti-coagulants

2.11.1. Anti-coagulants – Archana Panickar

What are anti-coagulants?

Anti-coagulants are drugs that reduce or prevent coagulation by interfering with the process of fibrin plug formation.

How do you classify anti-coagulants

There are four main classes:

- Anti-platelet drugs
- Heparins
- Oral anti-coagulants
- Fibrinolytic agents.

What do you know about the structure of heparin?

This question comes up in the MCQs as well as in the structured oral examination.

Heparin is an anionic mucopolysaccharide glycosaminoglycan organic acid containing sulphate residues. In the body, heparin naturally occurs in the lungs, liver, mast cells and arterial walls. Unfractionated heparin has a molecular mass of 5000–25 000 Da.

How does heparin act?

Try to go through the physiology of coagulation before doing the anti-coagulant drugs module, as it is will help you understand the mechanism of action better.

Heparin has four main effects:

1. Inhibition of coagulation by enhancing the formation of anti-thrombin III–thrombin complex, leading to inhibition of factors IIa, Xa, XIIa, XIa and IXa
2. Inhibition of platelet aggregation
3. Release of lipoprotein lipase from tissues, which reduces plasma turbidity
4. Increased vascular permeability.

Dr Podcast Scripts for the Primary FRCA, ed. Rebecca A. Leslie, Emily K. Johnson and Alexander P. L. Goodwin.   Published by Cambridge University Press. © R. A. Leslie, E. K. Johnson and A. P. L. Goodwin 2011.

What are the uses of heparin?

Heparin is used in the prophylaxis and treatment of deep vein thrombosis and pulmonary embolism, treatment of unstable angina, critical peripheral arterial occlusion, and priming of extra-corporeal circuits.

How is heparin administered?

Heparin can be administered intra-venously or subcutaneously.

The typical adult dose for thrombo-prophylaxis is 5000 IU subcutaneously every 8–12 hours. For full anti-coagulation as during cardiopulmonary bypass, the dose is 300 IU/kg, or 3 mg/kg. It can also be given as an infusion. Heparin has an immediate effect, and has a half-life of 40–90 minutes.

What are low molecular weight heparins? What are their advantages?

Low molecular weight heparins (LMWHs) are fragments derived from depolymerisation of heparin, and have a molecular mass of 2000–8000 Da. Compared with unfractionated heparin, LMWHs are more effective in inhibiting factor Xa, and less effective in potentiating anti-thrombin III. LMWHs are administered subcutaneously.

Advantages include:

• Single daily dose due to longer half-life
• Require less monitoring
• Less effect on platelets and reduced risk of heparin-induced thrombocytopenia
• Reduced affinity for von Willebrand factor.

How is heparin therapy monitored?

Heparin prolongs activated partial thromboplastin time (APTT), and thrombin time. APTT measures the intrinsic system factors (VIII, IX, XI and XII) in addition to factors in the common pathway (II, X and fibrinogen).

On cardiopulmonary bypass, anti-coagulation with heparin is monitored using the activated clotting time.

LMWHs have a more predictable plasma level, and do not need monitoring routinely. If monitoring is essential, factor Xa assay has to be done, as APTT is not prolonged by LMWHs.

What are the side effects of heparin?

The most common and obvious side effect is haemorrhage. Other side effects include heparin-induced thrombocytopenia, hypotension following a rapid infusion, osteoporosis and alopecia.

What do you understand by heparin-induced thrombocytopenia?

Heparin-induced thrombocytopenia may be of two types.

Type I is a non-immune based thrombocytopenia, which occurs within 4 days of starting therapy, and the platelet count returns to normal without stopping therapy. This is rarely of clinical significance.

Type II is an immune-mediated thrombocytopenia, which is more severe and occurs 5–14 days after starting therapy. Half of these patients develop serious thrombosis and mortality is high, most commonly from PE. This is due to formation of a complex between heparin, platelet factor 4 and IgG, causing platelet aggregation and thrombosis.

How is the effect of heparin reversed?

Protamine is used to reverse the anti-coagulant effect of heparin. Protamine is a basic cationic protein obtained from fish sperm. One milligram reverses the effect of 100 IU heparin.

Protamine is not fully effective in reversing LMWHs.

How does warfarin act?

Warfarin is a coumarin derivative oral anti-coagulant. It acts by inhibiting the γ-carboxylation of vitamin K-dependent clotting factors (II, VII, IX and X) by preventing the return of vitamin K to its reduced form.

Warfarin has no effect on the circulating clotting factors, therefore takes up to 3 days to exert its full effect.

What are the side effects of warfarin?

Side effects include haemorrhage, teratogenicity and drug interactions.

What are some of the drug interactions of warfarin?

Other drugs that have anti-coagulant effect such as NSAIDs and heparin potentiate the effect of warfarin. Highly protein bound drugs such as NSAIDs, oral hypoglycaemic agents, diuretics and amiodarone displace warfarin from the protein binding sites, resulting in higher free drug levels and potentiation of its effect. Broad spectrum antibiotics, reduced vitamin K intake and cimetidine potentiate the effect of warfarin.

The effect of warfarin may be reduced by induction of hepatic enzymes by barbiturates and phenytoin. Oestrogens increase the production of vitamin K-dependent clotting factors and decrease effectiveness.

How is warfarin therapy monitored?

Warfarin causes prolongation of the prothrombin time, which is a measure of factor VII from the extrinsic pathway, and the factors in the common pathway.

The international normalised ratio (INR) is the ratio of a patient's prothrombin time to a normal (control) sample, raised to the power of the International Sensitivity Index value, which is provided by the manufacturer.

How is the anti-coagulant effect of warfarin reversed?

After stopping warfarin, it takes 3–5 days for the INR to return to normal.

The anti-coagulant effect of warfarin can be reversed with fresh frozen plasma, vitamin K or prothrombin complex concentrate (PCC).

Fresh frozen plasma rapidly corrects warfarin-induced coagulopathy in the presence of bleeding or before surgery.

Vitamin K reverses the anti-coagulation more slowly.

PCC, or Beriplex, is a combination of blood clotting factors II, VII, IX and X, as well as protein C and S. PCC corrects clotting factor deficiencies more rapidly and completely than plasma, they also reduce the risk of fluid over-load, viral transmission, anaphylaxis, and other transfusion related reactions. It is indicated for the peri-operative prophylaxis and treatment of bleeding associated with congenital and acquired deficiencies of vitamin K-dependent clotting factors, when rapid correction is required. It is very expensive; hence its use is restricted to these indications.

What are the mechanisms of action of anti-platelet drugs?

Aspirin irreversibly inhibits cyclo-oxygenase enzyme within the platelets resulting in reduced production of thromboxane A_2. This leads to reduced platelet aggregation.

Dipyridamole inhibits platelet adhesion by inhibiting adenosine uptake and inhibits platelet phosphodiesterase activity, resulting in increased cAMP levels.

Ticlopidine and clopidogrel irreversibly prevent ADP from binding to its receptor on the platelet surface. This prevents transformation of glycoprotein IIb/IIIa into its active form.

The glycoprotein IIb/IIIa inhibitor abciximab is a monoclonal anti-body, which blocks the final common pathway of platelet aggregation.

How do fibrinolytic agents work?

The fibrinolytic agents streptokinase, urokinase and alteplase activate the fibrinolytic system by forming a complex with plasminogen. This facilitates conversion of plasminogen to plasmin. Plasmin causes enzymatic degradation of the fibrin clot.

What are the guidelines for central neuraxial block if a patient is on anti-coagulant medications?

There is no contraindication to regional block if the patient is on aspirin or NSAIDs. In elective cases, it is generally stopped 3–7 days pre-operatively.

Clopidogrel has to be stopped 7 days pre-operatively.

Unfractionated heparin subcutaneous injection should be given at least 4 hours before instituting the regional block, or 1 hour after.

Intra-venous heparin infusion should be stopped 4 hours before giving the regional block, or instituted 1 hour after the block. The catheter should be removed 4 hours after the last dose.

LMWH should be withheld for 12 hours before regional anaesthesia, and the next dose can be given 2 hours after the block.

With a treatment dose of LMWH, regional block should not be done for 24 hours.

Regional technique is contraindicated in patients on warfarin, unless it has been stopped 3–5 days prior, and the INR is less than or equal to 1.5.

What information can be gained from thromboelastometry monitoring? What are the advantages of this test?

Classical thromboelastometry is performed by filling a curette with native whole blood and lowering a pin suspended by a torsion wire into the sample. The cup is rotated and the torque of the cup is transmitted to the pin through the sample in the cup. Bleeding disorders can be characterised based on the trace produced. The measurement is displayed as a graph from the beginning of clot formation to fibrinolysis. The thromboelastograph looks at the whole process of blood coagulation using whole blood. It measures the time taken for the clot to form, the kinetics of clot formation and the tensile strength of the clot. Thromboelastometry analysis is able to identify the majority of coagulation disorders within a few minutes. Interventions can be made faster, and often with fewer blood products or other expensive therapies.

Statistics

2.12.1. Statistical data – Rebecca A Leslie

It is common for candidates to panic as soon as statistics is mentioned, but as long as you know the basics you will do well in these questions.

Which different types of data are you aware of?

Classify your answer, and then describe each different type of data in a logical manner.

The two main types of data are quantitative data and qualitative data.

Qualitative data are not numerical and are usually just names or labels. Examples of qualitative data include ASA grade, type of operation, pain scores or hair colour. Qualitative data can be further classified in to nominal data and ordinal data. Nominal data are mutually exclusive with no logical order, such as hair colour and type of operation. Ordinal data, as the name suggests, have an intrinsic order such as pain scores and ASA grades.

Quantitative data are numerical in value, and the variable represents a value on a continuous scale. Examples of quantitative data are heart rate, blood pressure and height. There are further sub-classifications of quantitative data, such as discrete data, continuous data, interval data and ratio data.

Discrete data can only vary by a set amount, such as the number of children you have, as it is not actually possible to have 2.4 children. This is in contrast to continuous data, which can take any number, such as height, blood pressure and age. After all it is possible to have a heart rate of 75.45 bpm or a systolic blood pressure of 120.38 mmHg. Interval data occurs when the zero point on the scale is simply another point and doesn't mean no measurement. An example of interval data is temperature using the degrees Celsius scale where $0°C$ does not mean no temperature but describes how cold the substance is. In contrast if zero truly does mean no measurement, such as with heart rate or height then the data are described as being ratio data.

How would you display qualitative data in graphical form?

As qualitative data are not numerical but each variable has a label it is best displayed initially in a frequency table before being depicted as a bar chart or pie chart. Each variable can be given a percentage of overall observations, see Figure 2.12.1a.

Dr Podcast Scripts for the Primary FRCA, ed. Rebecca A. Leslie, Emily K. Johnson and Alexander P. L. Goodwin.   Published by Cambridge University Press. © R. A. Leslie, E. K. Johnson and A. P. L. Goodwin 2011.

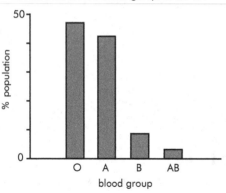

Occurrence of ABO blood groups in the UK

Figure 2.12.1a. Bar chart of categorical data. Reproduced with permission from Smith, T., Pinnock, C. and Lin, T. 2009. *Fundamentals of Anaesthesia.* Cambridge: Cambridge University Press. © Cambridge University Press 2009.

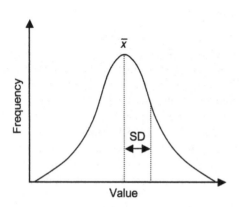

The curve is symmetrical around the mean, which is numerically identical to the median and mode. The SD should be indicated; 1SD lies approximately one third of the way between $\bar{x}$ and the end of the curve.

Figure 2.12.1b. The normal distribution curve. Reproduced with permission from Cross, M. and Plunkett, E. 2008. *Physics, Pharmacology and Physiology for Anaesthetists: Key Concepts for the FRCA.* Cambridge: Cambridge University Press. © M. Cross and E. Plunkett 2008.

In general how do we describe quantitative data?

To describe quantitative data we usually quote the central tendency of the data and the scatter of the data from this central point.

In data that are normally distributed we tend to use the mean to describe the central tendency and the variance or the standard deviation is used to describe the variation. Whilst in data that follow a non-normal distribution the central tendency is described by the median and the interquartile range gives an idea of the scatter about this point.

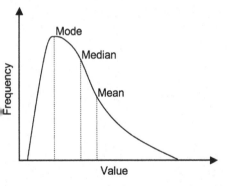

> The curve is asymmetrical with a longer tail stretching off towards the more positive values. The mean, median and mode are now separated so that $\bar{x}$ is nearest the tail of the curve; the mode is at the peak frequency and the median is in between the two. This type of distribution can sometimes be made normal by logarithmic transformation of the data.

Figure 2.12.1c. Positively skewed distribution. Reproduced with permission from Cross, M. and Plunkett, E. 2008. *Physics, Pharmacology and Physiology for Anaesthetists: Key Concepts for the FRCA.* Cambridge: Cambridge University Press. © M. Cross and E. Plunkett 2008.

What do you mean by a normal distribution and a non-normal distribution of data?

A distribution curve can be created by plotting the observed values on the x axis and the frequency on the y axis.

If data are normally distributed the distribution curve is symmetrical and bell shaped, see Figure 2.12.1b. In a normal distribution the mean, the mode and the median are all the same. These data can also be described as parametric.

Data are described as being non-normal or non-parametric if the distribution curve is not a symmetrical bell shape. Instead the curve may be skewed in either direction or may be bimodal. If the tail of skewed data extends to the right, this is called a right or positive skew, see Figure 2.12.1c. On the other hand if the tail of the skewed data extends to the left it is called a left or negative skew, see Figure 2.12.1d. If data are skewed, the mean, the mode and the median are no longer the same. The mode, which is the most frequently occurring value is always the peak of the curve. The median, which is the value where there are equal numbers or results both below and above it, moves towards the tail of the skewed data. The mean, which is the average of all the results, is also pulled in the same direction as the tail of skewed data because of the few erroneous results.

How do you calculate the variance?

To answer this question, don't just write out the formula, you also need to demonstrate a good understanding about how you actually calculate it.

The variance is the spread of data around a central point.

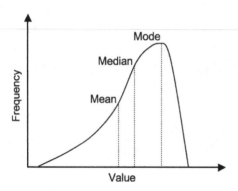

The curve is asymmetrical with a longer tail stretching off towards the more negative values. The mean, median and mode are now separated in the other direction, with $\bar{x}$ remaining closest to the tail. This type of distribution can sometimes be made normal by performing a power transformation (squaring or cubing the data).

Figure 2.12.1d. Negatively skewed distribution. Reproduced with permission from Cross, M. and Plunkett, E. 2008. *Physics, Pharmacology and Physiology for Anaesthetists: Key Concepts for the FRCA.* Cambridge: Cambridge University Press. © M. Cross and E. Plunkett 2008.

To calculate the variance of data, first you must work out the mean, $\bar{x}$.

Next you need to subtract each individual result from the mean to find the difference between the values.

$(\bar{x} - \chi)$

Next square all the results to make sure all the values are positive:

$(\bar{x} - \chi)^2$

Now add all the results together:

$\sum (\bar{x} - \chi)^2$

Next divide this number by the degrees of freedom, which is the number of observations minus 1, or n – 1:

$$\text{Variance} = \frac{\sum (\bar{x} - \chi)^2}{n - 1}$$

What is standard deviation?

As we have already mentioned, the central tendency of parametric data is described by the mean, and the variation around the mean described as the variance or the standard deviation. The standard deviation is calculated by the square root of the variance, and is used more frequently because it describes the data very conveniently. Sixty-eight percent of the population will fall within one standard deviation either side of the mean, 96% within 2 standard deviations of the mean and 99% within 3 standard deviations of the mean.

$$\text{Standard Deviation} = \frac{\sqrt{\sum (\bar{x} - \chi)^2}}{n - 1}$$

What is the standard error of the mean?

It is easy to get confused about the standard error of the mean (SEM), take some time to read about it, and understand it fully as it is key to statistical data interpretation.

The SEM is used to determine whether the mean of the sample reflects the mean of the true population. For example, imagine you have calculated the mean height of one hundred 8-year-old girls, yet the true population of 8-year-old girls is 10 000. By calculating the SEM you are able to show how the mean of your small sample reflects the mean of the whole population.

It is inherent that the larger the sample size, the more likely the mean is to reflect the mean of the true population. Also if the standard deviation is small, and hence the variance around the mean is small, then again you can be more confident that the mean of the sample is close to the mean of the true population.

The SEM is calculated by dividing the standard deviation by the square root of the degrees of freedom:

$$SEM = \frac{Standard\ Deviation}{\sqrt{(n-1)}}.$$

The SEM can be thought of as the standard deviation of the mean. So it can be said that 68% of sample means lie within one standard error of the true population mean, and 96% of sample means will lie within 2 standard errors of the true population mean.

What are confidence limits?

Confidence limits are related to the SEM. A sample mean will only lie outside 2, or more accurately 1.96, standard errors 5% of the time, therefore we can be 95% confident that the sample mean does in fact reflect the population mean. The range between two standard errors below the mean and two standard errors above the mean is called the confidence interval, and the values at either end the confidence limits. The confidence limits have the same value as the data measurements, which make them much easier to interpret.

Can you use standard error of the mean for non-parametric data?

This question is clearly non-sense, and they are just trying to confuse you. Don't let them!

No. For data that are skewed, the standard deviation does not accurately reflect the variation of the data around the mean, therefore it is impossible to calculate the SEM.

Instead for non-parametric data, we tend to quote a range that contains 50% of the results. The median is the value at which 50% of the results are above and 50% are below. The 25% centile is a point at which 25% of the subjects lie below and the 75th centile is the value at which 25% of the results are above. The range between these two values is called the interquartile range.

2.12.2. Statistical analysis – Rebecca A Leslie

In statistical terms what do we mean by the *p* value?

The *p* stands for probability, and it represents the probability of an event occurring. Therefore, if $p = 1$ the event always occurs and if $p = 0$ the event never occurs.

We use p values when we are comparing the difference between a sample population and the true population. In general the sample size is normally significantly smaller than the true population size, and we need to determine that any difference between the two groups has not occurred purely by chance.

It is accepted that if there is only a probability of 1 in 20 (which equates to $p = 0.05$) that the difference between the two groups has occurred by chance. This is considered to be small enough to be disregarded and therefore the difference between the two groups is statistically different.

If the $p > 0.05$ then the difference between the two groups is not statistically significant and it occurred purely by chance.

What is the null hypothesis?

When statistical tests are performed an assumption is made at the beginning that there is no significant difference between the means of the samples or that they originate from the same parent population. This is called the null hypothesis.

If the result of the statistical test produces a $p < 0.05$, which means that the probability that the two samples originate from the same population is less than 1 in 20. Therefore the null hypothesis can be rejected and there is considered to be a statistically significant difference between the samples.

If the result of the test gives a $p > 0.05$, then there is a higher probability that the difference has occurred purely by chance and the null hypothesis that there is no difference between the samples is accepted.

What is a type 1 error?

It is important you know the difference between type 1 and type 2 errors. It is easy to get confused between them, so make sure you take the time to learn their definitions.

A type 1 error is also called an α-error or a false positive. It occurs when a null hypothesis is wrongly rejected, so a difference between samples is found when there is none. The lower the p value and the larger the sample size the smaller the chance of making a type 1 error. By convention, we accept a p value of 0.05, which means that we accept the risk of making a type 1 error at a probability of 1 in 20.

What is a type 2 error?

A type 2 error is also known as a β-error or a false negative. A type 2 error occurs when the null hypothesis is accepted even though there is actually a difference between samples.

There are three factors that increase the chance of making a type 2 error:

- Small sample size
- A large variation in the study population
- Situations when a small difference is clinically important.

In contrast to a type 1 error where only a 5% chance of making an error is accepted, more leniency is allowed for type 2 errors. It is considered acceptable to allow a 20% chance of making a type 2 error. This means that the study is said to have a power of equal to or less than 0.2.

What do you mean by the power of a study?

The power of a study is a measurement of its likelihood of detecting a difference between groups if that difference really does exist. The power of a study is related to the type 2 error.

Power $= 1 - \beta$ (where β is the β error or type 2 error)

The power is effectively the probability of avoiding a type 2 error.

In a study, if no difference between two groups is detected, it can only be concluded that there is no clinically important difference in the samples providing the power of the study is adequate. If a type 2 error has been made, which is the same as saying the power of the study was insufficient, then all you can conclude is that the sample size is too small.

To ensure that if no differences are found between samples at the end of a study, meaningful conclusions can still be made, the power of a proposed study must be calculated prior to starting the study. The number of patients who must be included in the study to ensure a sufficient power can be determined by using equations or normograms.

How do you choose which statistical test to use to analyse data?

A number of considerations need to be taken prior to choosing the most appropriate statistical test. Firstly, the nature of the data must be considered; the data qualitative or quantitative?

If the data are quantitative then the type of distribution must be considered. Are the data parametric or non-parametric? Next you must take into account the number of different groups. Are there only two groups or are there more than two groups? Finally consider if the data are paired or unpaired.

So in summary there are four considerations that must be taken into account.

- Are the data qualitative or quantitative?
- Are the data parametric or non-parametric?
- Are there two groups or are there more than two groups?
- Are the data paired or unpaired?

Which test would you use to analyse qualitative data?

The chi-square test is one of the few statistical tests that is easy to calculate and as a result you should know in a bit more detail to the others.

Qualitative data, such as ASA grades, pain scores and hair colour, are typically analysed by using the chi-square test (χ^2):

$$\chi^2 = \Sigma \frac{(O - E)^2}{E}$$

where O is the number of observed occurrences and E is the number of expected occurrences.

The chi-square test compares the frequency of observed results against the frequency that would be expected if there was no difference between the groups.

For ease of explanation lets discuss the chi-square test with use on a 2×2 contingency table. A contingency table is created which has the two different sample groups and the two possible outcomes. For example, imagine two different drugs, drug A and drug B, are given and the number of patients who vomited after each drug and the number that did not vomit are recorded, see Table 2.12.2a.

Table 2.12.2a. Example contingency table for χ^2 test

	Vomiting	No vomiting	Total
Drug A	30	60	90
Drug B	70	20	90
Total	100	80	180

Table 2.12.2b. Example contingency table for χ^2 test showing expected values in brackets

	Vomiting	No vomiting	Total
Drug A	30 (50)	60 (40)	90
Drug B	70 (50)	20 (40)	90
Total	100	80	180

Next you need to calculate the number of patients who you would have expected to either vomit or not vomit if there was no difference between the two drugs. This must be calculated for each box in the table using the following formula:

$$\text{Expected value} = \frac{\text{Column total} \times \text{Row total}}{\text{Overall total}}$$

To calculate the number of patients you would expect to vomit after drug A if there was no difference between drug A and drug B using the above formula:

$$\text{Expected value} = \frac{100 \times 90}{180} = 50$$

Repeat this calculation for each box in the contingency table (Table 2.12.2b).

Next for each box in the contingency table, you apply the formula: $(O - E)^2/E$. The results of the four calculations are added together to give the chi-square result.

The p value depends on the chi-square and the degrees of freedom and can be determined from statistical tables.

When would you be unable to use the chi-square test?

If the expected occurrence in any of the boxes in the contingency table is less than five the chi-square test cannot be used accurately and the Fisher exact test should be used instead.

The Fisher exact test is difficult to calculate and only understood by statisticians. However there are computer packages that make analysis using Fisher exact test much easier.

What is the difference between paired and unpaired data?

Data are considered to be unpaired if two different groups of patients are being studied, whereas data are considered to be paired if the two variables which are being tested are from the same patients. An example of paired data is the anti-hypertensive effects of two different drugs that are being studied on the same group of patients.

If your data are parametric which statistical test would you use?

If you know your data are parametric then first you must determine how many groups there are.

If there are two groups of data then you would use either the paired student t test or the unpaired student t test depending on whether the data are paired or unpaired.

If you have more than two groups you would use the paired analysis of variance (ANOVA) or unpaired ANOVA.

Tell me a bit more about the student *t* test

A much dreaded question, but just keep it simple. The examiners are not expecting PhD level knowledge of all the different statistical tests, a basic overview of the more popular ones such as the chi-square and the student t *test is more than adequate.*

The student t test is used to analyse normally distributed data and relies on knowledge of the difference between the means of the two samples and the standard error of the difference.

$$t = \frac{\text{Difference between sample means}}{\text{Estimated standard error of the difference}}.$$

The p value is then read from statistical tables using the t value and the sample numbers.

What is ANOVA?

ANOVA is the analysis of variance, and it is used to compare parametric quantitative data when there are more than two different groups. The mathematics of ANOVA is complicated and computer software is used to handle the data.

Which statistical tests would you use if the data are non-parametric?

As with parametric data, first it is important to decide how many groups of data there are.

If there are two groups you would use the Wilcoxon signed rank test if the data are paired and the Mann Whitney U test if the data are unpaired.

If you have more than two groups you would use the Friedman test if the data are paired and the Kruskal–Wallis test if the data are unpaired.

Chapter

3.1

SI units

3.1.1. SI units – Emily K Johnson

There are many definitions to be learnt in this topic. It is tedious but there is no option. Study again and again until the definitions roll off your tongue with ease. They are frequently asked at the beginning of a question and you will not get off to a good start if you cannot comfortably remember them.

Once this material is covered there are some examples of the types of question you are more likely to be asked.

What are the fundamental SI units?

A mnemonic to help remember the base units is SMMACKK.

There are seven fundamental or base SI units.

- S for seconds is the unit of time
- M for meters the unit of length
- M for moles the unit of amount of substance
- A for amperes the unit of electric current
- C for candela the unit of luminous intensity
- K for kelvin the unit of temperature
- K for kilograms the unit of mass

Do you know the origins of the base SI units?

- A second is based on frequency of radiation emitted from caesium-133.
- A metre is the length light travels in a vacuum during a specified fraction of a second.
- The mole is the amount of substance which contains as many elementary particles as there are atoms in 0.012 kg of carbon-12.
- An ampere is the current which produces a force of 2×10^{-7} newtons per metre between two conductors one metre apart in a vacuum.
- The candela is the luminous intensity of a perfect black body at a specified high temperature.
- The kelvin is the fraction 1/273.16 of the thermodynamic temperature of the triple point of water. (The triple point of water is the point at which water, water vapour and ice all exist in equilibrium.)

Dr Podcast Scripts for the Primary FRCA, ed. Rebecca A. Leslie, Emily K. Johnson and Alexander P. L. Goodwin.   Published by Cambridge University Press. © R. A. Leslie, E. K. Johnson and A. P. L. Goodwin 2011.

- A kilogram is defined by the international prototype kilogram held at Sevres near Paris.

All units but the kilogram are based on physical properties of defined systems, which are reproducible over time. The kilogram is based on a prototype which is at risk of changing over time.

What are the derived SI units?

Although it is unlikely you will be asked this particular question in a structured oral examination it is useful to try and learn which are derived SI units. It is also a common MCQ question. The definition of any unit may be asked.

Derived units are those expressed in terms of multiplication or division of fundamental units. Some derived units are further combined to give other units. They are easier to consider as derived electrical units and derived non-electrical units.

There are four derived electrical units:

- **Volt** is the unit of electrical potential. One volt is the difference of electrical potential between two points of a conductor carrying a constant current of 1 ampere, when the power dissipated between these points is 1 watt.
- **Ohm** is the unit of electrical resistance. If a potential of 1 volt is applied across a conductor and produces a current of 1 ampere, the resistance of this conductor is 1 ohm.
- **Coulomb** is the unit of charge or quantity of electricity. One coulomb is the quantity of electricity transported in 1 second by a current of 1 ampere.
- **Farad** is the unit of capacitance. A capacitor has 1 farad of capacitance if a potential difference of 1 volt is present across its plates, when a charge of 1 coulomb is held by them.

There are seven derived non-electrical units:

- **Hertz** is the unit of frequency. One hertz is a frequency of one cycle per second.
- **Newton** is the unit of force. A force of 1 newton will give a mass of 1 kilogram and acceleration of 1 metre per second per second.
- **Pascal** is a unit of pressure. A pascal is the pressure of 1 newton per square metre.
- **Joule** is a unit of energy or work. A joule is the energy expended when the point of application of a force of 1 newton moves 1 metre in the direction of the force.
- **Electronvolt** is another unit of energy used for certain types of electromagnetic radiation. An electronvolt is the energy required to move one electron through a potential difference of 1 volt in a vacuum and equals 1.6×10^{-19} joules.
- **Watt** is the unit of power. Power is the rate of energy expenditure so 1 watt is 1 joule per second.
- **Celsius** is a unit of temperature. The size of one degree Celsius is identical to one degree kelvin. The relationship is 1 Celsius equals 1 kelvin minus 273.15.

Which commonly used units are not in the SI system?

Many different units are used for measuring pressure. Pascal is the derived SI unit. The mmHg, cmH_2O and atmospheres or bar are all units of pressure commonly used but do not belong to the SI system. They relate to each other as follows:

- 1 kilopascal equals approximately 7.5 mmHg.
- 1 centimetre of water equals 98 pascals, or 1 kilopascal equals 10.2 cmH$_2$O.
- 1 standard atmosphere is 101.325 kPa which is approximately 1 bar.
- 1 bar is therefore approximately 750 mmHg.

Energy is measured in several units; joule and electronvolt are derived SI units. Calorie is another unit of energy measurement and is not an SI unit. A calorie is 4.18 joules.

Force also has more than one unit, the derived SI unit of force is newton, the unit not in the SI system is kilogram weight. The kilogram weight or the kilopond, is the force of gravity on the mass of 1 kilogram. Gravity gives acceleration of 9.81 metres per second; hence 1 kilogram weight equals 9.81 newtons.

What are the commonly used prefixes to denote multiples of SI units?

Again this specific question is unlikely but a test of this knowledge may come into questions so it is just one of those things you must learn.

Starting from small to large the commoner multiples used are:

- Pico- which is 10^{-12}
- Nano- which is 10^{-9}
- Micro- which is 10^{-6}
- Milli- which is 10^{-3}
- Kilo- which is 10^3
- Mega- which is 10^6
- Giga- which is 10^9.

Some questions that you are more likely to encounter will now be asked.

What is standard temperature and pressure (STP)?

Standard temperature and pressure is 273.15 K which is equivalent to 0°C, and 101.325 kPa which is equivalent to 1 atmosphere, 1 bar and approximately 750 mmHg.

When expressed in SI units STP is 273.15 K and 101.325 kPa.

What is the definition of a mole?

A mole is the amount of substance which contains as many elementary particles as there are atoms in 0.012 kg of carbon-12.

Tell me about Avogadro's hypothesis

Avogadro's hypothesis states that equal volumes of gases at the same temperature and pressure contain equal numbers of molecules.

The molecular weights of the gases may be different but Avogadro's hypothesis states the number of molecules will be the same so although the mass will be different it is more useful to express quantity of gas in terms of numbers of molecules, which is the mole.

What is Avogadro's number?

Avogadro's number is the number of particles there are in 0.012 kg of carbon-12 and therefore the number of particles in a mole. This number is 6.022×10^{23}.

What is the volume occupied by 1 mole of gas at STP?

One mole of any gas will occupy the same volume, at the same temperature and pressure, according to Avogadro's hypothesis. This volume is 22.4 litres.

What volume of oxygen, molecular weight 32, would you obtain from a full cylinder containing a mass of 0.97 kg?

As the molecular weight of oxygen is 32, 1 mole of oxygen equals 32 g.

Therefore 32 g of oxygen would occupy 22.4 litres volume, so 970 g of oxygen would occupy $22.4 \times 970/32$.

So at STP the volume of oxygen obtained would be $22.4 \times 970/32$ which equals approximately 680 litres.

What are the units of pressure and how are they related?

There are several units of pressure. The derived SI unit is pascals. Also used frequently are the millimetre of mercury, centimetre of water, atmosphere and bar.

- A pascal is the pressure of 1 newton per square metre.
- A bar is 100 kilopascals and is roughly equivalent to an atmosphere which is precisely 101.325 kilopascals.
- 1 kilopascal is equivalent to 7.5 mmHg, so 1 bar is 750 mmHg and 1 atmosphere is roughly 750 mmHg.
- 1 centimetre of water pressure is 98 pascals, or 1 kPa equals 10.2 cmH_2O.

Chapter 3.2

Biological signals and their measurement

3.2.1. Biological signals – Adrian Clarke

Detecting biological electrical signals has become the cornerstone of many of the clinical measurements we use in anaesthesia today. Different organs produce different signals, which can be detected and used to monitor the function of that particular organ.

This script will cover the different types of signals produced by different organs, how each is detected and the necessary electrical methods of amplifying and filtering the signals so that they may be recorded in a meaningful fashion.

The exam demands a broad based knowledge – MCQ questions may concentrate on specific numbers, or require more general principles and understanding in the OSCE or structured oral examination.

Which biological signals do we frequently measure in anaesthetic practice?

Three organs which produce signals that we frequently measure are the heart, brain and skeletal muscle. Since each has very disparate cell types, the signals they produce differ in terms of their frequency and voltage. This is useful because different monitors can filter the signals, specific to a frequency range, so a clear output signal can be displayed.

Tell me more about the specific biological signals that occur in the heart

The heart produces signals when each cell membrane depolarises with each contraction. The electrical currents of each cell combine and produce a field of high amplitude. Along with a prolonged action potential, this depolarisation can be detected on the surface of the body, by an electrocardiogram (ECG). At the surface, this usually has a voltage of approximately 1 mV, and a frequency in the range of 0.05–100 Hz.

How does this compare with the biological signals of brain and muscle?

The brain produces smaller and more complex signals, and is harder to detect at the surface. Fewer neurones depolarise in synchrony, and the action potential is much shorter. Therefore, the electroencephalogram (EEG) is generated by the combined potential of many

Dr Podcast Scripts for the Primary FRCA, ed. Rebecca A. Leslie, Emily K. Johnson and Alexander P. L. Goodwin.   Published by Cambridge University Press. © R. A. Leslie, E. K. Johnson and A. P. L. Goodwin 2011.

post-synaptic potentials from sheets of large, symmetrically arranged pyramidal cells in the cortical layers III and IV.

The EEG signals tend to have an amplitude of 50–200 μV, and a frequency between 0 and over 13 Hz. Conventionally, the frequency content can be classified into four categories:

- δ-waves, 0–4 Hz
- θ-waves, 4–8 Hz
- α-waves, 8–13 Hz
- β-waves, 13 Hz and above.

Visual analysis of an EEG is difficult and requires significant knowledge and experience.

The electromyograph (EMG) measures electrical signals given off from skeletal muscle. It can use electrodes either on the skin, or embedded within the muscle itself. It operates at a frequency of 1–20 000 Hz and a voltage of around 1 mV. It can be used to investigate spontaneous or evoked electrical activity from skeletal muscle, and along with nerve conduction studies can differentiate between primary muscular disorders, neuromuscular junction abnormalities, and nerve disease or lesions.

Do you know of a monitor used in anaesthesia which measures the EEG?

A simplified version of EEG monitoring is becoming more widely available. The Bispectral Index (BIS) monitor receives input from a few electrodes placed on the patient's scalp. By analysing different components in the EEG signal an estimate of the degree of hypnosis, or depth of anaesthesia can be estimated. It produces a lower number for a patient at a greater depth of anaesthesia, and a higher number for a patient under a lighter general anaesthetic or sedation.

What is an amplifier, and why are they necessary when measuring biological signals?

Amplifiers are devices that convert a small weak electrical signal to a more powerful signal output. They are essential for interpreting biological electrical signals because the amplitude of the biological signal at the skin is too small, with too much noise and interference to interpret meaningfully.

Along with increasing the amplitude of any signal they receive, most amplifiers also filter certain frequencies of signal, thereby concentrating on the range most likely to contain the signal desired. The range of frequencies that an amplifier works over most efficiently is called the bandwidth.

What is a differential amplifier?

A differential amplifier works by measuring the difference between two separate inputs (for example two electrodes; one placed over the chest and one at the feet). Any signal which is the same at both sources (for example 50 Hz from main interference) will be eliminated, and the remaining signal will be amplified – hopefully the signal you are interested in measuring. This is known as "common mode rejection". This works effectively for eliminating mains interference when measuring the ECG, but the same principle applies to eliminating any ECG signals when measuring the EEG.

The common mode rejection ratio (CMRR) is the ratio of the unwanted signal to the wanted signal. For example a CMRR of 10 000 to 1 (fairly typical of most biological amplifiers) would require an interference signal at both electrodes 10 000 times greater than the desired signal applied at one electrode to achieve the same output.

What are filters?

Despite common mode rejection, some interference may still be present in the signal to be amplified.

Filtering is therefore essential to enhance the quality of the signal to be analysed, and reject all other currents. The terms used most frequently are "high-pass" and "low-pass" filters. High-pass filters eliminate all currents with a low frequency, thereby allowing the high-frequency currents to pass through. Low-pass filters eliminate high-frequency currents, and allow the low-frequency currents through to be analysed. A "Notch" filter is one which rejects a specific band of frequencies. For example, ECG machines sometimes use notch filters to eliminate frequencies between 48 and 52 Hz, to reduce the amount of interference from mains electricity. Using a combination of filters, a monitor can analyse just the desired signal and reduce the impact of noise or interference, allowing a pure output signal to be displayed.

What are the most common sources of interference?

There are many sources of interference with the clinical monitors used in theatre or an intensive care setting.

Electrical interference is probably the most common, and may originate from the main supply, radio or mobile phone signals. The main supply has a frequency of 50 Hz, and may interfere with the ECG or EMG, unless filters are used to eliminate it.

Surgical diathermy operates at a very high frequency (0.5–1 MHz), and therefore is easy to eliminate with a low-pass filter.

What are the problems posed by obtaining clinical measurements in an MRI scanner?

If ever asked about problems faced with anaesthesia in an MRI scanner, then it is imperative to classify first into "patient" factors and "anaesthetic" factors (e.g. an isolated site, limited visibility and access to the patient whilst being scanned, errors and interference with all clinical monitoring). For the purposes of this structured oral examination, this section will only discuss the problems with patient monitoring in MRI scanners.

MRI scanners pose a particular problem with regard to monitoring patients for two reasons. Firstly, they use a powerful magnet, so magnetic metals must not be taken within close range of the scanner, because they will interfere with the image the scanner produces. In addition powerful attraction to the magnet may make metal objects move dangerously (either outside or within the body). Secondly, scanners use a radio transmitter and receiver, to communicate with the control room, and these may interfere with the patient monitoring.

Some of these problems can be overcome relatively easily. For example, pulse oximetry is possible by using long leads with fibre-optic cables; however the electrical fields generated may degenerate the quality of signal produced. Sometimes another small radio transmitter is used (at a non-interfering frequency) to transmit the ECG signals from the patient in the

MRI to the control room. However, the entire MRI room is encased within a Faraday cage of conductive copper mesh which prevents radio waves getting in or out.

3.2.2. Electrocardiogram – Adrian Clarke

The electrocardiogram, or ECG, is an important topic because it is used so widely, either for monitoring or diagnostic uses. It is most likely to come up as part of a question on a broader topic – for example about biological signals, or standards of monitoring in anaesthesia.

The ECG was first recorded through an intact chest in 1887. Since then there have been many modifications to both the electrodes and analytical monitors, such that very detailed information is available instantly, and can be used to monitor and diagnose high-risk patients effectively.

What equipment is needed to monitor an ECG?

A question like this provides an ideal opportunity to show your general knowledge of components required for any clinical monitor, and it may allow you to steer a structured oral examination towards a topic you are more comfortable with. If you do try this, you MUST NOT show the examiners you are less comfortable talking about ECGs – otherwise they might pounce for a kill! They may also have a relatively closed marking scheme, so beware you will not score any points for talking about a subject that they cannot score you on.

Any biological signal requires a number of components before it can be displayed in a meaningful fashion, and the ECG is no exception. These components are:

- A detection device
- A transducer
- An amplifier
- A display device.

In the ECG, the electrodes act as the detection device. A transducer is unnecessary in an ECG as the energy does not need to change form. Other monitors (e.g. arterial or venous pressure or temperature measurement) need an input transducer to convert the signal energy into electrical energy. Next the signal is amplified, before passing to a display device. The display is usually able to be stored either on paper or in computer memory.

What are the electrodes used for ECG monitoring made of?

Adequate skin electrodes are essential for recording electrical signals, and reduce interference from other sources. Most ECG electrodes are composed of a silver electrode surface, in contact with silver chloride. This is in contact with chloride ions embedded in a gel, which is in direct contact with the skin. The electrode is secured to the skin by an adhesive disc. Significant dirt, hairs or skin diseases (e.g. psoriasis, erythroderma) may make electrode placement difficult.

There can be problems using certain electrodes. The water and electrolytes present on the skin surface, and the metal in the electrode can produce an electrical cell which generates its own potential. When the biological signal passes through the electrode, the distribution of ions within the electrode changes, and this is known as polarisation. This polarisation will affect the electrode potential, and affect the signal produced by the recording system. The silver/silver chloride choice of electrode is least likely to be affected by these problems.

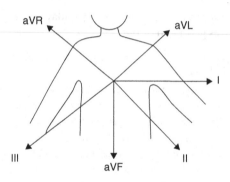

Figure 3.2.2a. Orientation of electrocardiograph leads relative to the chest wall.

Are similar electrodes used for any other purposes?

Similar electrodes can be used for either detection or transmission of electricity to or from the patient. Other monitoring electrodes include Bispectral Index monitors, or situations where electricity is conducted to the patient include neuromuscular blockade monitors, diathermy pads and defibrillator pads. If a defibrillator pad is used to monitor an ECG, there is a massive polarisation after a shock is delivered, which may mean that there is a delay in monitoring the ECG until the charges have realigned.

How are ECG signals produced?

The signals recorded by the ECG are produced directly by depolarisation of the heart muscle with each contraction. A small proportion of the energy required for cardiac contraction spreads into the surrounding tissues, which can be detected at the surface of the body.

The configuration of electrodes on the surface then allows analysis of electrical signals from different parts of the heart.

What are different ECG leads used for?

For monitoring, only three electrodes are necessary, and these are called the limb leads. These monitors will produce a continuous recording, which can be displayed. Electrodes are placed on the right shoulder, left shoulder and left costal margin (or leg). The signal produced is the difference in the electrical signals that each of the electrodes detects at the skin surface. The combination of different leads produces a signal from a different part of the heart. For example, lead I analyses signals between the right arm and left arm, lead II analyses signals between the right arm and left leg, and lead III between the left arm and left leg (see Figure 3.2.2a). Lead II is most commonly used for monitoring in anaesthesia and intensive care, because it gives a good signal across the left atrium, making it easiest to see atrial and ventricular dysrhythmias in this lead.

Another three leads can be derived from the three electrodes. These are called the augmented unipolar leads, and use a reference electrode of all three electrodes combined. Lead aVR analyses signals from the right arm, aVL from the left arm, and aVF from the left leg.

For diagnosis (usually of arrhythmias, ischaemia, or other pressure or anatomical abnormalities) then a 12-lead ECG is used. This uses the three limb leads, and another six electrodes placed across the anterior chest wall. V1–2 measures activity from the right side of the heart, V3–4 from the interventricular septum and V5–6 from the left ventricle.

Using a combination of different leads, analysis of separate areas of the heart is possible:

- The inferior portion of the heart is demonstrated in leads aVF, 2 and 3.
- The anterior heart is given by leads I, II and V1 and V2.
- The lateral part of the heart is given by aVL, I, V5 and V6.

Are there any other electrode configurations?

The electrodes can be placed anywhere on the body, but the positions described tend to give the most accurate results. It is essential that similar lead positions are used for diagnostic ECGs otherwise the detected signals will change, and interpretation of the ECG difficult.

The chest electrodes can be placed over the left posterior chest wall, and this will give a posterior ECG. This is useful to investigate right ventricular myocardial ischaemia.

Another configuration is the CM5 (central manubrium 5) configuration. This moves the standard electrode positions so that:

- The right arm electrode is positioned in the supra-sternal notch.
- The left arm electrode is positioned at the apex (V5 position).
- The left leg electrode is positioned on the left shoulder or leg, and acts as the ground or reference electrode.

If lead I is selected on the monitor with the leads in this position, it will display the "CM5" configuration, which gives more detailed information about the left ventricle, allowing detection of arrhythmias and ischaemia more easily.

There are other, more modern ECG systems available. One system often seen in coronary care units is the Philips EASI 12-lead system. This uses four electrodes positioned over the praecordium and one reference electrode which can be positioned anywhere on the patient. From these 5 leads it can derive a 12-lead ECG in the usual familiar format. This is useful so that patients requiring continuous monitoring, for example for acute coronary syndromes, can have instant 12-lead ECGs available. It may also be used for high-risk patients during angiography.

Please interpret this ECG for me

If shown an ECG during any part of the OSCE/structured oral examination, it is essential to show that you have a systematic approach, that you think clearly and logically, and make the right diagnosis. Not all the marks will be on getting the exact answer, there will be some specifically for your approach to interpreting the ECG. Do not panic, stay calm and stick to your well-rehearsed method of interpreting ECGs. The example given below is one possible method of ECG interpretation.

1. State the patient's name and date of ECG.
2. Check the speed of recording and the calibration. The speed is usually 25 mm/s, and is printed on the bottom of the ECG. The calibration is 1 mV/cm. A vertical rectangular shape at the edge of the ECG line allows calculation of the calibration.
3. Check the heart rate. Count the number of 5-mm squares in between successive QRS complexes, and divide this number into 300. This will give you beats per minute.
4. Check the axis. A normal axis is between −30 and +90 degrees. Left axis deviation is seen in left bundle branch block, and left ventricular hypertrophy. It can also occur in healthy patients (especially if pregnant, or have large volume ascites). Right axis

deviation may be seen in right ventricular hypertrophy, right bundle branch block and left posterior hemiblock. Remember right axis deviation can also be a normal variation.

5. Check the rhythm. Firstly, is it regular or irregular. Mark the QRS complexes on another edge of scrap paper if allowed. An irregular rhythm may be irregularly irregular (AF), or regularly irregular (e.g. missing every third QRS).
6. Check for P-waves. These are usually easiest seen in V1 or aVR.
7. Count the P-R interval (usually 3–5 small squares, i.e. 0.12–0.2 seconds).
8. Check the QRS complex. The width should be less than 3 small squares (0.12 seconds). It should be positive in leads I, II and V4 to V6. There should be a stepwise increase in height of the chest leads from leads V1 to V4. The size of the complexes may increase or decrease between leads V5 and V6.
9. Look for Q-waves, which might indicate previous myocardial infarctions.
10. The height of the QRS complex is important – the amplitude of all the leads I, II and III should be more than 5 mm. If there is left ventricular hypertrophy, then the R-wave in V6 and S-wave in V1 may be more than 35 mm tall. Right ventricular hypertrophy is shown by positive R-waves in lead V1, especially if they are taller than the S-waves in V2.
11. Look for extra waves such as J-waves in hypothermia or δ-waves in Wolff–Parkinson–White syndrome.
12. Look at the S-T segment. It should be within 1 mm of the baseline and relatively flat.
13. Look at the T-waves. They should have the same orientation as the QRS complexes.
14. Look at the QT interval. This is often calculated for you at the top of the ECG. The normal range is 0.35–0.43 seconds.
15. Look for U-waves. These are small waves following the T-waves. They may represent slow repolarisation of the papillary muscles, and are more prominent in hypokalaemia.
16. Look for recognisable patterns, for example, S1Q3T3 in pulmonary embolism or acute pulmonary hypertension, bundle branch blocks, or a stepwise decline in height through the chest leads in dextrocardia.
17. If you cannot see anything wrong with it, then remember it may be a normal ECG.

Are there any other situations that ECG monitoring may be useful?

Portable, external ECG monitors can be worn for 24 hours (a 24 hour tape), and help in diagnosis of palpitations or syncope.

Implantable devices are used to detect arrhythmias over a longer period (e.g. detection of VT before implantation of an internal defibrillator, or other more unusual arrhythmias).

Are there any standards for clinical monitoring during anaesthesia?

These standards are available on the AAGBI Web site, and only take 5 minutes to read. If you can recall them during an exam, it will demonstrate that you are a responsible and diligent practitioner, which is what the examiners need to let you pass.

The Association of Anaesthetists of Great Britain and Ireland published the fourth edition of their guidance "Recommendations of standards of monitoring during anaesthesia and recovery" in 2007. This states many important principles, but highlights are:

1. Continuous presence of an anaesthetist.
2. The following monitors must be available for induction and their use continued until the patient has recovered from the effects of anaesthesia:

    a. Pulse oximetry
    b. Non-invasive blood pressure monitoring
    c. ECG
    d. Airway gases
    e. Airway pressure.

3. Pulse oximetry and non-invasive blood pressure monitoring must be applied during recovery from anaesthesia. ECG, nerve stimulator, capnography and temperature measurement do not need to be attached, but must be immediately available if their use is required.
4. For regional anaesthesia, local anaesthesia, or sedation, pulse oximetry, non-invasive blood pressure and ECG monitoring must be applied as a minimum.

3.2.3. Neuromuscular monitoring – Dana L Kelly

How can you monitor the neuromuscular junction?

The degree of blockade of the neuromuscular junction can be assessed by clinical observation or, more precisely, by response to electrical stimulation.

Clinical assessment at the end of anaesthesia allows the crude estimate of adequate neuromuscular function. The most useful clinical indicator of adequate reversal is the ability to perform a sustained head lift for 5 seconds. This suggests under 30% receptor blockade is present. Other indicators include the ability to generate a tidal volume of approximately 10 ml/kg, protrude the tongue, maintain a sustained handgrip or cough. However these may be possible with 50–80% receptors blocked.

Neuromuscular blockade can be also be assessed by electrical stimulation using a peripheral nerve stimulator. Monitoring can be visual, tactile, mechanical or electrical.

Discuss the components of a peripheral nerve stimulator

The components include a battery powered stimulator that consists of an on/off switch and a facility to deliver a variety of simulator patterns, and two electrodes (either ECG electrodes or ball electrodes) that are positioned over the chosen peripheral nerve.

What is the mechanism of action of a peripheral nerve stimulator?

The stimulation is a unipolar square waveform. A supra-maximal stimulus is used to stimulate a peripheral nerve, and then the response of the muscle supplied by this nerve is observed. The muscle contraction can be observed visually, palpated or measured.

What is a supra-maximal stimulus?

It is important to eliminate variation in muscle response caused by partial depolarisation of nerve fibres. The stimulus supplied must activate therefore all the nerve fibres on each occasion. This so-called "supra-maximal stimulus" ensures 100% recruitment of nerve fibres and therefore a reproducible response.

What muscle groups do we commonly use to assess neuromuscular blockade?

Firstly, it is important to consider that any assessment will only determine the function of the particular muscle group tested, and that neuromuscular blockade may vary considerably in different muscular groups. In general, the smaller the muscle, the more sensitive it is to muscle relaxants.

If the ulnar nerve is used to assess neuromuscular block, electrodes are placed along the ulnar border of the wrist, and thumb adduction is assessed. The ulnar nerve is more sensitive to neuromuscular blocking drugs than the diaphragm and vocal cords.

Using the facial nerve for assessment involves placing electrodes anterior to the tragus of the ear. An assessment of facial muscle contraction is then made. Under-estimation of the degree of blockade is common with this site, both because of direct muscular stimulation and because the facial nerve is relatively insensitive to neuromuscular blocking drugs.

If the common peroneal nerve is used to assess neuromuscular block, the electrodes are placed lateral to the neck of the fibula, and an assessment of foot dorsiflexion is made.

What types of nerve stimulation patterns are commonly used?

Five different types of nerve stimulation patterns are commonly used: single twitch, tetanic stimulation, post-tetanic count, train of four (ToF) and double burst. I will discuss these stimulation patterns in detail individually.

Let's start with the **single-twitch** stimulation pattern. This involves a short duration (i.e. 0.1–0.2 msec) square wave stimulus of 0.1–1.0 Hz being applied to a peripheral nerve. A comparison between the measured twitch height after relaxant administration and the control twitch height before muscle relaxation is made. There is normally no reduction in twitch height with less than 75% receptor occupancy at the neuromuscular junction.

When using **tetanic stimulation,** tetanus of 50–100 Hz is applied to detect any residual neuromuscular block. A tetanic burst of 50 Hz for 5 seconds produces a muscle response comparable with maximal voluntary effort. Absence of fade following this stimulus can be interpreted as the return to full muscular power. This stimulation pattern is very unpleasant for a conscious patient, and even if applied during anaesthesia, may leave some residual pain.

Another nerve stimulator pattern commonly used is the **post-tetanic count,** also known as post-tetanic potentiation or facilitation. Intense muscle blockade can completely abolish the response to the ToF count. The post-tetanic count is used to produce a response at high levels of receptor occupancy. It works as tetanic stimulation increases the mobilisation of acetylcholine in the pre-synaptic membrane. Subsequent electrical stimulation will release supra-normal concentrations of acetylcholine, which may be sufficient to overcome the effect of the non-depolarising blockade. The number of resultant twitches depends on the degree of neuromuscular blockade present (as well as the frequency, amplitude and duration of the tetanic stimulus).

The **train of four (ToF)** is used to assess recovery from non-depolarising blockade. This stimulation pattern refers to four identical stimuli at 2 Hz 0.5 seconds apart therefore of a total of 1.5 seconds duration. It is applied no more often than every 10 seconds. The acetylcholine receptor occupancy can be estimated based on the number of detectable twitches. Four twitches suggests less than 75% receptor blockade, three twitches suggests 75% blockade, two twitches suggests 80% blockade, one twitch suggests 90% blockade and no twitches

Normal neuromuscular junction

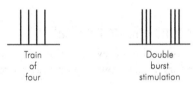

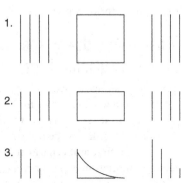

| Train of four | Double burst stimulation |

Non-depolarising agent present

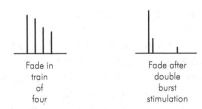

| Fade in train of four | Fade after double burst stimulation |

Figure 3.2.3a. Response patterns after double burst stimulation. Reproduced with permission from Smith, T., Pinnock, C. and Lin, T. 2009. *Fundamentals of Anaesthesia*. Cambridge: Cambridge University Press. © Cambridge University Press 2009.

Figure 3.2.3b. A drawing of response patterns following train of four stimulation, tetanus, and then further train of four stimulation: 1. normal; 2. partial depolarising block; 3. partial non depolarising block.

suggests 100% receptor occupancy. A comparison is made between the ratios of the fourth to the first twitch, known as the ToF ratio. For adequate respiratory function, the ToF ratio must be greater than 70%.

Finally, *double-burst* stimulation is used again to assess recovery from non-depolarising blockade, see Figure 3.2.3a. It allows a more accurate visual assessment than ToF for residual neuromuscular blockade. The stimulation pattern consists usually two 50-Hz tetanic stimuli (each made up of three square wave impulses of 20 msec) applied with a 750-msec interval.

Can you differentiate between depolarising and non-depolarising agents using a peripheral nerve stimulator?

A drawing of response patterns following train of four stimulation, tetanus, and then further train of four stimulation is the easiest way to answer this question, see Figure 3.2.3b.

There are characteristic stimulation patterns observed with depolarising and non-depolarising agents.

To start by looking at the "unblocked" response, the observed response with normal neuromuscular function is equal twitches in response to single electrical pulses or ToF. Sustained tetanic contraction is demonstrated.

With depolarising neuromuscular block, equal but reduced twitches are seen in response to ToF (i.e., ToF ratio is 1). Sustained but reduced tetanic contraction is demonstrated, with neither fade nor post-tetanic facilitation. This is known as phase 1 block.

With non-depolarising neuromuscular block, progressively decreasing twitches are seen with ToF. Tetanic contraction exhibits fade and post-tetanic facilitation is evident. This is known as phase 2 block.

Notably, if repeated doses of suxamethonium are given, the twitch response may change from a phase 1 to a phase 2 block pattern.

What is the suggested value of the ToF count prior to reversal?

ToF count of 3–4 should be present prior to administration of reversal. This represents 75% or less receptor occupancy of acetylcholine receptors by neuromuscular blocking agents.

What devices do you know of to accurately monitor neuromuscular blockade?

You may be shown an example of a device used to monitor neuromuscular blockade, commonly an accelerometer, and asked to discuss how it works.

There are several devices available to accurately monitor neuromuscular blockade. These include mechanical force transducers, accelerometers and electromyography.

Looking first at **mechanical force transducers**. These devices work on the principle that tetanic stimulation of peripheral nerve causes tension to develop within the muscle. The force of this isometric contraction is measured using a strain gauge transducer, allowing a measure of neuromuscular function. A control response prior to administration of neuromuscular blocking drugs must be obtained.

Accelerometers are electronic devices that act to transduce acceleration into electrical potentials that can be measured and displayed. The accelerometer is usually attached to the thumb. We know that force equals mass times acceleration, so for a given mass of thumb the acceleration is proportional to applied force.

Finally, **electromyography** uses EMG responses to assess neuromuscular function. This technique requires placement of five ECG dots (two stimulating, two recording, one neutral). The height of the EMG response or the area under the response curve can then be measured, and degree of neuromuscular blockade calculated.

Chapter 3.3

Gas flow and its measurement

3.3.1. Gas laws – Rebecca A Leslie

You will be expected to be able to competently discuss the gas laws. They are very straightforward but are the sort of thing that you can get confused about when you are put under pressure (pardon the pun!). Make sure you read them through the night before your exam.

What are the differences between a solid, a liquid and a gas?

All substances are composed of atoms or compounds of atoms called molecules.

In solids the atoms or molecules are arranged in a tight lattice. There are strong forces between all the molecules in the lattice. All the molecules are continuously in motion, oscillating about a mean position.

In a liquid the molecules have much more energy than in a solid and the molecules are free to move throughout the liquid. There are still forces between the molecules; however these forces are much weaker than in a solid. These forces of attraction are called Van der Waal forces.

If heat is added to a liquid the molecules gain more kinetic energy. As more heat is added enough energy is gained so that the molecules can escape the Van der Waal forces. This creates a gas or vapour where the molecules are free to move individually.

What is Boyle's law?

This perfect gas law, like all the others, needs to roll off your tongue.

Boyle's law is the first perfect gas law. It states that at a constant temperature, the volume of a fixed mass of a gas is inversely proportional to its pressure. This can be rearranged so that volume multiplied by pressure is equal to a constant.

Therefore at a constant temperature:

$V \alpha 1 / P$ or $PV = K$ where K is a constant.

Can you tell me a clinical application of Boyle's law?

Knowledge of Boyle's law allows us to calculate the amount of oxygen available from an oxygen cylinder.

Dr Podcast Scripts for the Primary FRCA, ed. Rebecca A. Leslie, Emily K. Johnson and Alexander P. L. Goodwin.   Published by Cambridge University Press. © R. A. Leslie, E. K. Johnson and A. P. L. Goodwin 2011.

Boyle's law states that pressure multiplied by volume is equal to a constant. From this it follows that:

$$P1 \times V1 = P2 \times V2.$$

When a size E oxygen cylinder is full it has a pressure of 13 700 kPa and an internal volume of 10 litres. This pressure is gauge pressure, so the atmospheric pressure of 100 kPa must be included to make the absolute pressure. Remember absolute pressure equals gauge pressure plus atmospheric pressure. So P1 equals 13 800 kPa, whilst V1 equals 10 litres. When the oxygen is released from the cylinder it is released at atmospheric pressure, 100 kPa, this is P2.

Therefore:

$$13\,800 \text{ kPa} \times 10 \text{ L} = 100 \text{ kPa} \times V2.$$

So:

$$V2 = (13\,800 \times 10)/100$$

$$V2 = 1380 \text{ L.}$$

In summary at atmospheric pressure the volume of oxygen available from a full size E oxygen cylinder would be 1380 litres.

What is Charles' law?

Charles' law is the second perfect gas law. It states that at a constant pressure the volume of a gas is proportional to the absolute temperature.

$V \alpha T$ or $V/T = K$ where K is a constant.

What is the universal gas law?

Boyle's and Charles' laws can be combined together to form the universal gas law. The universal gas law states that pressure multiplied by volume is equal to number of moles of a gas multiplied by the universal gas constant multiplied by the temperature.

$PV = nRT$ where R is the universal gas constant and n is the number of moles of gas.

What is the third perfect gas law?

The third perfect gas law is sometimes called Gay–Lussac's law. This law states that at a constant volume, the absolute pressure of a given gas is directly proportional to the absolute temperature.

$P \alpha T$, or $P/T = K$ where K is a constant.

What is a clinical application of the third perfect gas law?

A hydrogen thermometer relies on the third gas law for temperature measurement. When a constant volume of hydrogen is heated, it results in a rise in pressure. This pressure change can be accurately recorded and it gives a measure of the absolute temperature increase.

What is the definition of critical temperature?

The critical temperature is the temperature above which a gas cannot be liquefied regardless of how much pressure is applied.

What is the critical pressure?

It is the pressure needed to liquefy the gas at its critical temperature.

What is the difference between a gas and a vapour?

A gas is above its critical temperature, whilst a vapour is a substance in its gaseous form at a temperature below its critical temperature. This means a gas cannot be liquefied no matter how much pressure is applied, whereas a vapour can be liquefied if enough pressure is applied.

What is Dalton's law of partial pressures?

Dalton's law of partial pressures states that in a mixture of gases the pressure each gas exerts is the same as it would exert if it alone occupied the same volume.

For example, a cylinder filled with air is composed of 20.93% oxygen and 79.07% nitrogen. The full cylinder of air has an ambient pressure of 100 kPa. According to Dalton's law it is clear that the oxygen exerts 20.93 kPa whilst the nitrogen exerts 79.07 kPa.

Dalton's law is also relevant for the partial pressures of the different gases in the alveoli.

What is Henry's law?

When a liquid is placed in a closed container an equilibrium will be established between the vapour of the liquid and the liquid itself. In addition there is normally another gas present above the surface of the liquid, often nitrogen. Again, with time an equilibrium will form between molecules of nitrogen dissolved within the liquid and as a gas.

Henry's law states that at a particular temperature the amount of gas dissolved in a liquid is proportional to the partial pressure of the gas in equilibrium with the liquid.

When is Henry's law important?

Henry's law is important when considering hyperbaric oxygen therapy. According to Henry's law the amount of molecules of gas, in this case oxygen, that will dissolve in the solvent, in this example the plasma, is directly proportional to the partial pressure of the gas in equilibrium with the liquid. At atmospheric pressure and breathing air the amount of dissolved oxygen carried by the blood is very low and normally insignificant. However if the patient is exposed to 3 atmospheres of pressure the amount of oxygen dissolved in the blood increases dramatically according to Henry's law.

Henry's law is also important for divers. Recreational divers use compressed air mixtures, which they breathe at hyperbaric pressures, because every 10 meters they descend the pressure increases by 1 atmosphere. Breathing these gases under pressure causes the tissues to become saturated with nitrogen. Then if the diver ascends too quickly, the partial pressure of the nitrogen in the tissues will exceed the ambient pressure, so the nitrogen will come out of solution as small bubbles into the joints and circulation causing a condition called decompression sickness or "the bends".

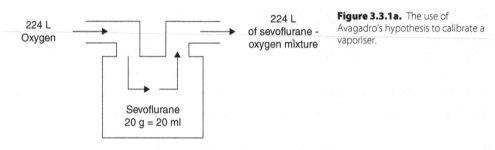

Figure 3.3.1a. The use of Avagadro's hypothesis to calibrate a vaporiser.

What is Avogadro's constant?

Avogadro's constant states that equal volumes of all gases under standard temperature and pressure will contain the same number of molecules.

However because the molecular weight of different gases varies, the actual mass of the different gases is different.

A mole is the quantity of a substance that contains the same number of molecules as there are atoms in 0.012 g of carbon-12. This number is 6.022×10^{23} molecules and is known as Avogadro's number. So, 1 mole of any gas at standard temperature and pressure will contain 6.022×10^{23} molecules and will occupy 22.4 litres.

How many molecules are there in 32 g of oxygen?

The molecular weight of oxygen is 32.32 g so according to Avogadro's constant this will contain 1 mole, or 6.02×10^{23} molecules.

When is Avogadro's hypothesis used in anaesthetic practice?

Avogadro's law is used to calibrate an anaesthetic vaporiser. Imagine you have a simple vaporiser containing 20 ml of sevoflurane with a steady stream of oxygen flowing into the vaporiser completely vaporising the sevoflurane into 224 litres of oxygen, see Figure 3.3.1a.

The density of sevoflurane is 1 g/ml, and the molecular weight is 200. Knowing the molecular weight is 200 allows us to calculate that 1 mole of sevoflurane is 200 g and according to Avogadro's hypothesis will occupy 22.4 litres. The vaporiser contains only 20 g (20 ml) of sevoflurane, which is equivalent to one tenth of a mole of sevoflurane, so will occupy one tenth of 22.4 litres, which is 2.24 litres. However, this 2.24 litres of sevoflurane is vaporised into 224 litres of oxygen, so the concentration of sevoflurane will be 2.24 divided by 224 which is 1%.

3.3.2. Flow – Caroline V Sampson

Define flow

Flow is a very important topic and will come up either in an OSCE or a structured oral examination or both. Have a definition that you know so well it just rolls off the tongue without you even having to think about it!

Flow is the quantity of fluid passing a point per unit of time. Fluid can be either gas or liquid. The units normally used in medicine are litres or millilitres per minute or hour.

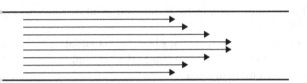

Figure 3.3.2a. Laminar flow.

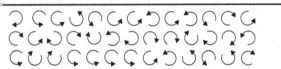

Figure 3.3.2b. Turbulent flow.

Discuss laminar and turbulent flow profiles. Draw a diagram for each

If you get stuck just remember a calm river for laminar flow – the fastest flow is in the middle, with the slowest flow next to the banks – and a set of rapids for turbulent flow. The diagrams are easy. First draw two tubes – these need only be parallel lines. Your laminar flow diagram will consist of a number of parallel lines, the longest in the middle representing the fastest flow and the shortest at the edge representing the slowest flow. The arrows form a bullet shape at their tips. The turbulent flow profile consists of lots of little curly arrows going in all directions.

In laminar flow, fluid moves smoothly with molecules moving in parallel. It is usually present in smooth tubes at low flow rates. The fluid can be thought of as moving in concentric rings whereby the fluid in the centre of the tube moves twice as fast as the fluid at the sides, see Figure 3.3.2a. This is due to the frictional forces between the sides of the tube and the fluid molecules slowing down the fluid closest to the edge.

Turbulent flow is disordered and molecules swirl in eddies and vortices, see Figure 3.3.2b. Turbulent flow is most likely in irregular tubes at a constriction, a corner or a narrowing, or with fast flow rates. Turbulent flow is less efficient and conversion from laminar to turbulent flow in a tube will reduce the flow for a given pressure drop.

Discuss the Hagen–Poiseuille equation. Why is it clinically relevant?

You must know this equation, so write it down repeatedly until it is firmly stuck in your head.

Laminar flow in Newtonian fluids (which have constant viscosity) in a tube is governed by the Hagen–Poiseuille equation. This states that flow equals the change in pressure $\times \pi \times$ the radius to the power of four divided by eight times the viscosity times the length of the tube. The formula is written like this:

$$\text{Flow} = \frac{\Delta P \Pi \Gamma^4}{8\eta|}.$$

Therefore flow is directly proportional to the change in pressure along the tube and inversely proportional to the length of the tube and the viscosity. This is why if we wish to infuse intravenous fluids rapidly we use a compression bag and increase the height of the fluid above the patient, which increases the pressure difference, and we shorten the length of the tubing. Likewise it is easier to infuse normal saline than blood as the former is less viscous. However the factor making the greatest difference in flow rates is the radius of the tube as flow is directly proportional to the fourth power of the radius. Doubling the radius will increase the flow rate by 16 times. Therefore the most important factor if you want to infuse fluid quickly is a wide bore intra-venous cannula.

This is also important in the airways. Secretions partially blocking an endotracheal tube in a neonate will have a far greater effect on air flow to the lungs than it would in the adult patient as the reduction of radius is much more marked.

What does gauge stand for on IV cannulae and what are the different flow rates possible through different cannulae?

It is important to talk about different gauge cannulae here rather than their colours as these can vary depending on the manufacturer. You have to just learn the numbers parrot fashion I'm afraid!

Gauge is an abbreviation for standard wire gauge and refers to the cross-sectional area of the cannula. It actually refers to the number of wires with the same diameter as the cannula in question that would fit into a certain sized hole; therefore the higher the gauge number the smaller the cannula diameter.

The flows for different gauge cannulae are as follows:

- 22G cannula is 20–40 ml/min
- 20G cannula is 40–80 ml/min
- 18G cannula is 75–120 ml/min
- 16G cannula is 130–220 ml/min
- 14G cannula is 250–330 ml/min.

What is Reynold's number?

Reynold's number is a dimensionless number which predicts whether flow will be laminar or turbulent within a particular tube. The formula to calculate Reynold's number is the linear velocity of the fluid times the density times the diameter, divided by the viscosity. A Reynold's number of less than 2000 predicts laminar flow, whereas a number greater than 4000 confidently predicts turbulent flow. Between 2000 and 4000 flow is usually turbulent, but there is still a chance it could be laminar.

$$\text{Reynold's number} = \frac{vpD}{\eta}.$$

How can you decrease the work of breathing using flow?

Turbulent flow is much more inefficient than laminar flow. Airflow in the upper airways is classically turbulent. Therefore to decrease the work of breathing the aim would be to reduce Reynold's number within the airway. An example of how this is done clinically is in the use of heliox in cases of upper airway obstruction. Heliox is a mixture of 30% oxygen in 70% helium and is five times less dense than 30% oxygen in 70% nitrogen, it therefore improves flow. As the viscosities of the two gas mixtures are similar it would not make any difference if flow were laminar.

The most important factor in laminar flow is radius, therefore always use the biggest endotracheal tube that will fit without causing mucosal damage as this will decrease the work of breathing spontaneously through a tube. This is most important in neonates and infants, although it would be rare to let this age group breathe spontaneously through a tube for any length of time.

What is the Bernoulli principle?

It is important not to get too mixed up between the different terms. Bernouilli's principle states that an increase in the speed of the fluid occurs simultaneously with a decrease in pressure or a decrease in the fluid's hydraulic potential energy. The Venturi effect is the drop in fluid pressure that results when an incompressible fluid flows through a constricted section of pipe. A Venturi pipe (or just a Venturi) is a tube which decreases in cross-sectional area and then increases again; that is gets narrower then wider. So Venturi demonstrated Bernouilli's principle with a narrowed tube.

Bernouilli's principle states that an increase in the velocity of a fluid must occur simultaneously with a decrease in pressure difference. The Bernoulli effect is demonstrated when fluid flows through a constriction in a tube or over an aerofoil surface. The first law of thermodynamics states that in any process, the total energy of the universe remains the same. Fluid flowing down a tube displays two different types of energy – the kinetic energy of the fluid as demonstrated by how quickly it is flowing and the potential energy of the pressure drop across the tube. At any narrowing in a tube fluid velocity will increase, therefore the fluid's kinetic energy increases. To compensate and keep the total energy the same the potential energy must therefore decrease manifesting as a pressure drop.

What is the Venturi principle and when is it used clinically?

The Venturi principle utilises the Bernoulli effect by having a constriction in a tube that gradually decreases in cross-sectional area then increases again. The pressure drop created can be used to entrain another fluid into the tube. This is used in fixed-performance oxygen masks, which are also called Venturi masks. Oxygen is passed through a narrow orifice creating a jet; the pressure drop entrains a constant proportion of air through holes in the side of the mask, delivering a fixed oxygen concentration. Different masks have different sized holes and require a different oxygen flow, for example the 24% oxygen mask requires a flow rate of 2 L/min. They then deliver a fixed fractional inspired oxygen concentration of 24 to 60% oxygen that is independent of the patient's minute volume. This is very useful in certain situations, for example in chronic obstructive pulmonary disease patients. The Venturi principle can also be used in the Sanders injector, in scavenging equipment, to humidify gases and to entrain liquid in nebulisers.

What is jet entrainment and what is meant by the entrainment ratio?

Jet entrainment occurs when a high-speed jet of gas, for example oxygen, pulls air along with it due to the frictional forces created by the fast moving oxygen molecules. In essence the injected gas drags the surrounding air with it. This is the main principle behind the Sanders injector. The total entrained flow is due to both the Bernoulli effect and jet entrainment. The entrainment ratio is defined as the ratio of entrained flow to driving flow.

What is the Coanda effect and what is its clinical relevance?

If this sounds a little far-fetched just run a tap and bring the curved surface of a spoon slowly towards it – the water will bend towards and around the spoon deflecting from its original path.

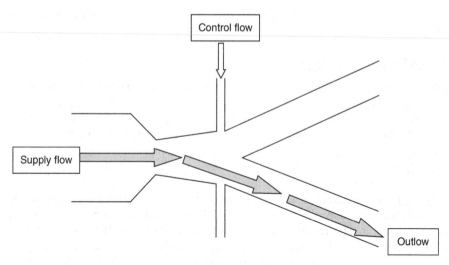

Figure 3.3.2c. Coanda effect – fluid logic valve mechanism.

The Coanda effect describes the fact that any fluid coming into contact with a curved surface will cling to this surface rather than follow a straight line in its original direction of flow. This is due to the solid stationary curved surface creating friction between itself and the fluid and therefore having a drag effect on the layer of fluid closest to the solid surface. This in turn has a drag effect on the next layer of fluid and so on, pulling the layers into the line of the curved surface. The Coanda effect is also seen with gases, when the flow of gas reaches a narrow part of a tube the low pressure created causes the gas to stick to one side of the tube. If the tube divides into two via a Y connector the gas will flow down one limb of the Y only. It is therefore due to a combination of the Venturi effect and surface tension.

The Coanda effect is said to explain the maldistribution of air in the pulmonary tree after a constricted portion of bronchiole, as the flow will stream along one fork of the division, leading to unequal distribution of gas flow. It has also been implicated in myocardial infarction – where narrowed coronary arteries proximal to a bifurcation cause blood to flow down one limb of the bifurcation, causing the cardiac muscle supplied by the other limb to infarct even though there was never a complete occlusion of either limb.

Where is the Coanda effect used in ventilators?

The Coanda effect can be used to make a valve mechanism with no moving parts if two tubes connected to a separate fluid supply are inserted at right angles before a Y junction in a tube. Fluid will naturally flow down one limb of the Y due to the Coanda effect, but can then be forced to flow down the other arm of the Y diversion by being pushed to this side by a flow of gas down one of the extra right angle tubes, see Figure 3.3.2c. Once the direction of flow is altered the fluid will remain travelling down this limb of the tube again due to the Coanda effect. Devices of this kind are known as fluid logic and can be introduced into ventilators to reduce the number of moving parts and valves needed. An example of a ventilator using fluid logic is the Penlon–Nuffield ventilator.

Tell me about rotameters

Rotameters are fixed-pressure variable orifice flowmeters. A bobbin or ball is supported in a tapered glass or plastic tube by the gas flow being measured. An equilibrium is reached at each different flow rate where the force of gas pushing up on the bobbin is matched by the weight of the bobbin. A gap exists between the bobbin and the tube wall. At low flows the gap is small, the tube walls are essentially parallel and the gas flow is laminar. As flow is laminar it depends upon viscosity. At higher gas flows the gap is much larger; however flow is turbulent and depends upon density. It is therefore important to know the viscosity and density of the gas being measured when calibrating the tube.

Do you know of any safety features used in rotameters?

Although positioned farthest from the common gas outlet, the oxygen is the last gas to be added to the fresh gas mixture. This is to avoid a hypoxic mixture being delivered to the patient in the event of a cracked rotameter.

Similarly the oxygen and nitrous oxide rotameter knobs are linked, so that nitrous oxide cannot be delivered to the patient without a safe concentration of oxygen also being delivered.

What can make rotameter readings inaccurate?

Electrostatic charges can build up on the bobbin especially at low flows, which could result in the bobbin sticking and giving an inaccurate reading. The bobbin therefore has small slits cut diagonally so it rotates in the gas flow to indicate free movement. Likewise the inside of the tubes are coated with a clear conductive coating or have a conductive strip to conduct away any electrostatic forces that build up.

Rotameters are gas specific – they cannot be used for different gases unless they are recalibrated.

The tubing must be vertical and flow rates should be read from the top of the rotating bobbin and the centre of the rotating ball.

3.3.3. Measurement of gas volume and flow – Rebecca A Leslie

Why do we measure gas flow?

When answering this question try to think about the occasions when we as anaesthetists measure gas flow.

As anaesthetists we measure gas flow to monitor respiratory flow in the patient's breathing circuit, to monitor the gas flow through the anaesthetic machine and as part of pulmonary function tests.

What is a Benedict–Roth spirometer?

Draw a simple and clear diagram whilst explaining the principles of the Benedict–Roth spirometer, see Figure 3.3.3a.

A Benedict–Roth spirometer is a light bell that is up turned in a water bath and contains a known quantity of air. As the subject breathes in and out of the air in the bell, the bell falls and rises. The movement of the bell is recorded by a pen moving over a rotating drum, which produces a spirometry trace.

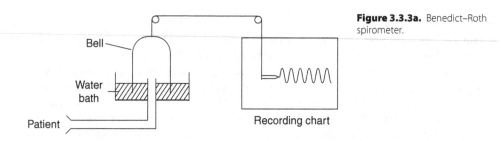

Figure 3.3.3a. Benedict–Roth spirometer.

Does the Benedict–Roth spirometer measure gas flow?

No. The Benedict–Roth spirometer does not measure gas flow it measures gas volume. However, gas flow can be derived from the spirometry trace because volume and flow are related. The volume of gas recorded over a given time is the gas flow.

What does a Vitalograph measure?

A Vitalograph is a set of bellows that are used to measure gas volume. The top plate of the bellows pivots and the motion is recorded by a pen on to a chart. The chart is motor driven and automatically starts moving as soon as the bellows fill up. This means that volume–time graphs are recorded. The gas flow rate can then be calculated from the volume–time graphs.

What are the advantages and disadvantages of the Vitalograph?

An advantage of the Vitalograph is that it is much smaller and therefore more portable than the Benedict–Roth spirometer. A disadvantage is that the Vitalograph only actually measures expiratory volume however from this, gas flow can be derived. Also the Vitalograph is only suitable for measuring limited gas volumes up to a few litres, which limits its use in anaesthesia. Another disadvantage of the Vitalograph is that the results are very dependent on the subject's technique.

What do you know about Wright's respirometer?

Questions on the Wright's respirometer often come up at an OSCE station. They may show you one and expect you to know what it is. Try and find one, so you are familiar with what it looks like. If you are presented with an unusual piece of equipment in the exam have a good long look at it before you start to panic because they often have their name written on!

Wrights respirometer allows you to measure tidal volumes in anaesthesia. It consists of an inlet and an outlet port, and a rotating vane that is surrounded by slits that direct the air in a circular motion to rotate the vane. The vane is attached to a pointer, which displays the gas volume. See Figure 3.3.3b.

Gas flow rates can be derived by averaging the tidal volumes over a period of time.

What are the limitations of the Wright's respirometer?

The Wright's respirometer is a one-way system that only allows the measurement of the tidal volume if the gas flow is unidirectional. Therefore it can only measure either inspiration or

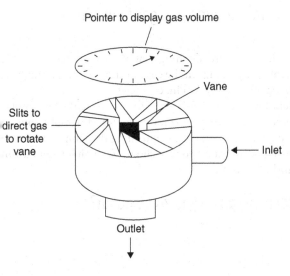

Pointer to display gas volume

Vane

Slits to direct gas to rotate vane

Inlet

Outlet

Figure 3.3.3b. Wrights respirometer.

expiration. For measurement of tidal volume in anaesthesia it should be placed in the expiratory limb of the breathing circuit as close to the patient's trachea as possible.

The Wright's respirometer is only accurate to approximately 5–10%, and its accuracy varies with the flow. It tends to over-read at high gas flows due to high flow inertia and under-read at low gas flows due to low flow friction.

Another problem with Wright's respirometer is that water condensation from exhaled gases may cause the pointer to stick and prevent it from rotating freely, leading to inaccuracies in the measurement.

Wright's respirometer does not give electrical output for analysis and recording which is an obvious disadvantage of its use in clinical practice. However it pre-dates electronic systems and was a very high quality mechanical system of its time.

What does a pneumotachograph measure?

A pneumotachograph measures gas flow and from this the gas volume can be calculated by integrating the flow signal over the duration of the inspiration or expiration.

What is the principle behind the screen pneumotachograph?

Give a simple and succinct description of how a pneumotachograph works. You may also find it helpful to draw a diagram.

A pneumotachograph is a "constant resistance, variable pressure" flowmeter. The screen pneumotachograph contains a gauze screen that has a sufficient diameter for the gas to move through with laminar flow. When the gas flows through the screen gauze there will be a pressure drop that is measured by two pressure ports, one on either side of the gauze screen. Because the resistance is constant, any change in pressure is proportional to gas flow. The pressure change is measured by a transducer, which converts the pressure change into an electrical signal.

A pneumotachograph can be incorporated into the breathing circuit and can measure rapid changes in the patient's respiration.

What could cause inaccuracies in measurement of gas flow with a pneumotachograph?

Laminar flow depends on fluid viscosity, therefore anything that alters the viscosity of the gas will affects its accuracy. Consequently, any change in the composition of the gas mixture, such as the addition of an anaesthetic agent, may lead to inaccuracies.

In addition, changes in the temperature of the gas mixture will also make the pneumotachograph inaccurate. In order to overcome this problem, some pneumotachographs contain a heating element that maintains a constant temperature. Controlling the temperature also prevents water vapour from condensing on to the pneumotachograph, which would again disrupt the laminar flow and cause turbulent flow.

What other types of pneumotachograph do you know about?

There are four different types of pneumotachographs:

- Screen pneumotachographs
- Fleisch pneumotachographs
- Hot-wire pneumotachographs
- Pitot tubes.

A Fleisch pneumotachograph consists of a bundle of fine bore parallel tubes that ensure laminar gas flow resistance. Again the pressure drop through the tubes is measured and is directly proportional to the gas flow as per the Hagen–Poiseuille equation. Heating the parallel tubes prevents condensation of water vapour. The Fleisch pneumotachograph is more bulky and much larger than a screen pneumotachograph.

A hot-wire pneumotachograph contains two hot wires that are mounted at right angles to each other in the lumen of the pneumotachograph. The gas flow results in cooling of the wires which is dependent on the gas flow. Cooling of the wires varies their resistance so a small electrical signal is produced. A disadvantage of the hot-wire pneumotachograph is that it requires energy to heat the wires.

The pitot tube pneumotachograph consists of two pressure sampling tubes which are mounted in the centre of the gas flow. One sampling port faces downstream, whilst the other faces upstream. The upstream port measures a higher pressure reading because it receives the full impact of the gas flow, whilst the downstream port measures the static pressure. A differential pressure transducer measures the difference between these two ports, and is dependent of gas flow. The pitot tube pneumotachograph is commonly used because it is small, cheap, simple and does not lead to the addition of a large volume of dead-space into the breathing circuit.

Gas supply and delivery

3.4.1. Cylinders and gas supply – Rebecca A Leslie

The following question may take the form of an OSCE station rather than a structured oral examination question. It is crucial you have a good level of understanding about the supply of the gases that we rely on every day.

How are medical gases supplied to the anaesthetic machine?

Gases such as oxygen, air and nitrous oxide are supplied from cylinders stored on the back of the anaesthetic machine or from the pipeline gas supply.

How can you identify different cylinders?

This question gives you the opportunity to demonstrate good knowledge of the equipment you are using every day.

Cylinders are colour coded for easy identification. In the UK a two part colour-coding system is used with the body and the shoulders different colours.

For example, oxygen cylinders are black with white shoulders, whilst air has a black body with black and white chequered shoulders. Nitrous oxide has both a French blue body with French blue shoulders, in contrast to Entonox which has a French blue body with blue and white chequered shoulders. Helium is stored in a cylinder with a brown body and shoulders.

What information is engraved on the gas cylinder?

There are a number of pieces of information engraved on gas cylinders. Firstly each cylinder has a unique serial number which is engraved onto it. The chemical formula of the gas is stencilled both on the shoulder of the cylinder and on the valve block. The tare weight, which is the weight of the cylinder when empty, is engraved on the cylinder. Finally, the test pressure and dates of tests performed are also engraved on the cylinder.

Dr Podcast Scripts for the Primary FRCA, ed. Rebecca A. Leslie, Emily K. Johnson and Alexander P. L. Goodwin. Published by Cambridge University Press. © R. A. Leslie, E. K. Johnson and A. P. L. Goodwin 2011.

What other information will you find on the cylinder?

The label on the cylinder states:

- The name
- Chemical symbol
- The batch number
- Hazards and safety notes
- Cylinder size code
- Maximum cylinder pressure
- The filling date
- Shelf-life and expiry date
- Directions for use
- Storage handling.

There is also a small plastic coloured ring around the cylinder neck which states the year when it was last tested.

What size cylinders do we commonly use in our anaesthetic practice?

Cylinders come in many different sizes, A to J. Size E cylinders are used on the anaesthetic machine. Size E cylinder will hold 680 L of oxygen, and 1800 L of nitrous oxide. As the letter of the cylinder size increases the volume also increases. Size J cylinders, the largest cylinders, can contain 6800 L of oxygen and 18 000 L of nitrous oxide and are normally used in cylinder manifolds.

What are the differences between an oxygen and nitrous oxide cylinder?

Oxygen is stored as a gas at a pressure of 13 700 kPa. In accordance with Boyle's law at constant temperature the pressure in an oxygen cylinder is inversely proportional to the volume of gas. So, for a cylinder of fixed volume a reduction in pressure will represent a reduction in the contents of the cylinder. Therefore if the cylinder is half full then the pressure exerted by the gas will be half of 13 700 kPa, i.e., 6850 kPa. All cylinders which contain only gas will act in a similar manner to oxygen cylinders.

Nitrous oxide however is stored in a liquid phase with its vapour on top of the liquid exerting a pressure of 4400 kPa. This is because the critical temperature of nitrous oxide is 36.5°C which is higher than room temperature. When nitrous oxide is used the vapour is released first. As a consequence of the vapour being used, liquid will vaporise to replace the used vapour. Thus the pressure exerted by the vapour is always the same, and the gauge will continue to read 4400 kPa. The pressure in the nitrous oxide cylinder will only drop when all the liquid has been used up, and only vapour remains. So unlike with oxygen cylinders the pressure in a nitrous oxide cylinder is not an accurate way of assessing how much nitrous oxide is left. Instead the weight of the cylinder is used.

You mentioned critical temperature, what do you mean by this term?

The critical temperature is defined as the temperature above which the substance cannot be liquefied no matter how much pressure is applied. Oxygen has a critical temperature of

−119°C, so in an oxygen cylinder at room temperature no matter how much pressure is applied to the cylinder it is impossible to turn the oxygen into its liquid form.

In contrast the critical temperature of nitrous oxide is 36.5°C, so it is below its critical temperature at room temperature. As a result it exists as both a liquid and a vapour.

What is the pseudocritical temperature?

The pseudocritical temperature rather than critical temperature is used for gas mixtures such as Entonox.

The pseudocritical temperature is the temperature when there is a risk that the gas mixture may separate out into its constituent gases. For example in Entonox cylinders there is a risk of liquefaction and separation if the temperature in the cylinder falls below −5.5°C. This is called the Poynting effect and results in a liquid containing mostly nitrous oxide with only approximately 20% oxygen dissolved in it, and above it a gas mixture containing a high concentration of oxygen. This means that when Entonox is used at a constant flow rate at a temperature below −5.5°C, initially a gas with a high concentration of oxygen is supplied. This is followed by a gas with decreasing oxygen concentration as the liquid nitrous oxide evaporates. It is possible under these circumstances to deliver a hypoxic gas mixture. Rewarming and mixing the constituents of the cylinder will reverse the separation.

What is the filling ratio?

Liquid is much less compressible than gas, so any increase in the ambient temperature could lead to a dangerous increase in pressure within the cylinder. To overcome this risk, the cylinders are only partially filled. The filling ratio is the weight of the liquid in the cylinder divided by the weight of water required to fill the cylinder. In the UK the filling ratio for nitrous oxide and carbon dioxide is 0.75. In hotter climates the filling ratio needs to be lower, often 0.67.

Sometimes when you use nitrous oxide you get ice forming on the outside of the cylinder, what causes this?

As the vapour in the nitrous oxide cylinder is used, liquid nitrous oxide vaporises to replace the used vapour. This process requires energy. The energy, called the latent heat of vaporisation, is supplied from the remaining liquid nitrous oxide and consequently the temperature of this liquid will drop. This drop in temperature can lead to the formation of ice on the outside of the cylinder.

What is the pin-index system and why is it used?

The pin-index system is a safety system which makes it almost impossible to connect a cylinder to the wrong yoke on the anaesthetic machine. There are specific pins on the yoke of the anaesthetic machine. These correspond to specific holes on the valve block of the cylinders. Unless these pins and holes match the cylinder cannot be fitted to the anaesthetic machine.

What are cylinders made of?

Cylinders are made of thin-walled seamless molybdenum steel. Lightweight cylinders can also be made from an aluminium alloy with a fibreglass covering in epoxy resin matrix. These are much lighter, tend to be smaller in size and are used to provide oxygen at home or on transport.

How are cylinders tested?

Cylinders in use are checked and tested by manufacturers at regular intervals, normally 5 years. This involves several different tests.

Internally endoscopic examination is carried out to look for cracks and defects in the inner surface.

Each cylinder is then subjected to high pressures, much higher than their normal working pressure, of normally approximately 22 000 kPa. This pressure is then stencilled on the valve block.

One out of every 100 cylinders undergoes tensile testing, where it is cut into strips and it is stretched to assess the yield point.

Bending, flattening and impact tests are also performed on 1 in every 100 cylinders.

What are the safety features of pipelined gases?

Pipelined medical gases and vacuum (PMGV) is a system where gases are supplied from a central store at a pressure of approximately 400 kPa.

The pipelines are made of special high quality alloyed carbon which prevents the breakdown of the gases it carries and also has bacteriostatic properties.

Outlet sockets are found throughout the hospital and the gas supplied is identified by name, shape and colour-coding.

Colour-coded hoses connect the outlet socket to the anaesthetic machine; these hoses have a quick connect/release Schrader valve, with an indexing collar for each gas. A single hose and tug test should be performed to check for misconnection or cross-connection.

The hoses should be permanently attached to the anaesthetic machine with a non-interchangeable screw thread.

Where are pipeline gases stored?

Pipeline gases come from a cylinder manifold, and in the case of oxygen it may be stored as liquid oxygen in a vacuum-insulated evaporator (VIE).

What size cylinders make up the cylinder manifold?

Size J cylinders are used, which can store 6800 litres of oxygen. The cylinders are divided into two groups, the primary and secondary group. All the cylinders in each group are connected to a common pipe through non-return and pressure-reducing valves. Initially all the cylinders in the primary group simultaneously empty, when the cylinders are nearly empty the gas supply automatically changes over to the second group of cylinders. The changeover is triggered by a pressure-sensitive device which senses when the pressure in the cylinders is getting low. The changeover also activates an electrical signalling system to alert staff to change over the primary group of cylinders.

Describe how a vacuum-insulated evaporator works

You may find it easy to explain about vacuum-insulated evaporators with the use of a diagram (see Figure 3.4.1a), if you volunteer to draw a diagram make sure you are confident in doing so

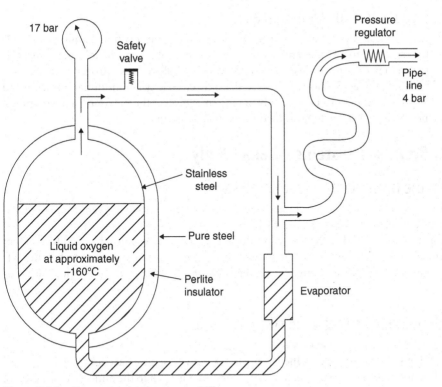

17 bar

Safety
valve

Pressure
regulator

Pipe-
line
4 bar

Stainless
steel

Pure steel

Liquid oxygen
at approximately
−160°C

Perlite
insulator

Evaporator

Figure 3.4.1a. Vacuum-insulated evaporator (VIE).

before you pick up the pencil. If you are not confident and they haven't specifically asked for a diagram just describe the salient features in words.

A vacuum-insulated evaporator (VIE) is the most economical way to store oxygen. The VIE consists of a thermally insulated double-walled steel tank with a layer of Perlite in a vacuum between the two layers acting as insulation. The inner wall of the tank is stainless steel whilst the outer wall is a pure steel jacket. The oxygen is stored in liquid form at temperatures well below its critical temperature, between −150 and −170°C. The vacuum shell helps maintain the low temperature. This is because as oxygen evaporates it requires heat, the latent heat of evaporation. This heat is taken from the liquid oxygen, helping to maintain its low temperature.

As oxygen is required it is passed through the main outlet at the top of the VIE. The cold oxygen gas is warmed by passing through a coil of copper tubing. An increase in the temperature of the gas causes an increase in the pressure of the gas, so it is also essential for the gas to subsequently pass through a pressure regulator to maintain a pressure of approximately 4 bar. If less oxygen is used than expected a safety valve opens at 17 bar to release the build-up of pressure.

If there is an increase in oxygen demand a control valve opens at the base of the VIE. This allows oxygen, in liquid form, to pass through a second outlet in addition to the main outlet at the top of the VIE. This liquid oxygen then passes through a super-heater made of un-insulated coils of copper tubing before joining the pipeline gas supply.

The VIE rests on a weighing balance to measure the mass of liquid oxygen.

How can you extract oxygen from air?

Oxygen concentrators extract oxygen from air by differential absorption. Ambient air is filtered and pressurised to 137 bar, and is then filtered through a Zeolite molecular sieve column, which has a very large surface area. The sieve selectively retains nitrogen which is then released back into the air. Concentrators require only electricity and minimal servicing and are reliable providing a continuous supply of oxygen. However the maximum concentration they can produce is 95% due to unwanted gases such as argon.

3.4.2. Breathing systems – Dana L Kelly

What is the function of a breathing system?

The basic functions of a breathing system are to maintain delivery of oxygen to a patient and to remove CO_2 excreted in the alveolar gas.

An anaesthetic breathing system, in addition to the above, must be able to conduct inhalational anaesthetic agents to the patient. It must also enable a patient to breathe satisfactorily without significantly increasing the work of breathing or the physiological deadspace.

How do you classify breathing systems?

Remember to first classify your answer.

Breathing systems can be classified as open, semi-open, semi-closed, or closed.

With an open breathing system, the respiratory tract is open to the atmosphere and there is no re-breathing within the system. The Schimmelbusch mask is an example of an open system.

With a semi-open breathing system, anaesthetic gases are carried by fresh gas but may be diluted with room air. Hudson masks and Venturi masks are examples of semi-open breathing systems.

With a semi-closed breathing system, anaesthetic gases are carried by fresh gas and there is no dilution with room air. Semi-closed breathing systems can be further sub-classified into the following:

- Re-breathing systems without CO_2 absorption
- Re-breathing systems with CO_2 absorption
- Non-rebreathing systems.

Examples of semi-closed breathing systems are Professor Mapleson's classification of breathing systems. Advantages of semi-closed breathing systems include the fact the system is more stable in that if the system fills to capacity the excess gas is simply lost via the pressure-relief valve. Also the higher flow rates allow use of a precision, out of circuit vaporiser. Disadvantages of a semi-closed breathing system are increased anaesthetic and oxygen usage and increased atmospheric pollution.

With a closed breathing system the system is closed to the atmosphere on both inspiration and expiration. Oxygen flows into the system to replace that consumed by the patient, and exhaled carbon dioxide is absorbed by the soda lime. An example of a closed breathing system is a circle system with APL valve entirely closed. Advantages of a closed breathing system include minimising anaesthetic and oxygen usage and also minimising atmospheric pollution. Disadvantages of a closed breathing system include the fact the system is inherently complex, in that if the fresh gas flow is not matched exactly to the patient's oxygen consumption, the system will over-fill or empty, and the patient will be unable to breathe. This is why the system is seldom used completely closed.

What are the features of an ideal breathing system?

The features that the ideal breathing system would demonstrate include efficient operation for both spontaneous and controlled ventilation, low dead-space and minimal resistance within the circuit. The ideal breathing system would allow economical use of the fresh gas supply and the volatile agent and effective removal of carbon dioxide. It would also limit pollution. It would be a light-weight system, be easy and failsafe to use, and have a wide patient application. The ideal breathing system would allow easy and reliable connection to monitoring equipment. Ideally it would be disposable and cost effective.

What factors determine re-breathing?

Re-breathing is defined as the inhalation of previously expired gases including carbon dioxide and water vapour. It depends on the design of an individual breathing system, the mode of ventilation (i.e. spontaneous or controlled), the patient's minute ventilation and the fresh gas flow rate

Discuss the Mapleson classification of anaesthetic breathing systems

The Mapleson classification refers to semi-closed re-breathing systems. It was introduced in 1954 by Professor W Mapleson. Breathing systems are classified into Mapleson A, B, C, D, E (and F) according to their configuration of several key components, see Figure 3.4.2a. These include a reservoir bag, an adjustable pressure-limiting expiratory valve, flexible tubing and face mask.

Tell me more about the Mapleson A breathing system

Mapleson A breathing system is also known as the Magill circuit. It is efficient for spontaneous ventilation due to conservation of exhaled dead-space gas within the reservoir bag and tubing and subsequent preferential venting of alveolar gas (containing CO_2) via APL valve due to increasing pressure within the breathing system. If the fresh gas flow is sufficiently high, all the alveolar gas is vented from the circuit before the next inspiration, and no re-breathing will take place.

In theory, fresh gas flow could fall as low as alveolar minute ventilation. In practice, a fresh gas flow equal to total minute ventilation is used to provide a margin of safety.

The Mapleson A system can be used for controlled ventilation but is relatively inefficient due to mixing of dead-space and alveolar gases. A fresh gas flow of 2–3 times minute ventilation is required to prevent re-breathing.

With the Magill system, the APL valve is near the patient. This reduces dead-space, but makes the circuit awkward to use, particularly when scavenging is used. This led to the development of the Lack circuit, which is a co-axial Magill circuit.

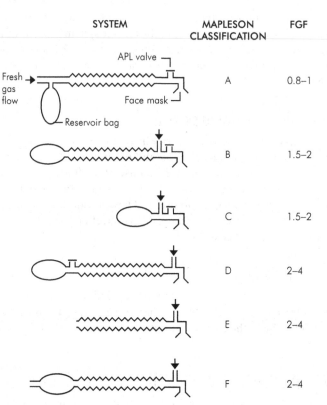

SYSTEM	MAPLESON CLASSIFICATION	FGF
	A	0.8–1
	B	1.5–2
	C	1.5–2
	D	2–4
	E	2–4
	F	2–4

Figure 3.4.2a. Mapleson Classification System from breathing systems. Reproduced with permission from Smith, T., Pinnock, C. and Lin, T. 2009. *Fundamentals of Anaesthesia.* Cambridge: Cambridge University Press. © Cambridge University Press 2009.

FGF is the fresh gas flow required to avoid rebreathing during spontaneous ventilation quoted as multiples of minute volume

The Lack circuit delivers fresh gas flow via an outer hose. The expiratory limb is via the inner hose, and the APL valve is placed next to the reservoir bag by the common gas outlet. The circuit is therefore less cumbersome to use, but there is high inspiratory resistance, and large apparatus dead-space.

Now tell me about Mapleson B and C breathing systems

These are practical circuits for resuscitation due to their simplicity. The Waters circuit is another name for the Mapleson C system. Both Mapleson B and C require a low-pressure oxygen supply and have low dead-space. However, re-breathing of exhaled gases occurs even when very high fresh gas flow rates are used, since inspiration is taken from the same space into which the previous breath was expired. These circuits are unsatisfactory for anaesthesia due to the high fresh gas flow rates required, but may be used for resuscitation.

Do we ever use a Mapleson D circuit?

Yes, the most commonly used Mapleson D circuit is the Bain circuit. This is a co-axial Mapleson D circuit, introduced in 1972 by Bain and Spoerel. Fresh gas flows down the central narrow bore tubing to the patient and exhaled gases travel in the outer corrugated tubing. This circuit has the practical advantage it can be of unlimited length, but notably the resistance within the circuit increases with increasing length. This is important as this system is often used in the MRI scanner. The reservoir bag may be removed and replaced by a ventilator such as the Nuffield Penlon 200 for mechanical ventilation, providing there is a long enough piece of tubing between the ventilator and the breathing system, otherwise the breathing gases are diluted by the driving gas (usually oxygen). The Mapleson D breathing system is inefficient for spontaneous ventilation; a fresh gas flow of at least 2 to 3 times minute ventilation is required. It is relatively more efficient for controlled ventilation; a fresh gas flow of 1–2 times minute ventilation is required.

Now tell me about the Mapleson E and T breathing systems

The Mapleson E breathing system is also known as the Ayre's T-piece. This system performs in a similar way to the Mapleson D, but has a smaller dead-space than other systems and because it has no valves there is less resistance to breathing. As a result it has proved very suitable for use with children. It is recommended as the circuit of choice for children weighing less than approximately 20 kg. The Mapleson E system is inefficient for spontaneous ventilation; a fresh gas flow of at least 2 times minute ventilation is required. It is relatively more efficient for controlled ventilation; a fresh gas flow of 1–2 times minute ventilation is required

The "Mapleson F" breathing circuit was not originally classified by Professor Mapleson, but the term Mapleson F is used to refer to Jackson–Rees' modification of Ayre's T-piece. The Jackson–Rees modification has an open bag attached to the expiratory limb. Movement of the bag can be seen during spontaneous breathing, and the bag can be compressed to provide manual ventilation. As in the Bain circuit, the bag may be replaced by a mechanical ventilator designed for use with children. Fresh gas flow rates are the same as for the Mapleson E system.

What is a Humphrey's circuit?

The Humphrey ADE circuit provides the ability to switch between the Mapleson A, D and E arrangements via a switch.

As discussed, the Mapleson A circuit is inefficient for controlled ventilation, as is the Mapleson D circuit for spontaneous ventilation. David Humphrey designed a single circuit that can be changed from a Mapleson A system to a Mapleson D by moving a lever on the metallic block which connects the circuit to the fresh gas outlet on the anaesthetic machine. The reservoir bag is situated at the fresh gas inlet end of the circuit, and gas is conducted to and from the patient down the inspiratory and expiratory limbs of the circuit.

Depending on the position of the control lever at the Humphrey block, gases either pass through the expiratory valve or the ventilator port. When the lever is "up" the reservoir bag and the expiratory valve are used, creating a Mapleson A-type circuit. When the lever is in the "down" position the bag and valve are by-passed and the ventilator port is opened creating a Mapleson D system for controlled ventilation. If no ventilator is attached and the port is left open the system will function like a Mapleson E circuit.

What are the basic components of a circle system?

The essential features of a circle system include a carbon dioxide absorber canister, a reservoir bag, unidirectional inspiratory and expiratory valves, a fresh gas supply, a pressure-relief valve, and connecting tubing, see Figure 3.4.2b.

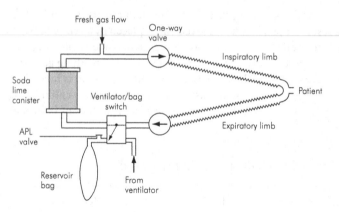

Figure 3.4.2b. A typical circle system. Reproduced with permission from Smith, T., Pinnock C. and Lin, T. 2009. *Fundamentals of Anaesthesia.* Cambridge: Cambridge University Press. © Cambridge University Press 2009.

3.4.3. Vaporisers – Rebecca A Leslie

What is a vaporiser?

A vaporiser is a device which allows controlled vaporisation of liquid anaesthetic agents into a vapour. A carefully controlled proportion of this anaesthetic vapour is then added to the fresh gas flow at a concentration suitable to produce anaesthesia.

Why is it necessary to use a vaporiser?

Try and think about basic principles. The key phrase that you must mention is saturated vapour pressure. If you do know the saturated vapour pressure of the commonly used volatiles mention them, but if you cannot remember them do not worry just explain the principles.

It is necessary to use a vaporiser because the saturated vapour pressure of volatile agents at room temperature is much higher than that required to produce anaesthesia.

The saturated vapour pressure is the partial pressure that the vapour of a liquid will exert if the liquid and the vapour of the liquid are in equilibrium. For example the saturated vapour pressure of sevoflurane at 20°C is 22.7 kPa. This means that it is able to reach a maximum concentration of 22.4%. This is calculated by dividing the saturated vapour pressure by the atmospheric pressure, which we know is 101.3 kPa.

Desflurane has an even higher saturated vapour pressure of 88.2 kPa which means it has a maximum achievable concentration of 87.1%.

At these concentrations these anaesthetic agents would be dangerous, so it is crucial we use a vaporiser which only allows a controlled amount of the anaesthetic agent into the fresh gas flow.

How would you classify vaporisers?

Vaporisers can be classified according to whether they are variable bypass vaporisers or measured flow vaporisers.

In variable bypass vaporisers the fresh gas flow is slit into two streams, one that enters the vaporising chamber and one that bypasses the vaporising chamber. The two streams then rejoin to give the required concentration of vapour to the patient. The vapour concentration is controlled by using a flow splitting valve which determines the fraction of the gas entering the

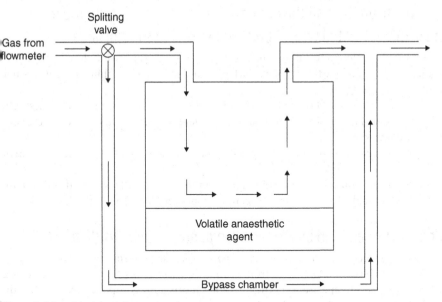

Figure 3.4.3a. Principle of plenum vaporisers.

vaporising chamber. Variable bypass vaporisers can be further classified as plenum vaporisers or draw-over vaporisers.

Draw-over vaporisers rely on sub-atmospheric pressure which is generated either mechanically or by the patient's respiratory effort to pull the gas through the vaporiser. Examples of a draw-over vaporiser include the Goldman vaporiser and the Oxford Miniature Vaporiser.

Plenum vaporisers are located on the back bar of the anaesthetic machine and the gas is forced through the vaporiser due to the positive pressure created by the gas supply. Examples include the Ohmeda TEC Mk 2, 3, 4 and 5.

Measured flow vaporisers produce a separate flow of vapour that is independently added into the patients fresh gas flow to produce the required concentration of volatile agent. An example of a measured flow vaporiser is the Ohmeda TEC 6 desflurane vaporiser.

How do plenum vaporisers work?

Keep this simple, if they want more details they can ask you. You should draw a simple diagram whilst explaining the principles, see Figure 3.4.3a.

The carrier gas is split into two streams as it enters the vaporiser, one stream enters the vaporising chamber, whilst the remainder passes through a bypass chamber. The exact amount that bypasses the vaporising chamber depends on the dialled concentration. The gas entering the vaporising chamber becomes fully saturated with vapour. The two different streams then rejoin as they leave the vaporiser, and a gas with only a small concentration of anaesthetic vapour is produced and passes to the patient.

When using a plenum vaporiser at low gas flows changes in the dialled concentration of the anaesthetic agent are reflected very slowly within the circle system. For this reason it is often necessary to increase the fresh gas flow rate in order to rapidly increase the depth of anaesthesia when using a plenum vaporiser.

How do we ensure that all the gas entering the vaporising chamber becomes fully saturated with vapour and why is this important?

We use a number of different techniques to ensure the gas in the vaporising chamber becomes fully saturated. These include the use of wicks, baffles and in the past bubbling the gas through the liquid anaesthetic agent.

Wicks are either metal or fabric and one end of the wick dips into the liquid anaesthetic agent. Due to the surface tension of the anaesthetic agent it is drawn up the wick, increasing the surface area for vaporisation.

Baffles act by repeatedly directing the gas flow onto the surface of the liquid anaesthetic agent.

It is important that the gas entering the vaporising chamber is fully saturated with volatile agent so that we are able to administer an accurate concentration of anaesthetic.

What do you understand by the term *temperature compensation*?

First describe the principle, then describe how we overcome the problem in practice.

In order for a substance to change from a liquid into a vapour heat is required, this is called the latent heat of vaporisation. The heat for vaporisation is supplied from either the liquid or from the surroundings. If there is no temperature compensation in a vaporiser the remaining liquid anaesthetic would get colder as some vaporises. This causes a fall in the saturated vapour pressure, and the concentration of anaesthetic vapour delivered to the patient would consequently fall. In order to make sure the patient continues to receive the same concentration of volatile agent the splitting ratio must be adjusted so that more of the fresh gas flow enters the vaporising chamber, and less bypasses it. In modern vaporisers this adjustment happens automatically by a temperature-controlled valve which adjusts the splitting ratio.

The temperature-controlled valve most commonly utilised is the bimetallic strip. This consists of two dissimilar metals which have different coefficients of thermal expansion. This means that if the temperature changes one of the metals expands or contracts more than the other, so the shape of the metal strip alters and it allows more gas into the vaporising chamber for a given dial setting.

A different type of temperature-controlled valve uses small flexible bellows which are filled with a liquid which has a high coefficient of thermal expansion. As a result when the temperature changes the bellows contract or expand and alter the amount of gas entering the vaporising chamber.

In addition to automatic, temperature-controlled valves, vaporisers are made of a metal with a good thermal conductivity. This allows heat to be transferred from the surroundings into the vaporising chamber maintaining the temperature of the liquid anaesthetic.

What is the actual definition of latent heat of vaporisation?

If you have just mentioned a term, don't be surprised if they then ask more details about it.

Latent heat of vaporisation is the amount of heat energy needed to convert 1 kg of a substance from the liquid form into a vapour at any given temperature. The SI unit for latent heat of vaporisation is joules per kilogram.

Can you put isoflurane in a vaporiser designed for halothane?

Vaporisers are carefully calibrated for individual agents depending on their saturated vapour pressure. If an anaesthetic agent is accidently put into the wrong vaporiser then it will deliver either a very high or a very low concentration of anaesthetic. For example if desflurane, with its very high saturated vapour pressure, is put in a sevoflurane vaporiser which has a much lower saturated vapour pressure then it will deliver an extremely high concentration of anaesthetic. Even a very small difference in saturated vapour pressure between agents could make a significant difference to the concentration of anaesthetic administered. The saturated vapour pressures of isoflurane and halothane are different by only 0.4 kPa but this can cause a difference in concentration of anaesthetic administered of up to 50% if isoflurane is used in a halothane vaporiser. So it is therefore advisable that anaesthetic agents are only put in vaporisers designed specifically for that agent.

What are the potential problems of a plenum vaporiser?

The original vaporisers were extremely flow dependent and the concentration of the anaesthetic agent depended on the gas flow. At high flows the gas concentration became much lower. Flow dependence has been overcome by ensuring that all the gas entering the vaporising channel becomes fully saturated with volatile agent and newer vaporisers are now independent of gas flow at rates of between 0.5 and 15 L/min. Outside these limits they will deliver less volatile agent than the dialled concentration.

Another potential problem with the plenum vaporiser is that overfilling the vaporiser may lead to the liquid volatile agent passing directly into the bypass chamber, leading to dangerously high anaesthetic concentrations.

If IPPV is used with a plenum vaporiser then it can increase the pressure and force air back into the vaporising chamber and saturated gas back into the bypass channel. This is called the "pumping effect". With forward flow of the gas when the ventilator cycles, a higher concentration of delivered vapour is given to the patient due to saturated gas being in the bypass channel.

In addition, if the pressure increases in the vaporising channel, for example when high gas flows are used with large vaporising chambers, then this may cause the gas to expand and then be forced both out of the inlet and outlet of the vaporising channel when the pressure again drops. This would result in fully saturated gas then passing through the bypass channel combining with the normal splitting ratio of saturated gas, and the vapour concentration being much higher than desired. This is described as the "pressuring effect".

If the plenum vaporisers were not temperature compensated then as the temperature of the liquid drops due to the latent heat of vaporisation the concentration of the volatile agent would also drop.

You mentioned the "pumping effect". How is this overcome?

The pumping effect is overcome by ensuring that there is a pressurising valve downstream of the vaporiser to ensure that the pressure in the vaporiser is constant and always greater than the ventilator.

How is the "pressurising effect" overcome?

The bypass chamber and the vaporising channel are designed to be the same size so that if gas expansion does occur, the expansion occurs equally in both routes so no retrograde flow occurs. Also a long inlet tube into the vaporiser ensures that if there is retrograde flow there is will never reach the bypass chamber.

What other safety features are incorporated into modern vaporisers?

Modern vaporisers have an anti-spill mechanism so that even if they are turned upside down liquid anaesthetic will not pass into the bypass chamber.

There is also an interlocking system between the vaporisers on the back bar, so that only one vaporiser can be used at a time.

The devices that are used for filling vaporisers are geometrically coded to only fit into the filling port of the correct vaporiser. They are also colour coded, for example sevoflurane vaporisers and filling devices are always yellow, isoflurane always purple and desflurane always blue. The filling devices also prevent the vaporisers from being overfilled which could potentially result in volatile agent entering the bypass chamber.

How is the desflurane vaporiser different from the rest?

Although the Tec Mk 6 vaporiser looks similar to the other Tec vaporisers it is completely different and is specifically designed for desflurane. Desflurane has a much lower boiling point than the other volatile agents and has a very high saturated vapour pressure of 88 kPa at room temperature. Because the boiling point of desflurane is 23.5°C and near room temperature, small changes in the operating theatre temperature could lead to very large changes in the SVP with an increase in depth of anaesthesia. To overcome this desflurane vaporisers contain a heating element which heats desflurane to a temperature of 39°C. An increase in temperature increases the saturated vapour pressure. When heated to 39°C desflurane has a saturated vapour pressure of 200 kPa. As the gas is now under pressure, a pressure-reducing valve is incorporated to reduce the pressure. Unlike in plenum vaporisers the fresh gas flow does not enter the vaporising channel, instead the desflurane is injected into the fresh gas flow, and the amount injected reflects the concentration of anaesthetic volatile agent delivered to the patient. A percentage control dial with a rotary valve controls the flow of desflurane vapour into the fresh gas flow.

What adjustments need to be made to vaporisers used at altitude?

Remember the saturated vapour pressure does not change with altitude, so the partial pressure of the vapour leaving the channel will not change. However the concentration of gas that leaves the chamber will be dependent on the ratio of that pressure to the atmospheric pressure. So if the atmospheric pressure drops, as it does at higher altitudes, the SVP is a greater proportion of the atmospheric pressure so the concentration increases.

Imagine that the atmospheric pressure halves, from 101.3 kPa to 50.65 kPa. A vaporiser set to deliver 1% concentration at sea level (101.3 kPa) will therefore deliver 2% at 50.65 kPa (101.3/50.65). A vaporiser set at 1% at sea level will produce a partial pressure of 0.1 multiplied by 101.3 kPa, i.e. 10.13 kPa. This is the same as 2% at 50.65 kPa;

0.2 multiplied by 50.65 which is also equal to 10.13 kPa. Therefore although the output of the vapour in volume increases at altitude, the partial pressure remains the same. Therefore vaporisers calibrated for sea level can be used normally at altitude or in hyperbaric conditions.

3.4.4. Soda lime and carbon dioxide absorption – Emily K Johnson

This topic is a common OSCE question but could arise in the OSCE or structured oral examination. You may be shown a canister of soda lime or some granules, or a photograph and asked about it. The question may lead onto breathing systems, specifically the circle system or carbon dioxide measurement and capnography. It is recommended you study the relevant podcasts to enhance your knowledge and understanding of the topic.

What is soda lime?

Soda lime is a granulated hydrated lime used for the absorption of carbon dioxide in anaesthetic breathing systems.

What is the composition of soda lime?

Soda lime is made up of more than 80% calcium hydroxide, less than 4% sodium hydroxide, approximately 16% water and a fractional concentration of an indicator dye. Also added in trace amounts are silicates that harden the granules. It used to contain potassium hydroxide but this was removed in January 2000.

What are the dyes used in soda lime, and what are the colour changes they undergo?

The indicator dyes used in soda lime are either phenolphthalein that has a colour change from red or pink to white or less commonly ethyl violet that has a colour change from white to purple. As the colours change in opposite directions it is important to know which dye is being used.

What are the series of reactions that occur in soda lime and can you draw them?

If this topic comes up then you will almost certainly be asked to write out the reactions that occur. You will fail if you are unable to do this. Practice writing it out swiftly and without any mistakes until it is easy. Once you can do this, explaining the reaction will be easy.

The first reaction to occur is carbon dioxide and water combine to form carbonic acid.

$$CO_2 + H_2O \Rightarrow H_2CO_3.$$

Then carbonic acid and sodium hydroxide combine to produce soluble sodium carbonate plus water and heat.

$$H_2CO_3 + 2NaOH \Rightarrow Na_2CO_3 + 2H_2O + heat.$$

Soluble sodium carbonate then combines with calcium hydroxide to produce insoluble calcium carbonate, sodium hydroxide which replenishes the original store and also produces heat.

$$Ca(OH)_2 + Na_2CO_3 \Rightarrow CaCO_3 + 2NaOH + heat.$$

As heat is produced in these reactions some calcium hydroxide breaks down to form calcium oxide and water.

$$Ca(OH)_2 + heat \Rightarrow CaO + H_2O.$$

Can you summarise the overall chemical reaction that occurs in soda lime?

The overall reaction that occurs in soda lime, in the presence of water and with sodium hydroxide as an activator is carbon dioxide and calcium hydroxide combine to form calcium carbonate and water.

$$CO_2 + Ca(OH)_2 \Rightarrow CaCO_3 + H_2O.$$

What are the benefits to using soda lime in a breathing system?

Soda lime is primarily used to absorb CO_2 therefore permitting low flows and re-breathing of gases without CO_2 accumulation. This technique allows for fresh gas flows equivalent to only the basal oxygen requirements resulting in a much more cost effective breathing system with less waste and pollution.

The reactions involved in the absorption of CO_2 produce heat and water, therefore gases passing through get heated and humidified.

What are the draw backs to soda lime?

Soda lime decomposes some inhalational anaesthetic agents. Sevoflurane is slightly decomposed by soda lime, and halothane even less so. The reaction between sevoflurane and soda lime produces a number of compounds, A, B, C, D, E and G. The compound of concern is Compound A, a pentafluoroisopropenyl fluoromethyl ether and has been shown to be toxic in rats, causing renal, hepatic and cerebral damage. There is no evidence to suggest it has these effects in humans, and even at very low flows the maximal concentrations are around 30 PPM with potential toxic levels as high as 150 to 200 ppm. However sevoflurane is not used with low flow anaesthesia for this reason in the United States.

If soda lime becomes dried out under warm conditions, and volatile agents containing the CHF_2 moiety, which includes isoflurane, desflurane and enflurane, are used with it, then carbon monoxide can be produced. This can happen as most anaesthetic machines continue to deliver 200 ml/min fresh gas flow even when the gases are turned off, therefore drying out the soda lime. Trichloroethylene is an old inhalational agent that when decomposed by soda lime formed a potent neurotoxin called dichloroethylene resulting in neurological damage particularly affecting the facial and trigeminal nerves.

The colour changes which occur in the indicator dyes can be misleading leading to the use of exhausted soda lime. This occurs when the soda lime becomes partially exhausted as CO_2 is absorbed and carbonic acid levels increase causing the pH to drop. The lower pH causes the indicator dye to change colour. However if at this point the soda lime stands unused then unused hydroxyl ions from the core of the granule migrate to the surface and neutralise the carbonic acid, raising the pH and reversing the colour change. Consequently the soda lime appears fresh even though it is partially exhausted.

Another drawback to soda lime is that it can be dusty to handle. This is less of a problem for patients due to the use of filters but can be more hazardous to staff handling the granules.

In which circuits do we use soda lime?

Soda lime was traditionally used in Water's circuit. This is a Mapleson C circuit with an added canister filled with soda lime, called a Water's canister. The Water's canister was added with the reservoir bag on one side and the fresh gas flow and expiratory valve at the patient end of the circuit. Exhaled gases were passed to and fro through the canister to eliminate the CO_2. This system is most efficient when the tidal volumes equal the contained air space. The deadspace equals the volume between the canister and the patient. This increased as the soda lime close to the patient became exhausted. The soda lime also required placement as close to the patient as possible for this reason, making the circuit bulky and difficult to use.

Currently soda lime is commonly used in the circle system. This is popular as it reduces cost and pollution.

What is the size of soda lime granules and why are they this size?

Soda lime granules are between 4 and 8 mesh. This means they will pass through a mesh with four to eight strands per inch in each axis. The granules need to be small enough to pack in tightly and avoid big spaces between them, which would allow gas channelling. They also need to have the largest possible surface area and provide the lowest possible resistance to flow. They should ideally be uniform size and shape to promote more uniform flow.

What other compounds are you aware of that can be used to absorb carbon dioxide?

There are several other compounds that absorb carbon dioxide: Baralyme and Amsorb.

Baralyme or barium lime comprises 80% calcium hydroxide and 20% barium hydroxide. Water is incorporated into the barium hydroxide. This is less efficient than soda lime and the reaction with sevoflurane producing Compound A is approximately five times more rapid.

Amsorb is a compound containing calcium hydroxide, calcium chloride and setting agents. Its absorption of CO_2 is similar to other agents and it is not associated with the formation of carbon monoxide or compound A.

3.4.5. Scavenging systems – Emily K Johnson

What methods are there to reduce pollution in the operating theatre?

Methods to reduce pollution in the operating theatre include the following:

- Theatre ventilation systems
- Scavenging systems
- The circle breathing system
- Total intra-venous anaesthesia
- Regional anaesthesia

What are the maximum levels permitted of anaesthetic gases in the UK and in other countries?

In the UK the recommended maximum acceptable concentrations set by the Health and Safety Commission in 1996 over a 8-hour period are as follows for:

- Nitrous oxide they are 100 ppm
- Enflurane and isoflurane they are 50 ppm
- Halothane they are 10 ppm.

In other countries they are 25 ppm for nitrous oxide and 2 ppm for any of the halogenated agents.

What are the potential implications of exceeding these concentrations?

An increased incidence of spontaneous abortions has been noted in staff working in the operating theatres. This could be due to increased exposure to trace quantities of anaesthetic agents in the air. Although there is no firm evidence to support this, it is reasonable to take measures to reduce pollution levels.

What is scavenging?

Define and classify.

Scavenging is the removal and safe disposal of waste anaesthetic gases. Scavenging systems can be divided into active and passive systems and open and closed systems.

Describe the features of a passive scavenging system

Passive scavenging systems are driven by the pressure the patient generates on expiration. A passive system consists of a collecting system which can be a shroud connected to the APL valve. This is connected to a receiving system by standard plastic tubing which is referred to as the transfer system. The tubing has 30-mm connectors to ensure it is not accidentally connected to the breathing system.

The receiving system consists of a reservoir to ensure adequate removal of the gases even if the removal rate is slower than the peak expiratory flow rate. The reservoir could be a rubber bag or a rigid bottle. If the system is closed there must be a dumping valve and a pressure relief valve to prevent excess negative or positive pressure being applied to the patient's airway.

The receiving system is connected to a disposal system which is often a wide bore copper pipe leading directly to the atmosphere or into the theatre ventilation system. If it leads directly to the atmosphere it is recommended that its outlet is above roof level to prevent re-entry of the scavenged gases into the building. There is no external energy supply involved in passive scavenging systems.

What are the advantages and disadvantages of a passive scavenging system?

The advantages of a passive scavenging system are that it is simple to construct and has no running costs. Theatre ventilation systems or extractor fans can assist it in extraction and disposal.

The disadvantages are that if it is connected to theatre ventilation systems recirculation or reverse flows can occur. It is also possible for excess negative or positive pressures to occur at the outlet where it connects to the atmosphere. Strong winds can cause this and could cause the flow to reverse. The outlet situated above roof level can result in dense vapour such as nitrous oxide giving back pressure into the breathing system. As the outlet is connected to the atmosphere it must be protected from insects with a wire mesh.

Describe the features of an active scavenging system

Active scavenging systems are driven by an external power source and the scavenged gases are drawn away from the patient by a vacuum. An active scavenging system consists of the same components as a passive system. There is a collecting system, transfer system, receiving system and a disposal system. The receiving system is commonly a valveless open-ended reservoir. The reservoir is commonly cylindrical with a vented base and connected to the anaesthetic machine in the vertical position. It contains a float to indicate flow and a bacterial filter between the receiving and disposal system.

An alternative reservoir is a bag with safety valves to prevent the risk of excess positive or negative pressure. This is connected to an active disposal system, which consists of a fan or an ejector flowmeter, used to generate a vacuum. The ejector flowmeter works using the venture principle. Oxygen or air flowing through the ejector causes entrainment of the waste anaesthetic gases. The rate of removal can be altered using a flowmeter until it is equal to the fresh gas supply rate. A low-pressure high-volume system is required for active scavenging, it is able to remove 75 L/min with peak flows around 130 L/min. Therefore the hospital suction system is not suitable as it is a higher pressure system with lower flow rates.

What are the advantages and disadvantages of an active scavenging system?

Advantages of active scavenging systems are that they can cope with a large range of flow rates, from 30 to 130 L/min. The receiving system can cope with changing flow rates which results in a steady flow being passed into the disposal system. They are a convenient way of scavenging for large hospitals with many theatres.

Disadvantages are that whilst older active scavenging systems used the hospitals centralised vacuum, it is now recommended an independent vacuum pump is used, which makes them more expensive.

It is possible that a blockage beyond the receiving system could result in excess positive pressure being delivered to the patient, causing barotrauma. Excessive negative pressure could occur if the vented end of the receiving system became blocked, resulting in collapse of the breathing system reservoir bag and possible re-breathing or negative pressure pulmonary oedema.

What is a dumping valve and at what pressure should it open?

A dumping valve is a device to prevent excessive negative pressure being applied to the patient's airway. It should open at a pressure of -0.5 cmH$_2$O allowing air to be drawn in.

What are the requirements for pressure limits and gas flows in scavenging systems?

The maximum negative pressure is 0.5 cmH$_2$O at a gas flow of 30 L/min.

The maximum positive pressure is 5 cmH$_2$O at a gas flow of 30 L/min and 10 cmH$_2$O at a gas flow of 90 L/min.

What are the features of theatre ventilation systems?

Theatre ventilation systems are important in scavenging as regardless of the scavenging system used it is inevitable some gases will escape. The recommendation is that ventilation should provide 15 air changes per hour in areas where volatile anaesthetics are used.

What is the difference between open and closed scavenging systems?

Open scavenging technique refers to suction being applied to a part of the system which is left open to the atmosphere, with no valves or bags present. Techniques include placing a funnel next to the expiratory valve to aspirate anaesthetic agents. These systems lack control and require high flows and placement of the funnel must be very close to the release point of the gases to be effective.

What is the aldasorber?

The aldasorber is a passive scavenging device. It is also known as the Cardiff aldasorber or a charcoal canister.

How does the aldasorber work?

The aldasorber consists of a canister containing activated charcoal particles. It is connected to the APL valve or ventilator expiratory valve by connector tubing. The waste gases pass through the canister and halogenated inhalational agents are absorbed by the charcoal particles.

What are the advantages and disadvantages of the aldasorber?

The advantage of the aldasorber is that it is a small and portable device that can be easily transported with the anaesthetic machine. It also has no set-up costs.

Disadvantages of the aldasorber are that the only way of telling if it is exhausted is the increasing weight and they tend to require replacement for every 12 hours of use so the costs add up. The charcoal only absorbs halogenated agents and not nitrous oxide. Any heating of the canister causes the release of agents back into the atmosphere.

Measurement of oxygen, carbon dioxide and anaesthetic agents

3.5.1. Measurement of anaesthetic agents – Caroline V Sampson

What different methods can be used to measure the concentration of anaesthetic gases and vapours and which of these are most common in your practice?

This is asking for a list without lengthy explanations. You should be aware of the different gas analysers used on common anaesthetic machines and be able to list the rarer mainly research-based analysers.

In practice oxygen is usually measured using a Clark or polarographic electrode, a fuel cell or a paramagnetic analyser. Carbon dioxide, nitrous oxide and volatile anaesthetic agents are most commonly measured using infrared absorption spectroscopy. Less common methods include using an ultraviolet light analyser to measure halothane, analysers containing quartz crystals which use the piezo-electric effect, analysers utilising Raman spectrometry and the mass spectrometer. Analysers used mainly in research include gas chromatography and analysers using photoacoustic spectroscopy, refractometers, the velocity of ultrasound through gas mixtures and katharometers which measure thermal conductivity.

How do infrared analysers measure different gases?

This will be covered in more detail in the capnography podcast. Draw a simple diagram of an infrared analyser to illustrate your point, see Figure 3.5.1a.

Infrared light is absorbed by molecules with two or more different atoms in the molecule, so can be used to measure carbon dioxide, nitrous oxide and the volatile anaesthetic agents, but not oxygen or nitrogen. It works on the principle that different molecules absorb infrared light at characteristic absorption spectra across a given bandwidth. For example the volatile agents demonstrate absorption peaks at a wavelength of 3.3 micro-millimetres, with peaks of 3.9 micro-millimetres for nitrous oxide and 4.3 micro-millimetres for carbon dioxide. Absorption is proportional to the concentration of gas present so the partial pressure of a gas can be determined by measuring the fraction of radiation absorbed by a gas mixture.

An analyser measuring a single gas consists of an infrared light source, a filter which only allows infrared radiation through at the peak absorption wavelength of that gas, a sample

Dr Podcast Scripts for the Primary FRCA, ed. Rebecca A. Leslie, Emily K. Johnson and Alexander P. L. Goodwin. Published by Cambridge University Press. © R. A. Leslie, E. K. Johnson and A. P. L. Goodwin 2011.

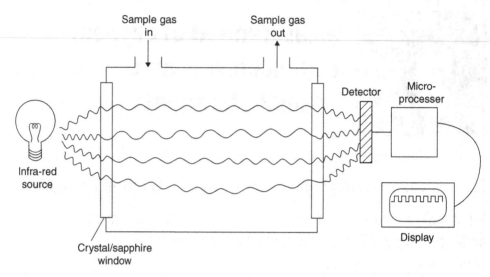

Figure 3.5.1a. Infra-red analyser.

chamber, a detector and a means of displaying the results. Multiple gases may be measured in the same sample chamber using a filter that is made up of a number of rotating windows, each allowing light of different wavelengths to pass through.

Do you know of any problems with infrared analysers?

Always try to classify your answer – give the examiner a list of problems and then explain them in more detail. That way hopefully you won't forget anything and the examiner can stop you if you go into too much detail.

Problems with infrared analysers include collision broadening, changes in output from the infrared source, changes in accuracy of the detectors and interference from other gases.

When different gas molecules collide their energy levels can alter slightly which affects the amount of infrared light absorbed at the characteristic wavelength, this is called the collision broadening effect. Therefore adding nitrous oxide to carbon dioxide can alter its absorption pattern. This is compensated for in newer machines.

Most analysers have a reference chamber which does not contain the gas being measured. This improves accuracy as any change in output from the detector reflects a change in concentration of the gas being measured rather than a change in output from the infrared source or a change in accuracy of the detector. These are known as double beam analysers.

Water vapour interferes with the infrared analyser, so gas samples must either be dried prior to being analysed, or a waveband chosen which is well away from water absorption maxima. Likewise alcohol can interfere with the analysers as it has a similar absorption spectrum to the volatile agents.

How does a mass spectrometer work?

The mass spectrometer is capable of separating and measuring many different gases including water vapour. It is versatile and has a fast response time of less than 100 msec but is bulky and very expensive. A sample of gas is drawn through a tube into a sample chamber where a few molecules of this gas mixture are allowed to leak out into an ionisation chamber. In the ionisation chamber the gas molecules are bombarded by a beam of electrons passing from a cathode to an anode. This causes some of the gas molecules to become charged. These charged particles are then accelerated by a negatively charged plate before being separated out and detected by one of two methods.

In the magnetic sector method the ions are deflected into an arc by a strong magnetic field which separates them into different particle streams according to mass. The lighter ions are deflected most and the heaviest ions are deflected least. These particle streams are then measured by a series of detector plates.

The second method is called the quadrupole method and uses four electrically charged rods. The electrical potential on the rods is altered so only ions of a specific mass are able to travel through the rods to a detector. This method only uses one detector but, by altering the electrical potential of the rods, ion streams of different masses can be analysed sequentially.

The mass spectrometer identifies compounds by their mass numbers; however molecules fragment in a predictable way during the ionisation process. This is how a mass spectrometer can differentiate between nitrous oxide and carbon dioxide which both have a mass number or 44. For example nitrous oxide is known to fragment into nitric oxide so the mass spectrometer can be set to measure the concentration of nitric oxide instead which has a mass number of 30.

What is the principle of gas chromatography?

Chromatography is the term used for a procedure that separates a mixture into its components by passing it through a column. In gas chromatography there is a stationary phase and a mobile phase. The mobile phase consists of an inert carrier gas such as nitrogen or helium. The stationary phase is packed into the chromatographic column and consists of very small particles coated with liquid such as polyethylene glycol. The gas mixture to be analysed is injected into the carrier gas. As this mixture passes through the column its component gases are slowed down by different degrees depending on their solubility in the stationary phase liquid and therefore appear separated out at the end of the column. At the outlet of the column a detector which is connected to a recorder monitors the appearance of the sample components as a series of peaks on a graph. The concentration of gas components is given by the height of the peaks and the component gases themselves are identified by comparison of the time lags of the different peaks with those for known gas samples.

There are several different types of detector including flame ionisation detectors which are better for measuring organic gases, thermal conductivity detectors which are better for inorganic gases and electron capture detectors which are more sensitive for halogenated compounds such as the volatile anaesthetic agents. Gas chromatography is very accurate and very sensitive but is expensive and requires some prior knowledge of the types of gases in the mixture. Continuous analysis is impossible. It is usually only used for research purposes.

What is the piezoelectric effect, and how is it used to measure volatile anaesthetic agents?

Gas analysers using the piezoelectric effect contain quartz crystals. When an electric potential is applied across a quartz crystal it contracts slightly, this is known as the piezoelectric effect. Quartz crystals can therefore be made to oscillate at their resonant frequency when placed in an alternating electric field. If a thin coating of oil is used to coat the crystals, volatile agents will dissolve in this oil. This will alter the resonant frequency of the crystal. The amount of volatile agent dissolved is proportional to its partial pressure in the gas mixture. Therefore the change in resonant frequency of the crystals will represent the partial pressure of volatile agent in the gas mixture. This change is measured electronically and displayed as a volatile concentration. These analysers cannot measure carbon dioxide or nitrous oxide and cannot distinguish between the different volatile agents.

What is the principle of Raman spectrometry?

When a photon of light hits a gas molecule a very small fraction of its energy is absorbed by the molecule, therefore it is re-emitted at a different (usually decreased) wavelength. This partial transfer of energy is known as the Raman effect, which was discovered by an Indian physicist, Rama, in 1928.

Absorption of radiation of a particular wavelength is determined by the bonds between the atoms in the gas molecule allowing different gases to be detected. In practice an intense source of light, classically an argon laser, is used to irradiate gases and vapours in a mixture. The new wavelengths given off are then passed through a set of filters, specific to each gas being measured, to identify the concentrations of each agent.

3.5.2. Oxygen measurement – Natasha A Joshi

How can we measure the fractional concentration of oxygen in a gas mixture?

(Top tips: Classify or fail! When there are a number of techniques, make sure you know most about the commonest one, and say this first in your list, as this is the one examiners will probably expect you to know most about.)

The fractional concentration of oxygen in a gas mixture can be measured using physical methods that are specific for oxygen measurement, and also using non-specific methods.

Physical methods specific for oxygen measurement include the following:

- The Clark/polarographic electrode
- The fuel cell and
- Paramagnetic analysis.

Non-specific methods for measuring the fractional concentration of any gas in a mixture include the following:

- Mass spectrometry.

How does a Clark/polarographic electrode work?

Draw a diagram as you are speaking, this will convey lots of information in a short space of time, and demonstrate understanding, see Figure 3.5.2a.

The Clark electrode consists of a platinum cathode and a silver/silver chloride anode. The cathode and anode are suspended in a potassium chloride electrolyte solution, and the whole apparatus is enclosed in a cylinder, which has a gas permeable plastic membrane covering its end. A potential difference of 0.6 volts is applied between the electrodes and current flow is measured.

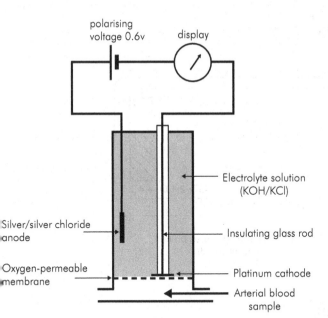

Figure 3.5.2a. Clark electrode. Reproduced with permission from Smith, T., Pinnock, C. and Lin, T. 2009. *Fundamentals of Anaesthesia.* Cambridge: Cambridge University Press. © Cambridge University Press 2009.

At the anode, silver reacts with the potassium chloride electrolyte solution, to produce silver chloride and liberate electrons.

(Useful to write down the chemical reactions taking place at the anode and cathode, on your diagram.)

At the cathode, oxygen combines with electrons and water, to produce hydroxyl ions:

$$O_2 + 4e^- + 2H_2O \rightarrow 4OH^-$$

(This reaction is the same as that occurring in the mitochondria of our cells, at the end of the respiratory chain.) Therefore the more oxygen there is available, the greater the number of electrons that can be taken up at the cathode and the greater the current flow in the circuit will be.

So the oxygen tension at the platinum cathode determines current flow through the cell.

What are the limitations of a Clark electrode?

There are a number of limitations with the Clark electrode:

Firstly, the electrode is temperature sensitive and should be kept at 37°C.

The plastic membrane covering the end of the electrode can easily become blocked with protein deposits from blood samples. It may also be contaminated or punctured and therefore needs to be checked and replaced regularly.

In the presence of halothane, the Clark electrode can give false high readings for the oxygen tension in a gas sample, but this can be avoided by using an electrode membrane that is impermeable to halothane.

How is the Clark electrode calibrated?

It is calibrated using standard gas mixtures.

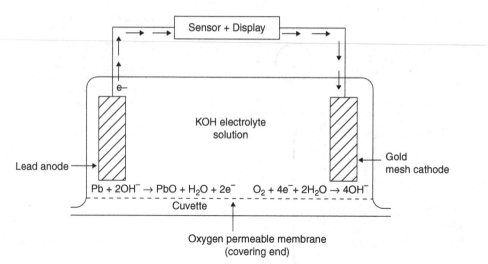

Figure 3.5.2b. Fuel cell.

How does a fuel cell work?

The fuel cell works in a similar manner to the Clark electrode, but it produces it own potential difference, hence its name.

The fuel cell consists of a lead anode and a gold mesh cathode, which are suspended in a potassium hydroxide electrolyte solution. The anode and cathode are connected in a circuit that also contains a sensor and a display. The whole apparatus is enclosed in a cylinder, with an oxygen permeable membrane covering its end.

(Again useful to draw a basic diagram of the fuel cell (Figure 3.5.2b) and annotate with the chemical reactions occurring at each electrode.)

At the anode, lead combines with hydroxyl ions from the potassium hydroxide electrolyte solution, to produce lead oxide, water and liberate electrons.

$$Pb + 2OH^- \rightarrow PbO + H_2O + 2e^-.$$

At the cathode, oxygen combines with these electrons and water, to produce hydroxyl ions:

$$O_2 + 4e^- + 2H_2O \rightarrow 4OH^-.$$

This generates a flow of electrons, or current through the circuit, which is proportional to the partial pressure of oxygen in the gas sample. (If more oxygen is available, more electrons will be taken up by the cathode.)

The fuel cell therefore produces its own voltage and acts like a battery. However, like any other battery, its shelf-life is limited. This largely depends on the duration of exposure of the fuel cell to oxygen.

How do you calibrate a fuel cell?

A fuel cell is calibrated for 21% oxygen by exposing it to room air. It is then exposed to 100% oxygen.

What are the advantages of a fuel cell?

It is compact and does not require a power supply.

What are the disadvantages of a fuel cell?

There are a number of disadvantages with a fuel cell. Firstly, it has a relatively slow response time, in the region of 20 seconds, and cannot be used for breath-by-breath analysis. Also, it has a limited life span, of around 6–12 months, and its accuracy may be affected by nitrous oxide, unless specialised cells are used.

What is the principle employed in a paramagnetic oxygen analyser?

Each oxygen molecule contains two unpaired electrons in its outer shell. As a result of this, oxygen is attracted towards a magnetic field. Substances attracted towards a magnetic field are referred to as paramagnetic, whereas those repelled by a magnetic field are referred to as diamagnetic.

Nitrogen and most other gases employed in anaesthesia are weakly diamagnetic. However oxygen and nitric oxide are paramagnetic, due to the unpaired electrons in the outer shells of these molecules. This principle can be employed in measuring the fractional concentration of oxygen in a gas mixture.

How does a paramagnetic oxygen analyser work?

Essentially, a paramagnetic oxygen analyser contains two nitrogen-filled glass spheres, in a gas-tight chamber. These are joined by a bar, which is suspended on a vertical wire, within a magnetic field. As oxygen is introduced into the analyser, it is attracted towards the magnetic field. This causes displacement of the glass spheres, which in turn rotates the bar, against the torque of the wire. The degree of rotation of the bar is proportional to the number of oxygen molecules present.

This may be measured by observing the deflection of a beam of light, reflected by a mirror mounted on the wire, or by measuring the current required to prevent rotation, when passing through a coil mounted on the bar.

What are the advantages of a paramagnetic oxygen analyser?

The newer paramagnetic oxygen analysers are very accurate and highly sensitive. This is because they have an alternating magnetic field (110 Hz) and a reference chamber. The membrane which vibrates between the two chambers produces an acoustic alternating pressure wave which is calibrated against gas concentration. These features make the newer devices much less prone to drift and to error due to small pressure changes, and also give a faster response time.

Paramagnetic oxygen analysers have a rapid response time, allowing breath-to-breath oxygen analysis. Therefore both inspired and expired oxygen concentrations can be measured.

What are the disadvantages of a paramagnetic oxygen analyser?

The accuracy of a paramagnetic analyser may be affected by the presence of nitrous oxide or water vapour in the gas sample. Water vapour may be eliminated by passing the gas sample through silica gel, before entering the analysis cell.

3.5.3. Pulse oximetry – Emily K Johnson

What is a pulse oximeter?

You may be shown a pulse oximeter in an OSCE scenario and asked what it is, or you could be asked about it in a structured oral examination question.

The pulse oximeter is a device used to determine arterial oxygen saturation. It measures the percentage of haemoglobin saturated with oxygen in the arterial blood.

What are the components of the pulse oximeter?

Pulse oximeters are normally probes which can be placed on a finger, toe, nose or ear. The probes consist of two high intensity monochromatic light emitting diodes on one side and a photodetector on the other side. The photodetector is connected to an electronic processor which uses the output to produce a pulsatile waveform.

What is Beer's law?

This is an important law you should know well.

Beer's law states that the absorption of radiation increases (transmission decreases) as the concentration of a substance increases.

What is Lambert's law?

This is an important law you should know well.

Lambert's law states that the intensity of transmitted light decreases exponentially as the distance travelled through the substance increases.

Describe the principles underlying the working of the pulse oximeter

The Beer–Lambert's law underlies the working of the pulse oximeter. The two laws are combined to describe the absorption of monochromatic light by a substance through which it passes. It states that light absorption and transmission vary as the concentration changes. It is these laws and the different absorption spectrums of oxy- and deoxyhaemoglobin that allow arterial oxygen saturations to be calculated.

How does the pulse oximeter work?

The light emitting diodes (LEDs) on one side of the probe emit light at particular wavelengths. One emits light in the red wavelength at 660 nm, and the other emits light in the infrared wavelength at 940 nm. The diodes are switched on and off in sequence then paused with both off, this sequence is repeated hundreds of times a second. This frequency of repetition allows the pulse oximeter to detect changes in the signal caused by arterial pulsations. The light passes through the finger or ear, and the photodetector picks up the signal. Some of the light gets absorbed by arterial blood, venous blood and the tissues. The light absorbed by blood depends on the amount of oxy- and deoxyhaemoglobin present in the blood and the wavelength of the light.

It would help explain your answer to draw the graph showing the absorption of light according to its wavelength with the curves for oxy- and deoxyhaemoglobin plotted (Figure 3.5.3a). Learn this graph and practice drawing it so you can do it quickly and correctly.

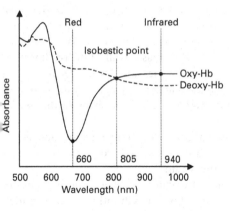

Figure 3.5.3a. Haemoglobin absorption spectra. Reproduced with permission from Cross, M. and Plunkett, E. 2008. *Physics, Pharmacology and Physiology for Anaesthetists: Key Concepts for the FRCA.* Cambridge: Cambridge University Press. © M. Cross and E. Plunkett 2008.

The absorbance of oxyhaemoglobin and deoxyhaemoglobin is different at wavelengths of 660 nm and 940 nm. At 660 nm, in the red region the absorbance of oxyhaemoglobin is lower than that of deoxyhaemoglobin, whereas at 940 nm, in the infrared region the absorbance of deoxyhaemoglobin is lower than that of oxyhaemoglobin. The LEDs emit light at these particular wavelengths to allow the photodetector to compare the absorbances and therefore calculate the oxygen saturation. The pause with both diodes off allows the photodetector and processor to pick up any ambient light signal and compensate for this in the calculations. The pulsatile component of the signal is analysed and the non-pulsatile component ignored so the absorbance of light by the venous blood and tissues is eliminated from the calculation. The signal is processed in the electronic processor and a pulsed waveform produced showing arterial oxygen saturations.

What is an isobestic point?

The graph showing absorbance against wavelength for oxy- and deoxyhaemoglobin would help you to illustrate your answer more clearly.

An isobestic point is the point at which two substances absorb a certain wavelength of light to the same extent. In the case of oxy- and deoxyhaemoglobin the isobestic points occur at 590 nm in the red spectrum and 805 nm in the infrared spectrum. At these wavelengths oxy- and deoxyhaemoglobin absorb the same amount of light.

The isobestic point can be used as a reference where absorption of light is independent of degree of saturation. Old oximeters used this principle.

What are the advantages of the pulse oximeter?

The pulse oximeter is a non-invasive, safe, continuous and reliable method of detecting arterial oxygen saturations. It is simple to apply and interpret and can be used in the majority of settings. It is an excellent tool to pick up hypoxaemia early allowing prompt treatment.

What are the limitations of the pulse oximeter?

There are several limitations of the pulses oximeter.

The range of accuracy is give or take 2%, between 70 and 100%. Below 70% the readings are less accurate and they are inaccurate below 50%. This is because the measurements are plotted against a curve which was determined by taking measurements of arterial saturations from healthy volunteers so the lower readings had to be extrapolated.

Hypoperfusion, low cardiac output and peripheral vasoconstriction affect the pulse oximeter readings. This is because the pulsatile element of the signal which is sensed is only between 1 and 5% of the total signal so if the arteries are vasoconstricted this is even smaller making it less accurate. Atrial fibrillation and other arrhythmias can affect the readings.

The oximeter measures oxygen saturations, it does not measure oxygen delivery to the tissues. It is also important to remember large changes in arterial partial pressure of oxygen may occur with only small changes in oxygen saturations due to the shape of the oxygen dissociation curve.

Excessive movement can interfere with readings and excessive ambient light causes inaccuracy, also diathermy can cause interference. Nail varnish or skin discolouration can cause inaccuracies although skin colour does not affect the readings.

Any venous pulsation causes inaccuracies. The pulse oximeter will assume any pulsatile flow is arterial therefore in cases with pulsatile venous flow the saturations may be underestimated. This may occur in impaired venous return such as high airway pressures.

Carbon monoxide poisoning can result in false high readings of the pulse oximeter. This is because carboxyhaemoglobin has an absorption spectrum similar to that of oxyhaemoglobin so the probe is unable to distinguish between the two.

A number of factors can cause a falsely low saturation reading. These include methaemoglobin and intra-venous dyes such as indocyanine green and methylene blue.

Factors such as hyperbilirubinaemia, foetal haemoglobins, anaemia and polycythaemia do not have any effect on the accuracy of readings.

The pulse oximeter probes can cause pressure sores and burns if used continuously and sites must be regularly inspected and altered.

Is the pulse oximeter a fast or slow monitor of oxygen saturations?

The pulse oximeter averages the readings every 10 to 20 seconds. This makes it a slow monitor of oxygen saturations as it is unable to detect acute desaturations. The response time is even longer when the finger probe is used, and can be more than 60 seconds.

3.5.4. pH and CO_2 measurement – Rebecca A Leslie

This podcast covers the pH and the Severinghaus electrode, for more information on capnography please read chapter on "Capnography".

How are pH and hydrogen ion concentration related?

Start your answer by stating the relationship between pH and hydrogen ion concentration. If you can remember, next give examples of hydrogen ion concentration at a certain pH or draw a simple graph.

The pH is the negative logarithm to the base of 10 of the hydrogen ion concentration. This means that for a decrease in the pH by one unit, there is a 10-fold increase in the hydrogen ion concentration. This can be shown nicely as on Figure 3.5.4a.

Important points on the graph are as follows:

- pH of 8 is a hydrogen concentration of 10 nmol/L
- pH of 7 is a hydrogen concentration of 100 nmol/L
- pH of 6 is a hydrogen concentration of 1000 nmol/L

The normal blood pH is 7.4 which represents a hydrogen ion concentration of 40 mmol/L.

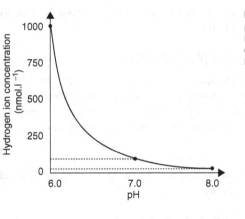

Figure 3.5.4a. Acid–base balance. Reproduced with permission from Cross, M. and Plunkett, E. 2008. Physics, Pharmacology and Physiology for Anaesthetists: Key Concepts for the FRCA. Cambridge: Cambridge University Press. © M. Cross and E. Plunkett 2008.

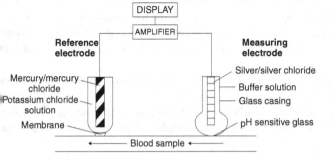

Figure 3.5.4b. pH electrode.

How do we measure the pH in a blood sample?

You may find it helpful to draw a simple diagram while describing how the pH electrode works, see Figure 3.5.4b.

Arterial blood gas machines measure arterial pH by using a pH electrode. The pH electrode consists of two electrodes; a measuring electrode and a reference electrode. The measuring electrode is made of silver/silver chloride which is surrounded by a buffer solution in a glass casing. The bulb of the glass at the tip of the electrode is made of special pH-sensitive glass which is in direct contact with the arterial blood sample.

The reference electrode is made of mercury/mercury chloride and is surrounded by a potassium chloride solution. The potassium chloride solution is in contact with the arterial blood sample via a membrane. The reference electrode maintains a constant potential despite changes in the arterial pH. At the measuring electrode, hydrogen ions move through the hydrogen sensitive glass, but the pH remains the same because of the action of the inner buffer solution. However a pH gradient does exist between the buffer solution and the blood sample. This gradient produces an electrical potential difference. The two electrodes create an electrical circuit so the potential can be measured and converted to a direct reading of hydrogen ion concentration.

How is the pH electrode calibrated?

The pH electrode is calibrated with two different buffer solutions each containing a known concentration of hydrogen ions. The first buffer solution has a pH which is the same as the buffer solution inside the measuring electrode and is taken as zero. The second buffer solution is used as a reference against which the blood pH is measured.

What are the potential problems with the pH electrode?

The pH electrode must be kept at a constant temperature to ensure it is accurate. This is because hypothermia increases the solubility of carbon dioxide, and therefore the $PaCO_2$ is proportionally reduced which results in an increased pH. Therefore the electrodes and the blood channel are surrounded by a thermal control system to maintain the temperature at 37°C.

In addition the electrodes must be carefully maintained to ensure that they remain accurate. There must not be any holes in the membrane and the electrodes need to be cleaned regularly to remove any protein material which may accumulate on it.

What is the principle behind the Severinghaus electrode?

This is not a difficult question, although it may throw you off balance initially. All the examiners want you to say is that the CO_2 electrode is based on the pH electrode because the partial pressure of carbon dioxide is related to the hydrogen ion concentration. Write the equation down as you give your answer.

The Severinghaus electrode is a modified pH electrode and is used to measure carbon dioxide partial pressure. It is based on hydrogen ion measurement because carbon dioxide reacts with water to produce carbonic acid which in turn dissociates into hydrogen ions and bicarbonate. Therefore the partial pressure of carbon dioxide is related to the hydrogen ion concentration.

$$CO_2 + H_2O \rightarrow H_2CO_3^- \rightarrow H^+ + HCO_3^-.$$

How does the Severinghaus electrode work?

Your answer should be supplemented by a simple, clear diagram, see Figure 3.5.4c.

The Severinghaus electrode consists of two electrodes; a glass electrode and a silver/silver chloride reference electrode. The glass electrode is made of hydrogen sensitive glass, and is covered in a nylon mesh which is coated in a thin film of bicarbonate solution. Both electrodes are contained within a plastic membrane which is in contact with the blood sample and is permeable to carbon dioxide but impermeable to blood cells, plasma and hydrogen ions.

Carbon dioxide diffuses from the blood sample through the plastic membrane into the nylon mesh which is impregnated with bicarbonate solution, and combines with water to produce hydrogen ions and bicarbonate. The glass electrode measures the change in hydrogen ions which is proportional to the change in carbon dioxide tension.

What are the advantages and disadvantages of the Severinghaus electrode?

Advantages of the Severinghaus electrode are that it is both accurate and stable.

However a disadvantage of the Severinghaus electrode is that the response time is approximately 2 to 3 minutes, which is slower than the pH electrode. This is because the carbon dioxide must have time to diffuse through the plastic membrane, and react with water to produce hydrogen ions and bicarbonate. The reaction can be sped up by the addition of carbonic anhydrase.

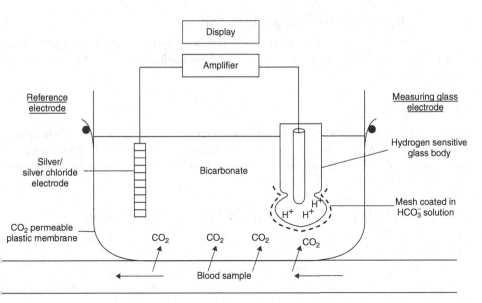

Figure 3.5.4c. Severinghaus electrode.

In addition, like the pH electrode, the Severinghaus electrode will become inaccurate if the plastic membrane is damaged therefore the electrode must be carefully maintained.

It is also essential that the Severinghaus electrode is maintained at 37°C and calibrated with two different gas mixtures with known partial pressures of carbon dioxide.

How can the arterial carbon dioxide concentration be measured in vivo?

Transcutaneous Severinghaus electrodes are available to measure carbon dioxide concentration in vivo. The Severinghaus electrode must be modified slightly for it to function as a transcutaneous electrode. These modifications include the addition of a heating element and a thermistor to the electrode, so that the skin can be heated to a temperature of between 40 and 42°C. This increases capillary blood flow, carbon dioxide production and carbon dioxide solubility. It is worth remembering that the transcutaneous carbon dioxide is usually higher than arterial carbon dioxide.

An advantage of the transcutaneous carbon dioxide electrode is that it allows continuous measurement of carbon dioxide concentration. However it does carry a risk of skin burns, the response time is slow, and the correlation between transcutaneous and arterial concentration is variable.

Another way to measure carbon dioxide concentration in vivo is to use an intra-vascular probe. These include a miniature carbon dioxide electrode that can be inserted through an arterial cannula.

The carbon dioxide concentration could also be estimated from the end-tidal carbon dioxide measurement. In normal individuals the end-tidal carbon dioxide usually measures 0.5 kPa less than the arterial carbon dioxide concentration, although in respiratory disease the magnitude of the difference of end-tidal and arterial carbon dioxide concentration increases.

3.5.5. Capnography – Emily K Johnson

This topic is very popular with examiners and could come up in the OSCE or structured oral examination. You will be expected to have good and thorough knowledge in this area and will not pass if you don't.

What is capnography?

Capnography is the continuous measurement and pictorial display of carbon dioxide concentration at the airway to allow the monitoring of end-tidal CO_2 tension. Capnometry refers only to the measurement of carbon dioxide concentration. The capnogram is the pictorial trace showing the end-tidal CO_2 measurement.

What methods do you know for carbon dioxide measurement?

There are several ways of measuring carbon dioxide concentration in the blood, they can be divided into direct and indirect.

Direct methods include the Severinghaus carbon dioxide electrode.

Indirect methods include measurement of end-tidal carbon dioxide concentration, most commonly using infrared spectroscopy, although other methods including mass spectrometry, Raman scattering and gas chromatography are available. Colorimetric techniques are available and can be used as portable devices to detect CO_2 thereby confirming endotracheal tube placement when formal capnography is not available. The Siggard–Andersen nomogram and van Slyke apparatus can also be used to estimate carbon dioxide concentrations in blood.

On what principle does capnography work?

Capnography most commonly works using infrared spectroscopy. Gases that have two or more different atoms in the molecule absorb infrared radiation at specific wavelengths. Therefore by selecting a specific wavelength and having some knowledge of the likely components of a gas mixture it is possible to measure a particular gas. In anaesthesia, expired gas is likely to contain nitrogen, oxygen, nitrous oxide, carbon dioxide and an inhalational agent. As carbon dioxide and nitrous oxide have two different atoms the bonds between these molecules will absorb light in the infrared spectrum. Carbon dioxide absorbs infrared radiation with a peak wavelength of 4.28 μm whereas nitrous oxide's peak absorption is slightly higher so can be avoided by adjusting the wavelength to 4.28 μm.

Describe how end-tidal carbon dioxide is measured

End-tidal carbon dioxide can be measured using a capnograph, which may be a side-stream or main-stream analyser.

A gas sample is extracted from the breathing system close to the patient. This is introduced into a sampling chamber made of sapphire. Glass cannot be used for the sampling chamber as it reflects infrared radiation. On one side of the chamber is a hot wire that emits infrared radiation. The radiation is then passed through a filter before it passes through the sapphire sampling chamber. The filter only allows radiation of around 4.28-μm wavelength through. The infrared radiation passes through the chamber and therefore through the gas sample. On the opposite side of the chamber is a lens to focus the radiation on a photodetector. The amount of radiation that reaches the photodetector is dependent on the concentration of carbon dioxide in the chamber. The higher the concentration of carbon dioxide in the chamber the more radiation is absorbed and the less falls on the photodetector.

The detector output is then processed and gives a measurement of the concentration of carbon dioxide in the sample chamber.

There can be fluctuations in the detector output, the infrared input, the detector sensitivity and the transmission of optical components that can lead to inaccuracies in the measured concentrations. Therefore a reference chamber is used. This is a chamber alongside the sample chamber that contains carbon dioxide–free air. Radiation from the same source is passed through the sample chamber and a reference detector picks up the signal. This signal is subtracted from the signal from the sample detector to remove these potential inaccuracies. This is known as a double beam capnometer.

What is the collision broadening effect?

The collision broadening effect is the process that occurs in a gas mixture resulting in slight variations in the absorption wavelengths of infrared radiation between molecules of the same kind.

Collision broadening is the broadening of the bandwidth of infrared absorption of carbon dioxide due to the proximity of nitrous oxide molecules, which interact with the carbon dioxide molecules, exchanging kinetic energy with them.

It is also known as pressure broadening.

Discuss the differences between side-stream and main-stream capnographs?

Side-stream capnography involves a sample being drawn from the expiratory limb of the breathing circuit as close to the patient as possible. The sample is then carried via a tube with a 1.2-mm internal diameter to the analyser. This tube is made of polytetrafluoroethane, more commonly called Teflon, so it is impermeable to CO_2 and doesn't react with volatile agents. This system contains a moisture trap so water does not interfere with the infrared absorption and shouldn't block the tube. The analyser has an exhaust post that allows return of gas either to the breathing system or the scavenging system.

The main-stream analyser consists of a special connector in the breathing system. This connector incorporates a sapphire windowed chamber through which the expiratory gases pass. The analyser sits over this chamber and passes the infrared beam through the chamber.

The main-stream analyser has no transit time so results are immediate. It avoids a sampling line when compared to the side-stream analyser which requires a flow of 150 ml/min through its tubing to achieve rapid response times. Provided the tubing is the correct size and this flow is achieved the side-stream analyser has a delay of less than 1 second which is not significant.

The side-stream analysers have the added benefit of being situated away from the patient so not weighing down the breathing system near to the patient and not contributing to the dead-space as the main-stream analysers do.

It is possible, despite the water trap, for side-stream analysers to become blocked with moisture causing inaccuracies. However the main-stream analyser has the additional problem of requiring heating to 41 degrees in order to prevent water condensing on the sapphire

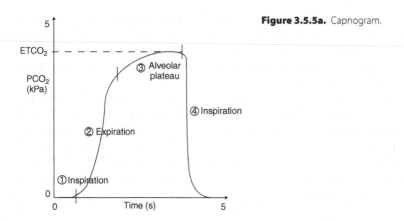

Figure 3.5.5a. Capnogram.

windows of the chamber. This adds expense and risk of burns to the patient. The side-stream analysers are used more commonly for these reasons and the fact they are able to measure other gases simultaneously, whereas the main-stream analysers only measure carbon dioxide.

Describe the end-tidal carbon dioxide waveform

You must be able to draw the capnogram quickly, whilst explaining it. Make sure you practice this and are able to do it easily (Figure 3.5.5a).

The end-tidal carbon dioxide waveform demonstrates the end-tidal carbon dioxide tensions throughout the respiratory cycle and is commonplace on most monitors in theatres and intensive care units. The capnogram is divided into four phases. The baseline is during inspiration when carbon dioxide should be negligible; this is phase 1. Initially on expiration the dead-space gas is exhaled which should not contain any CO_2. Then alveolar gas is expired. At this point there is a rapid rise in CO_2, which is phase 2. It then reaches a clear plateau in healthy lungs; this is called the alveolar plateau. The curve may rise very slowly and the highest point is termed the end-tidal CO_2 tension. It represents the final portion of gas involved in gas exchange in the alveoli. This plateau phase is phase 3. Then inspiration starts again and the trace drops back down to the baseline. The sudden drop back to baseline is phase 4.

What additional features may be seen on the capnogram?

You may be asked to draw the capnogram with any of the additional features and describe what is the problem and why. Be able to easily identify the different waveforms and reproduce them with ease.

A number of additional features may be seen on the capnogram. These can be normal or indicative of problems with the patient or equipment.

Regular superimposed oscillations may be seen that correspond to the heartbeat. Small additional or superimposed waves may be observed which could represent the patient starting to breathe and inadequacy of neuromuscular blockade. A raised baseline indicates rebreathing and may indicate failure of a breathing system component such as a valve or exhausted soda lime. Information can be derived from the shape of the trace. A progressive rise instead of the clear alveolar plateau can indicate bronchospasm or chronic obstructive pulmonary diseases due to uneven emptying of alveoli with different time constants.

What could cause an increased end-tidal CO_2?

An increased end-tidal CO_2 could be due to either decreased ventilation, increased production of CO_2 or increased inspired CO_2.

Decreased ventilation may be due to a low respiratory rate, a reduced tidal volume or increased dead-space in the breathing circuit. An increased CO_2 production would occur in hypermetabolic states and may indicate malignant hyperpyrexia or fever. An increased inspired CO_2 would be due to re-breathing, exhausted soda lime or an external source of added CO_2.

What could cause a decreased end-tidal CO_2?

A decreased end-tidal CO_2 may occur gradually or suddenly and the likely causes for each event differ.

A gradual decrease in end-tidal CO_2 could be attributable to increased alveolar ventilation, reduced CO_2 production such as in hypothermia or a hypometabolic state, increased alveolar dead-space or a sampling error. Increased alveolar dead-space indicates there are ventilated alveoli not being perfused. The causes for this could be hypotension due to a low cardiac output, pulmonary embolism or high PEEP during IPPV. A sampling error could consist of water blocking the sampling line, an inadequate tidal volume or air entrainment into the sample.

A sudden or complete decrease in end-tidal CO_2 warns of a failure of ventilation or circulation. Ventilation failure could occur due to a blockage or disconnection of the equipment or endotracheal tube displacement. Circulation failure may occur due to cardiac arrest or pump failure for another reason such as a massive MI. A massive PE or embolus of another origin would cause loss of lung perfusion and therefore a loss of end-tidal CO_2. This could be complete if the embolism was catastrophic or to a lesser degree if some of the lung remained perfused.

End-tidal CO_2 would be absent in cases of oesophageal intubation. It is said that if carbonated drinks have been ingested up to six waveforms of end-tidal CO_2 may be seen in the presence of oesophageal intubation. Therefore following intubation, capnography recorded for more than six breaths is the gold standard confirmation of endotracheal placement of the tube.

Explain the causes between the difference in measured end-tidal CO_2, alveolar CO_2 and arterial partial pressures of CO_2

The end-tidal CO_2 in normal lungs is 0.5 to 0.8 kPa less than the arterial partial pressure of CO_2. This difference is increased in patients with mismatched ventilation and perfusion. In such cases the end-tidal CO_2 may grossly under-estimate the arterial CO_2.

The partial pressure of alveolar CO_2 is less than arterial CO_2 because the blood from unventilated alveoli and lung parenchyma, with higher CO_2 tensions, mixes with the blood from ventilated alveoli bringing the overall CO_2 tension in arterial blood up. The end-tidal CO_2 is lower than the alveolar CO_2 due to the dilution of alveolar gases with dead-space gas and gas from un-perfused alveoli, which don't contain any CO_2. These differences account for the end-tidal to arterial CO_2 difference.

Chapter

3.6

Temperature and humidity

3.6.1. Heat loss – Rebecca A Leslie

Tell me about the mechanisms by which patients lose heat intra-operatively

Remember always start by classifying your answer. Then, if you are not interrupted with another question, go on and describe each process in more detail. The mnemonic to remember the main four processes starting with the most important and progressing to the least important process is Royal College Exam Room. Royal stands for radiation, College for convection, Exam for evaporation and Room for respiration.

The mechanisms of heat loss can be divided in to five different processes: radiation, convection, evaporation, respiration and conduction.

Radiation accounts for up to 50% of the heat loss that occurs in theatre. A hot object will emit radiation. This radiation takes energy away from the hot object reducing its temperature. If this energy is then absorbed by another object it will become hotter. This results in the transfer of heat energy from a hotter object to cooler objects, which are not in contact. Thus the patient acts as an efficient radiator. The process is accelerated in anaesthesia if cool objects surround the patient. In addition, the patients are often prevented from receiving heat from the environment. Further heat loss will occur by radiation if the body has to heat up cool infused IV fluids.

Convection accounts for 30% of heat loss in the anaesthetised patient. Convection is the process by which the air adjacent to the surface of the body is warmed. The warmed air then expands and it becomes less dense and rises. This provides a convection current which takes heat away from the patient. It is accelerated in theatre if large body areas are exposed to the convection currents. Heat losses are particularly large due to convection in laminar flow theatres.

Evaporation accounts for 20% of heat loss. As the moisture on the body surface evaporates it requires energy, the latent heat of vaporisation, and the body temperature drops. The amount of heat lost from this process is dependent on the water vapour pressure gradient between the skin and the air. It is an important mechanism for heat loss in health but becomes an undesirable process during surgery. It is increased in surgery where there is a large moist

---

Dr Podcast Scripts for the Primary FRCA, ed. Rebecca A. Leslie, Emily K. Johnson and Alexander P. L. Goodwin.   Published by Cambridge University Press. © R. A. Leslie, E. K. Johnson and A. P. L. Goodwin 2011.

surface area open such as during a laparotomy, a major orthopaedic case or reconstructive plastic surgery.

Respiration causes heat loss by evaporation and by heating of inspired gases. It accounts for 10% of total heat loss and can be reduced by using heat and moisture exchangers.

Conduction is heat loss due to direct contact with a cooler substance and is not a significant cause of heat loss in theatre. Metals are good conductors of heat whilst gases are poor conductors. Conduction is only a problem in theatre if the patient if lying directly on an efficient heat conductor such as a metal table. Conduction accounts for only 5% of heat loss.

What measures can we as anaesthetists take to avoid heat loss?

Loss by radiation can be minimised by increasing the operating room temperature and where possible covering exposed surfaces with warm blankets. Forced air blankets can also be used.

All intra-venous fluids that are given to susceptible patients should be warmed to prevent heat loss by radiation.

Fluids used for irrigation should be warmed, and exposed viscera should be covered or enclosed in plastic bags.

Inspired gases should be humidified, and heat exchangers used. Low flow circle systems help to keep gases well humidified by only introducing small flow rates of cold gas and by using the exothermic process of CO_2 absorption.

Why is it important to maintain body temperature?

Body temperature is tightly regulated because many transport systems and enzymes will not work outside a limited temperature range. The normal body temperature is 37°C and thermoregulatory mechanisms maintain this by 0.2°C.

What do you mean by thermoregulatory mechanisms?

Temperature information from the skin, central tissues and neural tissues are passed to the hypothalamus where the information is integrated and compared to temperature thresholds.

If the body becomes hot and the temperature exceeds the warm threshold then heat-losing responses are initiated, such as behavioural modification (removal of clothes), cutaneous vasodilation, sweating and panting.

If the body is cold and the temperature is less than the cold threshold then thermogenic activities are initiated. These include behavioural activities, such as putting on more clothes and turning on heat sources, cutaneous vasoconstriction, shivering and non-shivering thermogenesis. Non-shivering thermogenesis is an effective method of heat production in infants who utilise specialised brown fat to increase metabolic rate by fat oxidation.

What is the definition of hypothermia?

Hypothermia is defined as a core body temperature of less than 36°C. It is common in the elderly, drowning, hypothyroidism and prolonged surgery.

Why are patients at risk of hypothermia when they have an anaesthetic?

Anaesthesia has a number of effects on temperature control. Firstly the behavioural aspect of thermoregulatory control is completely abolished, they are unable to control the number of clothes they are wearing, their environment or the level of voluntary muscle activity. Also cutaneous vasoconstriction, which is normally responsible for heat preservation, is antagonised by vasodilatory anaesthetic agents such as propofol and volatile agents. In addition the temperature thresholds that are normally present are affected by anaesthesia. The hypothermic thresholds are markedly reduced by up to 3–4°C, so thermoregulatory mechanisms to heat loss are greatly impaired or even abolished.

What are the clinical consequences of hypothermia?

Remember always classify your answer. For this question it will probably be easiest to classify your answer into the effects on different body systems, starting with the most important.

The cardiovascular consequences of hypothermia are as a result of the slowing down of normal metabolic and physiological processes. This leads to hypotension, bradycardia and can in severe cases lead to dysrhythmias such as ventricular fibrillation. In hypothermia the cardiac output is also decreased and blood viscosity increases.

The oxygen–haemoglobin dissociation curve is shifted to the left, increasing oxygen affinity and consequently reducing oxygen delivery. In severe cases of hypothermia pulmonary oedema may occur.

Within the central nervous system there is progressive deterioration in mental function to the point where the EEG will record no cerebral activity.

The metabolic effects of hypothermia are also important. The metabolic rate drops by approximately 6% for every drop in temperature of 1°C. Enzymatic reactions throughout the body are slowed. Particularly of importance to the anaesthetist is the slowing of all the enzymes controlling the reactions of intermediate metabolism. This results in prolongation of the actions of most anaesthetic drugs, particularly neuromuscular blocking agents.

Renal function becomes depressed with hypothermia, and in time acidosis will develop. However the patient may have a diuresis due to the failure of active reabsorption of sodium and water in the renal tubules.

Hyperglycaemia can occur because there is a failure of glucose utilisation.

How would you manage severe hypothermia?

Always start with the basic generic approach of ABC before moving on to the specific management options for severe hypothermia.

Firstly it is important to assess the airway, breathing and circulation. As soon as these areas have been successfully managed it is important to initiate rewarming of the patient. Rapid rewarming is better for rapid onset hypothermia such as sudden immersion, whereas slow rewarming of approximately 1°C/hr is more appropriate for hypothermia of gradual onset.

Techniques used for rewarming of patients are from external heat sources and using internal warming methods.

External warming methods:
- Forced air blankets
- Radiant heaters.

Internal warming:
- Warm intra-venous fluids
- Warm intra-peritoneal fluids

- Warm intra-gastric fluids
- Bladder irrigation with warm fluids
- Cardiopulmonary bypass.

How do forced air warmers work?

Forced air warmers heat up the ambient air to a temperature of between 32 and 40°C. The air is then delivered via a hose to a thin-walled channelled bag positioned over the patient warming them by conduction, convection and radiation. They have been found to be effective even when only a limited surface area is covered.

What methods can you use to warm intra-venous fluids?

There are two methods of warming intra-venous fluids, the dry heat warmer and the co-axial fluid heating system, often called the hot line.

The dry heat warmer consists of a thin-walled PVC bag that is inserted between the two hot metal plates. Fluid passes through the bag and gets warmed.

The co-axial fluid warmer consists of an inner and outer tube. The outside tube carries heated sterilised fluid, whilst the inside tube delivers warmed fluids to the patient. The sterile water is heated to 40°C and stored by the heating case. The water is circulated through the outside tube to avoid it being cooled by continuous flow of cold IV fluids for the patient.

3.6.2. Temperature and its measurement – Rebecca A Leslie

What is heat?

Heat is a form of energy that is determined by how active the molecules of a particular substance are. Heat can be transferred from a hotter substance to a cooler substance. If heat energy is added to a substance, not only will the temperature increase but the physical properties will also change, for example the resistance may increase or it may expand or change state.

What is temperature?

Temperature is a measure of the average kinetic energy of the individual atoms and molecules that make up the substance. By measuring temperature we are able to quantify the thermal state of the substance.

What are the units of temperature?

The SI unit for temperature measurement is the kelvin. One kelvin is 1/273.15 of the thermodynamic temperature of the triple point of water.

In medicine we commonly use degrees Celsius (0 degrees Celsius is equal to 273.15 kelvin). The intervals on the kelvin and degrees Celsius scale are the same. Thus the temperature in kelvin is equal to the temperature in degrees Celsius plus 273.15.

What is the triple point of water?

The triple point of water is the temperature at which ice, water and water vapour are all in equilibrium.

How can temperature be measured?

Remember it is important to classify your answer; do not just start randomly mentioning different methods of measuring temperature. Stop, think and then classify.

There are three main types of device for measuring temperature: electrical, non-electrical and infra-red. Non-electrical methods include alcohol and mercury thermometers and dial thermometers. Electrical techniques include resistance thermometers, thermistors and thermocouples. Infra-red techniques include tympanic membrane thermometers.

What are the problems with using mercury thermometers?

Mercury thermometers work because the volume of mercury expands when the temperature rises. They are calibrated against fixed points, like the triple point and the boiling point of water.

There are several problems with mercury thermometers that limit their use in anaesthesia. Firstly, they are slow to equilibrate with the temperature and take 2–3 minutes for an accurate measurement. In addition, there are limited sites that can be used for measurement using a mercury thermometer, especially in anaesthesia. Rectal measurements with a mercury thermometer may be especially slow due to the presence of faecal material. In neonates there is a risk of rectal perforation if a mercury thermometer is used to take a rectal measurement. Mercury thermometers also carry the risk of breakage, trauma and toxicity.

What are the advantages of an alcohol thermometer?

In modern practice alcohol thermometers are used instead of mercury thermometers. This is because they are much cheaper and don't carry the risk of toxicity. They are also better suited to colder temperatures (mercury solidifies at $-39°C$), however alcohol thermometers are not accurate at high temperatures because alcohol boils at $78.5°C$.

What are dial thermometers?

Dial thermometers may consist of either a bimetallic strip or a Bourdon gauge.

A bimetallic strip thermometer is a coil comprising of two different metals that have different coefficients of expansion. As the temperature rises, the two different metals expand by different amounts causing the coil to tighten, and the pointer to move across the scale.

A Bourdon gauge is normally used to measure pressure, but it can also measure temperature if the gauge is attached to a small sensing element containing mercury or a volatile fluid. As the temperature increases the volume of the sensing substance increases, which causes a small increase in pressure which can be detected by the Bourdon gauge and measured in degrees Celsius.

Describe the different types of electrical thermometer

There are three types of electrical thermometer; resistance thermometers, thermistors, and thermocouples.

Describe in more detail how a resistance thermometer works

Resistance thermometers are based on the principle that when temperature increases it causes a linear increase in the electrical resistance of metals, see Figure 3.6.2a. Consequently resistance thermometers consist of a platinum wire, a source of electrical potential and an

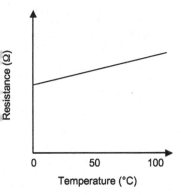

Figure 3.6.2a. Resistance wire graph.
Reproduced with permission from Cross,
M. and Plunkett, E. 2008. *Physics,
Pharmacology and Physiology for
Anaesthetists: Key Concepts for the
FRCA.* Cambridge: Cambridge University
Press. © M. Cross and E. Plunkett 2008.

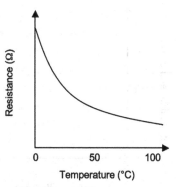

Figure 3.6.2b. Thermistor graph.
Reproduced with permission from Cross,
M. and Plunkett, E. 2008. *Physics,
Pharmacology and Physiology for
Anaesthetists: Key Concepts for the
FRCA.* Cambridge: Cambridge University
Press. © M. Cross and E. Plunkett 2008.

ammeter to measure the current. A change in resistance due to a change in temperature is measured by the ammeter and is then calibrated to show temperature. The addition of a Wheatstone bridge improves their accuracy. Resistance thermometers are not used in clinical practice.

How do thermistors work?

A thermistor contains a small bead of a semi-conductive material, usually a metal oxide that is incorporated into a Wheatstone bridge circuit. In contrast to the resistance thermometer the resistance of a thermistor falls non-linearly with an increase in temperature, see Figure 3.6.2b.

What are the advantages and disadvantages of a thermistor?

The beads of metal oxide within the thermistor can be made very small, and they are incredibly robust so can be used easily within the theatre set-up. They are used in the tips of pulmonary artery flotation catheters for thermodilutional techniques. Although the change in resistance is non-linear they can be manufactured so that over their working range the response is virtually linear.

A disadvantage with thermistors is that with time the calibration may drift, and it may become less accurate. Also if the thermistor is subjected to severe changes in temperature, for example during heat sterilisation, the calibration may change.

How do thermocouples work?

Thermocouple are based on the Seebeck effect, which states that at the junction between two dissimilar metals a voltage is produced, and that the voltage is proportional to the temperature, see Figure 3.6.2c. Copper and constantan, a copper and nickel alloy, are normally used in a thermocouple. Another junction is needed to complete the circuit and at this junction a temperature-dependent voltage will also develop. This junction is kept at a constant

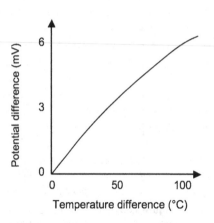

Potential difference (mV)

6

3

0

0   50   100

Temperature difference (°C)

Figure 3.6.2c. Thermocouple graph. Reproduced with permission from Cross, M. and Plunkett, E. 2008. *Physics, Pharmacology and Physiology for Anaesthetists: Key Concepts for the FRCA.* Cambridge: Cambridge University Press. © M. Cross and E. Plunkett 2008.

temperature as the reference junction whilst the other junction acts as a measuring temperature probe. Thermocouples are stable and accurate to 0.1°C.

What do you know about infrared temperature measurement?

The human body emits infrared radiation. The intensity and wavelength of this radiation is dependent on the temperature. A tympanic membrane thermometer uses a tube, which is inserted into the ear, and it directs the radiation, which is emitted from the ear, on to a pyroelectric sensor. The sensor comprises of a polarised substance, normally a ceramic crystalline material, whose polarity changes with temperature. The polarity can be detected as an electrical output, which is in turn proportional to temperature. The response time of a tympanic membrane thermometer is very rapid compared to other thermometers. Inaccuracies can occur with wax in the ear canal, or if the probe is not directed at the tympanic membrane, but at the side of the ear canal.

Where can core body temperature be measured?

Sites that allow the measurement of core body temperature include the nasopharynx, the distal oesophagus, the pulmonary artery, the rectum, the bladder and the tympanic membrane. There are advantages and disadvantages to all of them.

The best method is via pulmonary artery catheter but this is clearly too invasive for many patients. The nasopharynx offers an accurate measure of core body temperature provided a probe is inserted into the nasopharynx under direct vision and that gas leaking around the cuff of the endotracheal tube does not interfere with its reading. Oesophageal measurement is most stable in the lower quarter of the oesophagus where it is not affected by tracheal gases and where, due to its position, it accurately records cardiac temperature. The tympanic membrane accurately mirrors oesophageal temperature providing there are no drafts in the external auditory canal. The bladder temperature is determined mainly by urine flow, and unless there are at least 270 ml of urine a day the bladder temperature will not accurately reflect core body temperature. Rectal temperature is affected by the insulating properties of faeces, and blood returning from the lower limbs, so rectal temperature can be 0.5–1°C higher than elsewhere.

Skin temperature will allow the peripheral to core temperature gradient to be calculated and hence adequacy of peripheral perfusion.

So to conclude, areas used most commonly in anaesthesia for accurate core temperature measurement include the nasopharynx, the lower oesophagus and the tympanic membrane.

3.6.3. Humidification – Rebecca A Leslie

What is the clinical importance of humidification for an anaesthetist?

Humidification is incredibly important to anaesthetists because during anaesthesia the normal mechanism for humidifying inspired gases which is the nose, is often bypassed by an endotracheal tube or occasionally a tracheostomy. If gases supplied to the patient are not warmed and humidified there are major consequences on the tracheobronchial tree. The airway secretions become dry and tenacious and can lead to thick mucus plugs that can potentially block the airways.

There is also a reduction of ciliary activity and impairment of the mucociliary escalator. If the cilia are continually exposed to dry gases they soon disappear and the epithelium becomes keratinised. Another consequence of prolonged inspiration of dry gases is heat loss through latent heat of vaporisation, as the body has to humidify the gases in the respiratory tract.

Which patients are particularly at risk from airway damage if dry inspired gases are used?

High-risk patients include those who are undergoing prolonged anaesthesia and intensive care patients. Patients with underlying respiratory disease are also at risk as damage to the mucociliary escalator will have much more significance. Other patients at risk are those at the extremes of age.

How do we express humidity?

Humidity is normally described as either absolute humidity or relative humidity.

Absolute humidity is the mass of water vapour present in a given volume of air. The values of absolute humidity are normally expressed as milligrams per litre (mg/L) or grams per cubic metre (g/m^3), both of which have the same numerical value.

Relative humidity is the ratio of the mass of water in a given volume of air to the mass of water required to saturate that given volume of air at the same temperature. It is usually expressed as a percentage.

What methods are available to measure humidity?

Remember always classify. With this sort of question you really don't want to have to get in to the finer details of a hair hygrometer so start your answer with a clear classification. This way you show the examiner that you have a clear understanding of the topic, and you may escape without having to go into any further specific details of the different techniques.

Instruments to measure humidity can be divided into those that measure relative humidity and those that measure absolute humidity. Relative humidity can be measured using a hair hygrometer, a wet and dry bulb hygrometer or a Reynault's hygrometer. Absolute humidity can be measured using transducers or a mass spectrometer.

The simplest method of measuring relative humidity is to use a hair hygrometer. This instrument works on the principle that the hair gets longer as the humidity rises. The hair is

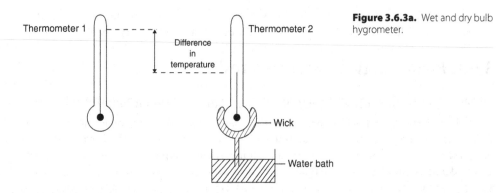

Figure 3.6.3a. Wet and dry bulb hygrometer.

attached to a spring and a pointer, and as the length of the hair changes the pointer moves over a scale.

The wet and dry bulb hygrometer is another instrument for measuring relative humidity, see Figure 3.6.3a. This technique uses two thermometers. One of the thermometers is in equilibrium with the ambient temperature of the room. A wick surrounds the bulb of the second thermometer, which is in contact with a water bath. The temperature displayed by this thermometer is consequently lower than the ambient room temperature because of the cooling effect of the evaporation of the water surrounding the bulb, the latent heat of vaporisation. The temperature difference between the two thermometers is related to the rate of evaporation of water, which in turn is related to the ambient humidity. A figure for the relative humidity is calculated from a set of tables from this temperature difference.

The third way of measuring relative humidity is using a Reynault's hygrometer. In this technique, air is bubbled through a solution of ether within a silver tube. As air passes through the solution it causes the ether to evaporate and consequently reduces the temperature of the remaining liquid. The point at which condensation or misting appears on the outer shiny surface of the tube is called the dew point, and represents the temperature at which the ambient air around the outside of the tube is fully saturated. The ratio of the saturated vapour pressure at the dew point to the saturated vapour pressure at ambient temperature gives the relative humidity. The result is determined from tables.

Absolute, rather than relative humidity can be measured using a transducer. The transducer detects a change in electrical resistance or capacitance as the substance absorbs water from the atmosphere, which is in turn dependent on the ambient humidity.

Mass spectrometry can be used to accurately measure humidity and has a quick response time. However the equipment is cumbersome, expensive and rarely ever used.

You mentioned the saturated water vapour pressure, what do you mean by this term?

It is the maximum attainable water vapour pressure at a certain temperature.

What is the simplest method we use to humidify inspired gases?

This is a simple question, just think about what you use every day.

We commonly use heat and moisture exchangers (HMEs) that provide a passive form of humidification. The HME contains a paper, foam or sponge element that is covered by hygroscopic material enclosed in a sealed unit with an inlet and an outlet. As the patient exhales, their warm, moist expired gases pass through the HME element. The gas is cooled and water condenses on the element. The element in turn is warmed by both the latent heat of the water condensing on it and by the specific heat of the expired gases. During inspiration as the cold, dry gases are inspired they become warmed as they pass through the HME. In addition the water, which condensed on the HME element during expiration, now evaporates and humidifies the inspiratory gases. After inspiration the transfer of heat and water to the inspiratory gases results in cooling of the HME so it is ready for the next expiration and the whole process can occur again.

How does the efficiency of an HME compare with the normal humidification of inspired gases in the nose and pharynx?

Under optimum conditions an HME will achieve an inspired air humidity of 25 g/m^{-3}. Normally, the air reaching the trachea is saturated with water vapour to a humidity of 34 g/m^{-3}. Therefore the HME gives a relative humidity of 60–70%.

What are the disadvantages of the HME?

The HME humidifier takes 15–20 minutes to reach its optimum ability to humidify dry gases. The performance of the HME is affected by inspired tidal volume and minute volumes, which affect the time that the gases are in contact with the HME medium. The performance is also affected by the water vapour content and temperature of the exhaled gases.

The efficiency of the system decreases with time, and an HME is only recommended for use for 24 hours. There is an increase in resistance to flow of approximately 0.1–2 cmH$_2$O as a result of use, and this resistance is increased more dramatically if the element becomes blocked with mucus or secretions.

HME increases the dead-space of the breathing circuit, which could increase PCO$_2$ unless alveolar ventilation is increased.

There is also a risk of infections with organisms such as pseudomonas.

What is a hot water bath humidifier?

A hot water bath humidifier is commonly used in intensive care units to deliver a relative humidity much higher than is possible with an HME. This is an active system where the hot water bath is heated to 60°C to inhibit microbial contamination. The fresh gas flow is channelled into the container and is directed to pass in close contact with the hot water, allowing it to gain maximum saturation. The saturated gases then pass out along tubing that has poor thermal insulation properties, which causes a decrease in the temperature of the inspired gases that is essential for safety. The temperature of the gases is measured by a thermistor at the patient end, which can trigger changes in the water bath temperature. When using a hot water humidifier it is possible to deliver gases at 37°C that are fully saturated.

What are the disadvantages of using a hot water bath humidifier?

A disadvantage of using a hot water bath humidifier is that it is an expensive and bulky piece of equipment. There is risk of scalding the patient, although thermostats are present which will automatically switch the power to the heater off if extreme temperatures are reached. There is also a risk of electrical shock. Another potential problem with a hot water bath humidifier is that vaporised water can condense in a redundant loop of tubing and can both obstruct the gas flow to the patient, or may get blown into the patient's airways. For this reason a water trap is always included in the circuit.

What is a cascade humidifier?

This is a variation of the hot water bath, where the gas is allowed to bubble through a perforated plate and through the water to maximise the amount of gas exposed to the water. The large surface area of the gas exposed to water ensures that the gas becomes fully humidified. It is more efficient than a hot water bath humidifier.

How do nebulisers work?

Nebulisers can also be used as humidifiers. A capillary tube embedded in a water container sits near to a high-pressure gas stream. As gas flows through a Venturi, creating a negative pressure, water is entrained through the capillary tube and broken into fine droplets. These droplets can be made even smaller by directing them at an anvil. Nebulisers are able to produce droplets of between 2 and 4 microns, these droplets tend to be deposited in the pharynx and upper airways.

There are also ultrasonic devices in which water is nebulised by a plate that vibrates at ultrasonic frequencies. These are not commonly used, because they can deliver gas that is 100% humidified so will easily overload the pulmonary tree with fluid.

Chapter

3.7

Pressure and cardiac output measurement

3.7.1. Pressure measurement – Archana Panickar

Can you define pressure?

Pressure is the force applied per unit area. The SI unit of pressure is pascal (Pa), but as this represents a very small pressure, pressure is commonly expressed in kilopascals.

How do you define a pascal?

One Pascal is defined as a force of 1 newton acting over an area of 1 square metre.

What is force?

Force is defined as that which changes or tends to change the state of rest or motion of a body.

How can force be measured?

Force is measured in newtons. One newton is the force that will accelerate a mass of 1 kilogram by 1 metre per second per second or 1 N is equal to 1 kg per square metre.

The force of gravity accelerates a body in free fall by 9.81 metre per square second. Therefore, the force of gravity on the body of 1 kg is 9.8 newtons. This force is known as one kilogram weight. One newton is equal to 1 divided by 9.81 kilogram weight, that is 102 gram weight.

What are the other units of pressure, and how are the units inter-converted?

In addition to the Pascal the other units of pressure are as follows:

- Bar
- Dynes per square cm
- Pounds per square inch
- Torr
- cmH_2O

- mmHg
- kg·cm^{-2}
- Atmosphere.

One bar is equal in pressure to the following:

- 100 kPa
- 14.5 pounds per square inch
- 750 torr
- 10^6 dynes/cm^2.

A standard atmosphere is the pressure of 101.325 kPa therefore 1 atmosphere is roughly the same as 1 bar.

1 kPa is equal to 7.5 mmHg and therefore 1 bar is equal to 750 mmHg.

1 kPa is also equal to 10.2 cmH$_2$O, therefore 1 cmH$_2$O is equal to 98 kPa.

Can you give some clinical implications of force and pressure?

This is a very commonly asked question and you should have a clear concept.

The first example is that of the relative difficulty of injecting a liquid from a large syringe and a small syringe.

$$\text{Pressure} = \frac{\text{Force}}{\text{Area}}$$

The pressure developed in the syringe depends on the force applied, and the area over which it is applied, that is, the area of the plunger. If the force exerted by the thumb on the two syringes is the same, a greater pressure is generated in the smaller syringe compared to the large syringe, as the area of the plunger in the small syringe is less than that of the large syringe.

If the diameter or radius of the plunger in the large syringe is twice that of the small syringe, the area of the large plunger will be four times more than the small plunger, as area is equal to the square of the radius. This means that the pressure in the large syringe will be four times less compared to the pressure in the small syringe, for the same applied force.

It is easy to produce accidental extravasations of drugs while injecting at high pressures using syringes with a lower diameter plunger. This is of relevance when performing intravenous regional anaesthesia, where a tourniquet is inflated above the systolic blood pressure to prevent systemic effects of the local anaesthetic injected into the limb. During injection, the pressures in the vein can be very high, and the protection from the tourniquet may be inadequate if a vein close to the tourniquet is used.

Can you give some other examples?

An example of pressure generated as a result of force acting over an area is the formation of bed sores in an immobilised patient. The patient's weight acting over a small area such as the sacrum can lead to high pressure. If this pressure is higher than the typical systolic blood pressure of 16 kPa, the blood supply to the area is cut off, and pressure sores develop.

To understand the following examples, you will need to have an understanding of expiratory valves and the oxygen failure warning device.

Pressure relief valves and expiratory valves on anaesthetic breathing systems are other examples. The pressure generated by gases in the breathing circuit act over the area of the disc of the expiratory valve, which exerts an upward force on the disc. If this force is greater than the downward force exerted by the spring of the expiratory valve, the disc rises, and releases gases.

It is important you have a good depth of knowledge about pressure reducing values as they are often asked about in the structured oral examination. Don't be surprised if you are asked to draw one, so do practice before taking the exam.

Pressure reducing valves or pressure regulators used in anaesthetic machines and Entonox valves also work by balancing the force of a spring against that from the pressure on a diaphragm.

The oxygen failure warning device works on the same principle. When the oxygen pressure falls below a set minimum value, the force acting on the diaphragm fails to hold it against a spring. This causes the diaphragm to move down, and oxygen leaks past a small valve to blow the whistle, warning of failing oxygen pressure.

What is the relationship between gauge pressure and absolute pressure?

Absolute pressure = Gauge pressure + Atmospheric pressure.

When the pressure is measured relative to atmospheric pressure, the value obtained is called gauge pressure. Absolute pressure is zero referenced against a perfect vacuum, so it is equal to gauge pressure plus atmospheric pressure. For example when an oxygen cylinder is full, the gauge reads 137 bar. When the cylinder is empty, the gauge reads 0 bar, but the cylinder still contains oxygen at atmospheric pressure of 1 bar, unless the cylinder has been completely emptied by applying a vacuum. Hence the true or absolute pressure in an empty cylinder is 1 bar, and for a full cylinder is 138 bar.

Ventilator and gas cylinder pressures, arterial blood pressure and venous pressure are all gauge pressures. The gauge pressure above or below the existing atmospheric pressure is recorded in all these cases. Atmospheric pressure is an absolute pressure measurement.

Atmospheric pressure on the surface of the earth is due to the gravitational force on the air molecules. Thus, the atmospheric pressure will depend on the density of air, which in turn, depends on the altitude and weather conditions at that point.

What is the principle of a manometer?

The manometer is a very basic device for measuring pressure (Figure 3.7.1a). A column of liquid in a tube is subjected to the unknown pressure. The column will rise or fall until its weight is in equilibrium with the pressure differential between the two ends of the tube. The height of the fluid column is independent of the cross sectional area of the tube.

The pressure exerted by a column of water 10.2 cm high is 1 kPa. The top of the manometer tube should be open to the atmosphere. Mercury manometers used for blood pressure measurement have a disc of permeable material at the top to prevent spillage.

What is the advantage of using a mercury manometer?

Mercury is 13.6 times denser than water, so the force exerted by its weight is 13.6 times higher (Figure 3.7.1b). Higher pressures can be measured with a shorter column of mercury,

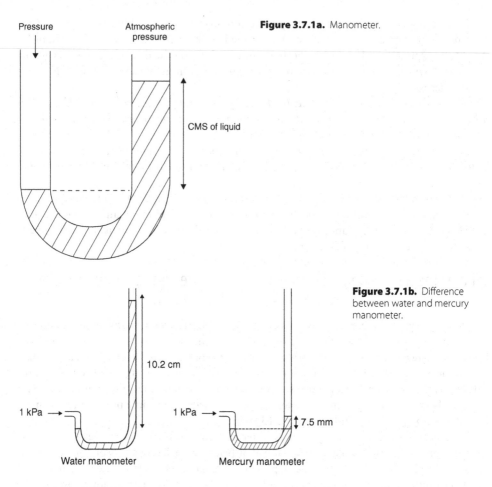

Figure 3.7.1a. Manometer.

Pressure

Atmospheric pressure

CMS of liquid

Figure 3.7.1b. Difference between water and mercury manometer.

10.2 cm

1 kPa ⟶

Water manometer

1 kPa ⟶

7.5 mm

Mercury manometer

compared with a column of water, because a pressure of 1 kPa, which supports 7.5 mm mercury, will support a 10.2 cm column of water.

A mercury manometer measuring 750 mmHg is equivalent to a pressure of 1 bar, 1 atmosphere or 101.3 kPa. The units of bar and kilopascal are not affected by changes in temperature or gravitational force.

What is the effect of a slope in the manometer tube?

If a manometer tube is tilted, the liquid rises along it, until the necessary vertical height is reached. A sloped manometer is used in sensitive pressure gauges.

What is the difference between a barometer and a manometer?

A mercury barometer is used to measure the atmospheric pressure. The column of mercury is sealed, and a vacuum is present above the column of mercury, so that the absolute atmospheric pressure is recorded.

The vacuum above the mercury column is also called Torricellian vacuum and contains mercury vapour at saturated vapour pressure.

What would happen to the meniscus of a mercury barometer if a few drops of isoflurane were introduced into the vacuum above it?

If a small amount of any liquid is introduced above the column, a pressure is exerted, due to the saturated vapour pressure of that substance, at the particular temperature. This will cause the meniscus to fall by a level which corresponds to the saturated vapour pressure of that substance.

At 1 atmosphere, the height of the mercury column is 750 mmHg. Isoflurane has a saturated vapour pressure of 250 mmHg. If a few drops of isoflurane are introduced into the vacuum, the mercury column would fall by 250 mmHg, thus the final height of the column would be 500 mmHg.

What is a Bourdon gauge, and how does it work?

A Bourdon gauge is an aneroid gauge (without liquid) and consists of a coiled tube with a pointer which moves on a calibrated scale when subjected to pressure. Increasing pressure causes the tube to uncoil, and this moves the pointer, via an amplification gear, over a scale on a dial. This type of gauge is used for measurement of high pressures, such as gas cylinder pressures, where the required height of the fluid column would be impractically high. The advantage of bourdon gauges over manometers is that there is no liquid to spill.

What is differential pressure measurement?

Differential pressure measurement is the measurement of the difference in pressure between two points, for example between two points in the anaesthetic breathing system. Differential pressure gauges have two inlet ports, each connected to one of the volumes whose pressure is to be monitored.

3.7.2. Blood pressure measurement – Rebecca A Leslie

How do we measure blood pressure?

Remember; always classify your answer.

Blood pressure measurement can be invasive or non-invasive.

Non-invasive methods for measuring blood pressure include the following:

- Simple cuff and manometer
- von Recklinghausen oscillotonometer
- Automated oscillometric techniques
- Doppler ultrasound techniques
- Volumetric clamp technique (Penaz technique).

Invasive blood pressure measure requires arterial cannulation.

If you were using a cuff and a manometer how would you measure the blood pressure?

I would place an appropriately sized cuff on the patient's upper arm with the centre of the cuff over the brachial artery. I would then pump the cuff up to a pressure higher than I expect the systolic blood pressure to be. Then, whilst listening over the brachial artery with my stethoscope I would slowly release the pressure by 2–3 mmHg per second.

What are the sounds you are listening for called?

The sounds I am listening for are called Korotkoff sounds after a Russian physician. The sound has five different phases. The first phase is the onset of the sound and is when blood starts to flow through the artery. This first phase correlates with the systolic blood pressure. The second phase is a slight muffling whilst the third phase is an increase in the volume of the sound. Next there is a further, dramatic fall in the sound level representing phase 4. Phase 5 is the loss of any sound. There is some controversy as to what indicates the diastolic pressure; some people believe it is at phase 4 although it is more widely accepted to be at phase 5.

You said you would use an appropriately sized cuff, what do you mean by this?

The width of the cuff should be approximately 20% greater than the diameter of the patients arm. A cuff that is not the right size will give an inaccurate blood pressure reading. If the cuff is too small for the patient the blood pressure over-reads, and if the cuff is too large the reading will be falsely low.

What is a von Recklinghausen oscillotonometer?

This method for measuring blood pressure uses two different cuffs; a proximal and a distal cuff. The proximal cuff is the occlusion cuff, and the distal cuff is used for detecting the pulsations. Each cuff is connected to a different aneroid barometer. The cuffs are pumped up to a pressure exceeding the expected systolic blood pressure. The pressure in the proximal cuff is then slowly released. When the systolic pressure is reached the pulsations in the brachial artery cause oscillations in the distal cuff and the aneroid it is connected to. These oscillations are transferred through a mechanical amplification system to a needle. The onset of the oscillations indicates the systolic blood pressure, the point of maximum oscillations is the mean arterial pressure and the diastolic pressure is when the oscillations diminish.

How does a DINAMAP differ from a von Recklinghausen oscillotonometer?

First define what a DINAMAP is then describe the differences.

DINAMAP stands for Device for Indirect Non-invasive Automated Mean Arterial Pressure. It works on a similar principle to the von Recklinghausen oscillotonometer; however it only has one cuff and instead of an aneroid barometer has a pressure transducer to measure the oscillations. The system contains a microprocessor to interpret the pressure changes and to control the timing of the inflations and deflations. The DINAMAP also contains a timing mechanism to adjust the frequency of measurements and a display to show the blood pressure result.

Initially the cuff is inflated to a suitably high pressure, normally around 160 mmHg. This pressure is then decreased in small increments. Similar to the von Recklinghausen oscillotonometer the return of blood flow causes oscillations in the cuff pressure. This is sensed by the pressure transducer and interpreted by the microprocessor. The mean arterial pressure corresponds to the maximum oscillation and the diastolic blood pressure corresponds to the rapid decline in the oscillations. For subsequent blood pressure readings the cuff is only inflated to 25 mmHg higher than the previous systolic blood pressure.

What are the problems with using an automated oscillometric technique?

One of the main problems with the DINAMAP is that it is not accurate in dysrhythmias such as atrial fibrillation, or at extremes of blood pressure. It will under-estimate the blood pressure when it is extremely high, and over-estimate the blood pressure when the blood pressure is too low.

Similar to the simple manometer methods there are erroneous readings if the wrong sized cuff is used.

The maximum frequency of blood pressure measurement using a DINAMAP is approximately 1 minute, and there are times during anaesthesia when this is not frequent enough.

There have also been reported cases where frequent cuff inflations have caused ulnar nerve palsies and petechial haemorrhages under the cuff.

Tell me about invasive blood pressure measurement?

The basic system for invasive blood pressure measurement comprises of an intra-arterial cannula in continuity with a column of heparinised saline, and a transducer. The heparinised saline is pressurised to 300 mmHg and connected to a flushing device.

The transducer converts mechanical energy from the movement of a diaphragm into an electrical signal that is then amplified and processed. The column of fluid that is in continuity with the arterial blood is responsible for moving the diaphragm in the transducer as the arterial pressure changes. The diaphragm in the transducer is connected to a strain gauge. As the diaphragm moves there is an alteration in the tension of the strain gauge and as a result the resistance changes. The changes of current through the resistor wire can be amplified and displayed as a pressure waveform.

To allow accurate measurement of these small changes in resistance a Wheatstone bridge circuit is often used, see Figure 3.8.1b in the next chapter. A Wheatstone bridge consists of four resistors, a galvanometer and a source of energy such as a battery. The resistors are arranged in two parallel branches; there are two constant resistors, a variable resistor and the unknown resistor which in this case alters according to changes in the pressure transducer diaphragm. The Wheatstone bridge circuit uses a null deflection system so no current flows through the galvanometer when the bridge is balanced. Changes in resistance are measured and electronically converted and displayed as an arterial pressure waveform.

In practice most pressure transducers used for arterial pressure measurement include four strain gauges which comprise of the four resistors of the Wheatstone bridge. It is designed so that the resistances of two of the strain gauges on opposite sides of the Wheatstone bridge increase as the pressure increases, while the resistances of the other two strain gauges decrease as the pressure decreases. This gives a larger change in potential at the galvanometer which can then be amplified and displayed as a pressure.

What information can be gained from an arterial pressure waveform?

In addition to the blood pressure and heart rate other information can be gained from the characteristics of the waveform. The slope of the systolic upstroke gives some indication to the contractility of the myocardium, with a slow rise indicating the need for inotropic support. The position of the dicrotic notch reflects the systemic vascular resistance; if the dicrotic notch is high it indicates peripheral vasoconstriction, if there is vasodilation the dicrotic notch moves down the curve. The stroke volume can be estimated by measuring the area under the curve from the beginning of the upstroke to the dicrotic notch. By looking at the waveform you can also see a respiratory swing.

What are the indications for an intra-arterial blood pressure measurement?

Arterial lines are used in three groups of patients:

- Patients where rapid changes in blood pressure are expected
- Patients where frequent blood gases are required
- Patients where non-invasive blood pressure measurements are inaccurate.

Rapid changes in blood pressure are expected in patients with cardiovascular instability, severe blood loss, hypovolaemia, and those undergoing intra-cranial surgery.

Non-invasive blood pressure measurements are inaccurate in patients with dysrhythmias, and in the morbidly obese.

Patients requiring inotropic support also require an arterial line for beat-to-beat blood pressure measurement.

What are the complications of arterial cannulation?

These can be early complications and late complications.

Early complications include ischaemia distal to the cannulae due to direct occlusion. Multiple attempts at insertion and haematoma formation increase the risk of ischaemia.

Late complications include distal ischaemia as a result of thrombosis formation and infection. Local infection is thought to occur in less than 20% of cases, whilst systemic cases occur in less than 5% of cases.

Other complications of arterial cannulation which can occur at any point include the risk of intra-arterial injection and the risk of exsanguination if disconnection occurs.

What is Allen's test?

Allen's test is carried out before arterial cannulation to ensure adequate blood supply to the distal limb if the radial artery is occluded. The patient clenches their fist and the doctor then occludes both the radial and the ulnar artery with their fingers. The patient then relaxes their clenched fist which is now white from lack of blood supply. The doctor then releases the patient's ulnar artery to ensure that the patient's hand quickly re-perfuses with blood from the ulnar artery. If the hand does not flush pink within 5 seconds then it suggests that collaterals from the radial to the ulnar artery are not adequate enough to perfuse the hand and another site for arterial cannulation must be found.

3.7.3. Resonance and damping – Henry Murdoch

This is a popular topic that is often asked in the both the OSCE and the structured oral examination. The key to any questions on this subject is a solid understanding of the basic principles and applying this to examples in practice. This topic is usually asked as part of a discussion on invasive pressure monitoring.

With any question, think before you speak (though not for too long!) about the best way to structure your answer. Often questions will be asked in such a way that this will be obvious. However if this isn't the case start with a simple structure, this gives you time to think and compose yourself and allows room for expanding your answers when asked.

Often the examiners will start with a straightforward introduction question to get things going. This will usually involve asking you to give a definition of something. If not, they usually will want you to start with a simple answer.

What is natural or resonant frequency?

The resonant frequency is the frequency that a system will oscillate at if disturbed and left alone.

Analogy: Imagine a jelly on a plate. If you disturb the plate, the jelly will wobble or oscillate at a unique frequency. This is its resonant frequency.

An invasive pressure monitoring system has a resonant frequency too. This is an important feature as it can influence its response as a monitoring system. Its natural frequency can amplify pressure signals by up to 40%. By designing the system with a natural frequency 10 times that of the fundamental frequency to be measured (i.e. heart rate) you can avoid the unwanted amplification and distortion of the signals associated with them coinciding. If the natural frequency falls below 40 Hz then it will start to coincide with that of the blood pressure range. This will result in a sine wave, which will cause distortion of the pressure waveform and affect the reading.

What affects the natural frequency of an invasive monitoring system?

This question looks for you to demonstrate that you know some of the key features in the design of invasive monitoring equipment.

The natural frequency increases with the diameter of the catheter lumen (they are directly proportional). The square root of the length of tubing, compliance and fluid density are inversely proportional to natural frequency.

This is why the arterial line set-up is relatively short, wide and stiff. This ensures the natural frequency is approximately 10 times the fundamental frequency and avoids distortion of the signals.

What do we mean by resonance and damping?

This appears a difficult question at first but by keeping it simple and providing definitions you can demonstrate a basic understanding that can be developed if asked. And they may not ask!

Resonance is the tendency of a system to oscillate whereas damping is the tendency to resist oscillations.

A system that is resonating will see an increase in the amplitude of its oscillations whereas in damping the stored energy in the system is dissipated resulting in a reduction in the amplitude of its oscillations.

Analogy: If you shake the jelly at a frequency that coincides with its natural frequency the jelly will start to resonate and the oscillation amplitude or wobble factor will increase. If you leave the jelly alone it will settle and the oscillations will eventually return to their starting point. The time taken for this is determined by damping. Steadying the plate with your hand reduces the amplitude of the oscillations and the jelly quickly returns to its resting state. Your hand is resisting or damping the oscillations by dissipating the energy in the system. An over-damped system will stop very quickly with minimal oscillations. An under-damped system will stop slowly.

Can you give me an example of where damping and resonance occur in your practice?

Invasive pressure monitoring is a good example of damping and resonance in practice. Both arterial and CVP monitoring have a diaphragm transducer that is disturbed by the blood pressure waves oscillating in a column of fluid. The oscillations are converted to an electrical signal that is displayed as a pressure trace on a screen. The accuracy of the monitoring signal is affected by both resonance and damping.

The effect of resonance should hopefully be removed by ensuring the natural frequency of the system is 10 times that of the fundamental frequency being measured. If the natural and fundamental frequencies approach one another the pressure waves coincide and amplify the waveform amplitude.

Damping will smooth out the trace displayed on the monitor as the oscillation amplitude is reduced. This can be caused by anything that affects transmission of arterial pressure to the transducer. Common causes include blood clots, air bubbles and kinked cannulae.

What are some of the main causes of damping in a system?

The main causes of damping include cannulae that are kinked or contain blood clots, as well as air bubbles in the tubing. Excessively compliant or long tubing and a soft diaphragm can also damp a monitoring system. Standard tubing length should not exceed 120 cm whilst diameter should be 1.5–3 mm. All these factors will dissipate the energy of the oscillations and smooth out the trace.

What would you see in a system that was over-damped?

An over-damped pressure trace will under-estimate systolic blood pressure and over-estimate diastolic pressure. Mean arterial pressure will be unaffected.

In over-damped pressure monitoring systems, a disturbance due to a pressure wave will have its energy dissipated and the extent of the oscillations will be reduced. The trace will appear smooth and flat.

What would you see in a system that was under-damped?

An under-damped pressure trace will over-estimate systolic blood pressure and under-estimate diastolic pressure. Mean arterial pressure will be unaffected.

In an under-damped pressure monitoring system, the disturbance by the pressure wave will take a long time to return to its steady state because the oscillations will have resonated creating large amplitude waves displaying extremes of pressure.

What is optimal damping? How would you check for this?

A balance needs to be established between resonance and damping. If a system is under-damped the time taken for the system to respond to a disturbance will be prolonged. It will be affected by resonance. If you flush an arterial line it should oscillate for 2–3 cycles before settling (these cycles are seen as transduced pressure sine waves on the monitor). This is optimal damping and is given a value of 0.64. An under-damped system will oscillate for >3 cycles before settling whereas an over-damped system may not oscillate at all. A flush should be with normal saline at 300 mmHg.

What is critical damping?

Critical damping occurs when there are no oscillations in response to a disturbance. It is given a value of 1.

This is the extreme extent of over-damping. It is seen when the arterial line is flushed or the connector is switched off. As all the energy of the arterial pressure oscillations is dissipated there is no pressure waveform displayed.

3.7.4. Intra-cranial pressure measurement – Caroline SG Janes

What is the Monro–Kellie doctrine?

The Monro–Kellie doctrine states that the skull is a closed box, therefore any increase in one of the components within it must result in a decrease in one of the other components for the pressure to remain constant. A small increase in one of the components without compensation can produce large changes in intra-cranial pressure (ICP) resulting in reduced blood flow to the brain and hypoxia.

The three components within the skull include 1.5 kg of brain tissue which makes up 80–85%, 50–120 ml of cerebrospinal fluid (CSF) which makes up 5–12% and 50–70 ml of blood which makes up the remaining 5–7%.

What is normal ICP?

Normal ICP is 8–12 mmHg when supine. ICP is related directly to intra-thoracic pressure and has a normal respiratory swing. It is increased by coughing, straining and positive end-expiratory pressure.

Please draw a graph of the relationship between ICP and intra-cranial volume

Make sure you begin all graphs by labelling the axis – for this graph ICP in mmHg is on the y axis and intra-cranial volume in ml on the x axis (Figure 3.7.4a). The graph should show a slow rise in pressure at first as the volume increases reflecting initial intra-cranial compliance. The pressure then suddenly rises exponentially with a small increase in volume as the skull can no longer accommodate it, at this point ischaemia starts to develop.

What role does autoregulation play in maintaining cerebral blood flow?

In health autoregulation plays a vital role in maintaining cerebral blood flow.

The brain is very sensitive to over-perfusion, and cerebral autoregulation plays an important role in maintaining an appropriate blood pressure to that region.

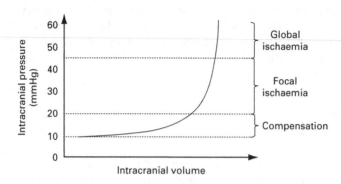

Draw and label the axes as shown. Note that the x axis is usually drawn without any numerical markers. Normal intracranial volume is assumed to be at the left side of the curve and should be in keeping with an ICP of 5–10 mmHg. Draw a curve similar in shape to a positive tear-away exponential. Demonstrate on your curve that compensation for a rise in the volume of one intracranial component maintains the ICP <20 mmHg. However, when these limited compensatory mechanisms are exhausted, ICP rises rapidly, causing focal ischaemia (ICP 20–45 mmHg) followed by global ischaemia (ICP >45 mmHg).

Figure 3.7.4a. Intra-cranial volume–pressure relationship. Reproduced with permission from Cross, M. and Plunkett, E. 2008. *Physics, Pharmacology and Physiology for Anaesthetists: Key Concepts for the FRCA.* Cambridge: Cambridge University Press. © M. Cross and E. Plunkett 2008.

What happens initially to compensate for a rise in ICP?

The principal buffers for increased volumes include both CSF and, to a lesser extent, blood volume. Initially there is movement of CSF into the spinal canal, there is also an increase in the venous absorption of CSF. Venous sinuses are then compressed reducing the total amount of blood present.

Eventually these compensatory mechanisms will be overwhelmed. The rise in ICP will start to exceed cerebral perfusion pressure (CPP) and impede cerebral blood flow. Unless CPP is increased or ICP reduced this will cause ischaemia.

Remember:

$$CPP = MAP - (ICP + CVP).$$

What are the clinical features of a raised ICP?

The signs and symptoms of raised ICP include headache, nausea and vomiting, papilloedema and reducing consciousness. In addition infants may have a bulging fontanelle. Symptoms are usually worse first thing in the morning and exacerbated by bending down or straining.

In severe cases raised ICP causes cerebral herniation – this most commonly affects the brainstem which is forced out through the foramen magnum. This stretches the cranial nerves and coning occurs. This causes hypertension and bradycardia – referred to as the

Cushing reflex and is a pre-terminal sign. Once the body is no longer able to maintain the Cushing reflex hypotension, apnoea and fixed, dilated pupils will follow inevitably resulting in death.

What are the causes of raised ICP?

ICP can be caused by an increase in the amount of one or more of the three components: CSF, brain or blood.

It can be due to an increase in CSF resulting from blockage, obstruction to absorption or overproduction – this is termed *hydrocephalus*.

The brain tissue itself can swell and cause mass effect – this can be caused by a tumour, oedema, contusions or an abscess.

Thirdly it can be due to an increase in blood from haemorrhage or venous obstruction – haemorrhage can be extra-dural, sub-dural, subarachnoid or intra-cerebral in location. Venous obstruction can be caused by venous sinus thrombosis. There is also a condition called benign intra-cranial hypertension which causes raised ICP of unknown cause.

What non-pharmacological methods are used to reduce ICP?

This is a key question – try to work through your management logically so that you don't miss anything out. It may help to think about what you do when you get ready to transfer a head injury patient.

The principles of treating raised ICP are to maintain oxygenation to the brain tissue and thus prevent secondary brain injury. Treatment should therefore be aimed at both decreasing ICP and optimising CPP. A raised ICP can be reduced with careful attention to ventilation, drainage and posture. In certain cases immediate neurosurgery may be the only definite treatment so prompt diagnosis is crucial in all neurological emergencies.

Ventilation should aim to maintain pCO_2 at low–normal levels between 4.5 and 5.0 kPa – this causes vasoconstriction thus reducing ICP. This is best achieved by increasing the respiratory rate, however, hypocapnia should be avoided as it can result in inadequate oxygen delivery. This is because hypocarbia causes cerebral vasoconstriction.

Optimum venous drainage should be ensured by keeping the head in the midline position, nursing the patient at 30° head up and removing tight fitting tube ties and neck collars. Positive end-expiratory pressure should only be used when absolutely necessary for improving oxygenation as it can impede venous drainage.

Cooling has been advocated in order to reduce cerebral metabolic rate but has not been shown to improve mortality in patients with raised ICP and is therefore not recommended unless patients are pyrexial.

CPP should be maintained at all times. In some cases of raised ICP the patient's autonomic system will stimulate the cardiovascular system and increase the mean arterial pressure (MAP); however, in most cases the MAP needs to be maintained by the use of vasoactive substances and adequate hydration – the most commonly used agent is noradrenaline.

Surgery should always be considered when there is a rise in ICP – even where surgery has previously not been deemed appropriate as new problems such as hydrocephalus can develop. The main surgical interventions include surgical decompression of haematomas or abscesses, debulking of tumours, drainage of CSF and in extreme cases craniectomy.

What are the effects of anaesthetic agents on ICP?

Many anaesthetic drugs are used to control ICP. Intra-venous induction agents such as propofol, etomidate and thiopentone cause a dose-dependent decrease in ICP, cerebral blood flow and cerebral metabolic rate. Propofol is the most commonly used with thiopentone only being used in refractory rises in ICP. Benzodiazepines decrease cerebral metabolic rate and blood flow but do not markedly alter ICP. Opiates do not decrease ICP but in large doses decrease cerebral metabolic rate.

Neuromuscular blockers do not alter ICP but are useful where ICP is exacerbated by coughing or straining. Suxamethonium causes a transient increase in ICP which can be attenuated by intra-venous anaesthetic drugs.

Volatile anaesthetics increase ICP due to cerebral vasodilatation although this is slightly offset by a reduction in cerebral metabolic rate. They are therefore best avoided in neurosurgery; however they can be used at low doses, with a MAC of less than 1. Nitrous oxide causes both vasodilatation and increases cerebral metabolic rate and therefore increases ICP. Ketamine also increases cerebral metabolic rate and ICP and is not used.

How does mannitol help reduce ICP?

Mannitol is an osmotic diuretic. It is filtered and not reabsorbed by the kidney and therefore causes a diuresis. This has the knock-on effect of withdrawing water from the intracellular fluid and interstitial spaces thus reducing brain volume. It also acts as a free radical scavenger and reduces CSF production. The recommended dose is 0.5–1 ml/kg of 20% solution.

What anti-convulsive is commonly used in patients with raised ICP?

Phenytoin is often used to prevent and treat convulsions. It is a membrane stabiliser which acts by decreasing Na and Ca influx during depolarisation. It has a narrow therapeutic window and levels need to be checked regularly. It is an enzyme inducer and has many side effects which can be divided into idiosyncratic and dose-related. Idiosyncratic side effects include gum hyperplasia, hirsutism, acne, blood dyscrasia and dose-related side effects include hypotension, nausea and vomiting, headache, confusion and drowsiness.

How can ICP be monitored?

ICP is usually measured continuously, ideally this is done in conjunction with mean arterial pressure so that a derived reading of CPP can be continuously displayed. It can be measured in a number ways.

An extra-dural fibreoptic probe can be inserted between the dura and the skull via a burr hole. The advantages of this method is that it is easy to position and has a low infection rate. However, CSF drainage is not possible and it is liable to drift.

A subarachnoid bolt can be used. This is also inserted via a burr hole, is easy to position and is more accurate but it has higher infection rates.

An external ventricular drain (EVD) can be inserted during craniotomy. This allows both drainage of CSF and can be transduced to measure ICP. It is associated with higher infection rates in the range of 3–5%.

The most commonly used device is the fibreoptic probe except where drainage of CSF is required when an EVD is inserted.

3.7.5. Cardiac output measurement – Rebecca A Leslie

What do you understand by the term *cardiac output*?

The cardiac output (CO) is the amount of blood that the left ventricle pumps around the body per minute. It is equal to the product of the heart rate and the stroke volume.

$$CO = HR \times SV.$$

With a normal heart rate between 70 and 80 bpm and an average stroke volume of 70–80 ml, the normal cardiac output of a 70-kg person is approximately 5–6 litres at rest.

How can we measure cardiac output?

Remember always classify your answer. It is less important how you classify it just make sure that you do. In this case it would be reasonable to classify into direct and non-direct or invasive and non-invasive.

Cardiac output can be measured using invasive techniques, semi-invasive techniques or non-invasive techniques.

Invasive techniques include the use of thermodilution or dye dilution techniques to measure the cardiac output using the Fick principle. Alternatively a PiCCO (pulsed induced contour cardiac output) can be used as an invasive technique to determine the cardiac output.

A semi-invasive technique for cardiac output measurement is the use of a trans-oesophageal Doppler.

Non-invasive techniques include trans-thoracic Doppler, magnetic resonance imaging and thoracic impedence.

You have mentioned Doppler techniques several times, could you explain this in more detail?

The Doppler effect describes the change in the frequency of sound if either the transmitter or the receiver is moving. An example of this is the change in pitch of sound emitted from a rapidly moving truck as it passes the observer. A change in pitch represents a change in frequency of the sound waves. Ultrasound is very high-frequency sound waves which exceeds the threshold of human hearing. Although we cannot hear it, the Doppler effect occurs with ultrasound too.

Doppler ultrasonography utilises the Doppler effect. Ultrasound waves from a vibrating crystal are directed at an artery and the reflected waves sensed by another crystal. The waves are reflected back by the moving red blood cells. The frequency of these reflected waves is proportional to the velocity of flow of red blood cells towards the receiving crystal. The faster the flow of red blood cells, the higher the frequency.

The Doppler ultrasound apparatus cannot provide quantitative measurements of blood flow because estimation of the vessel size may not be accurate or the flow throughout the vessel might not be uniform. Despite this the technique can be used to assess adequacy of blood flow through a vessel and can provide an estimate of cardiac output.

In cardiac output measurement using Doppler ultrasound the aortic arch cross-sectional area is estimated by knowledge of the patient's height and weight. The stroke volume is then estimated by integration of the velocity of the red blood cells and the cross sectional area of the aorta. Cardiac output is then calculated by multiplying the stroke volume by the heart rate.

Doppler ultrasound transducers can be incorporated into trans-thoracic probes, oesophageal probes and in pulmonary artery catheters.

What are the advantages and disadvantages of oesophageal Doppler techniques?

An advantage of the oesophageal Doppler is that it allows an estimate of cardiac output to be made quickly and using only a minimally invasive technique. It also allows the response to therapeutic techniques such as a fluid challenge to be rapidly assessed. The oesophagus is in close anatomical proximity to the aorta at the level of T5 to T6, so there is little interference from bone, soft tissue or from air in the lungs. In addition the smooth muscle tone of the oesophagus helps to hold the probe in position for repeated measurements.

A problem with the use of an oesophageal Doppler probe is that it can only be used in an adequately sedated, intubated patient due to the discomfort of passing the probe and maintaining it in position. Also, it must not be used in patients with pharyngo-oesophageal pathology such as oesophageal varices. Another problem with its use for repeated readings is that it is difficult to hold in the correct position for long periods of time and will need to be frequently repositioned.

You mentioned the Fick principle, what do you mean by this?

The Fick principle states that the uptake or the excretion of a substance by an organ or tissue must be equal to the difference between the amount of substance entering and the amount of substance leaving the organ. The amount of the substance entering the organ is equal to the product of the arterial blood flow and the arterial concentration, whilst the amount leaving the organ is equal to the venous blood flow multiplied by the venous concentration. If this formula is rearranged it can be seen that the blood flow to the organ is equal to the rate of uptake or excretion of the substance divided by the arterial–venous concentration difference.

$$\text{Organ blood flow} = \frac{\text{Rate of uptake or excretion of a substance by an organ}}{\text{Arterial} - \text{venous concentration difference}}.$$

This can be applied to oxygen content of the blood to determine the cardiac output. The cardiac output equals the pulmonary blood flow and we know that the lungs add oxygen to the blood. So firstly the steady state oxygen content of the arterial and venous blood is measured. This allows the arterial–venous concentration difference to be determined. Next the oxygen uptake in the lungs over 1 minute is measured. Using the Fick principle oxygen uptake divided by the arterial–venous oxygen difference is equal to the pulmonary blood flow, which in turn is equal to the cardiac output.

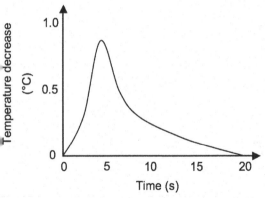

Figure 3.7.5a. Thermodilutional graph (bottom diagram). Reproduced with permission from Cross, M. and Plunkett, E. 2008. *Physics, Pharmacology and Physiology for Anaesthetists: Key Concepts for the FRCA.* Cambridge: Cambridge University Press. © M. Cross and E. Plunkett 2008.

It is important to note that the Fick principle can only be used when the arterial supply represents the only source of the substance that is taken up.

You said you would measure oxygen uptake in the lungs for 1 minute. How do you actually do this?

The patient must breathe through a spirometer which is filled with 100% oxygen. Included in the circuit is a carbon dioxide absorber, to remove all exhaled carbon dioxide. After 1 minute the amount of oxygen taken up by the lungs can be ascertained from the final concentration of oxygen in the spirometer.

From where would you take blood samples to measure arterial and venous oxygen content?

A peripheral arterial blood sample is thought to be accurate enough to estimate the oxygen content of the pulmonary veins.

In order to measure the venous oxygen content a pulmonary artery catheter must be inserted and a mixed venous sample taken from it.

Tell me about the thermodilutional techniques used to measure cardiac output

A pulmonary artery catheter is inserted via the internal jugular or subclavian vein. The pulmonary artery catheter is floated through the right atrium and ventricle, and as the name suggests the end sits in the pulmonary artery. Pulmonary artery catheters have several different lumens; the most proximal is positioned 30 cm from the tip of the catheter and opens into the right atrium. A thermistor is located 3.7 cm from the distal end of the pulmonary artery catheter. When the pulmonary artery catheter is in position the thermister sits in the pulmonary artery. To calculate cardiac output cold saline is injected through the proximal lumen into the right atrium. The thermistor in the pulmonary artery then measures the change in blood temperature. The recorded temperatures allow the generation of a temperature to time curve, see Figure 3.7.5a.

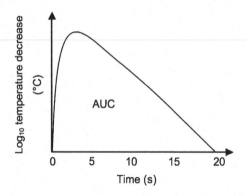

The semi-log transformation again makes the rise and fall of the graph linear. As the fall on the initial plot was exponential, so the curve is transformed to a linear fall by plotting it as a semi-log. The AUC is used in the calculations of cardiac output.

Figure 3.7.5b. Thermodilutional graph. Reproduced with permission from Cross, M. and Plunkett, E. 2008. *Physics, Pharmacology and Physiology for Anaesthetists: Key Concepts for the FRCA.* Cambridge: Cambridge University Press. © M. Cross and E. Plunkett 2008.

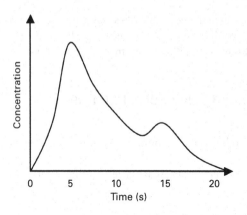

Draw a curve starting at the origin that reaches its maximum value at around 5 s. The curve then falls to baseline but is interrupted by a recirculation hump at around 15 s. This is caused by dye passing completely around the vasculature and back to the sensor a second time.

Figure 3.7.5c. Dye dilution graph. Reproduced with permission from Cross, M. and Plunkett, E. 2008. *Physics, Pharmacology and Physiology for Anaesthetists: Key Concepts for the FRCA.* Cambridge: Cambridge University Press. © M. Cross and E. Plunkett 2008.

This data then undergoes a semi-log transformation to make the rise and fall of the graphs linear, see Figure 3.7.5b. The area under the curve (AUC) is then entered into an algorithm, based on the Steward–Hamilton equation, to calculate cardiac output.

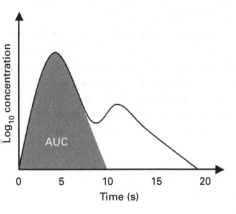

Demonstrate that the semi-log plot makes the curve more linear during its rise and fall from baseline. The recirculation hump is still present but is discounted by measuring the area under the curve (AUC) enclosed by a tangent from the initial down stroke. This is the AUC that is used in the calculations.

Figure 3.7.5d. Dye dilution graph. Reproduced with permission from Cross, M. and Plunkett, E. 2008. *Physics, Pharmacology and Physiology for Anaesthetists: Key Concepts for the FRCA.* Cambridge: Cambridge University Press. © M. Cross and E. Plunkett 2008.

How does this technique differ from dye dilutional techniques?

When using dye dilutional techniques a known quantity of indocyanine green is injected into a central vein while blood is continuously sampled from a peripheral arterial cannula. Indocyanine green is used because it is non-toxic and has a short half-life. The change in dye concentration measured by the samples taken from the arterial cannula, allows a concentration against time curve to be produced. The dye recirculates and produces a second peak in the dye concentration–time curve, see Figure 3.7.5c.

If the cardiac output is high the dye will be washed out quicker. In contrast if the cardiac output is low the dye will be washed out more slowly.

This curve is re-plotted on semi-logarithmic paper to make the rise and fall of the curve more linear. If a tangent is drawn from the initial down-stroke an enclosed area is formed, see Figure 3.7.5d. The cardiac output can then be calculated using this area.

How does a PiCCO differ from the thermodilutional techniques you have described?

A PiCCO avoids the risks associated with the insertion of a pulmonary artery catheter and instead uses a standard central line with a thermistor at its tip. A special arterial catheter is placed in the brachial or the femoral artery and has a thermodilution sensor incorporated within it. Cool saline is injected via the central line, and thermodilutional curves are produced by changes in temperature measured by the arterial line. The curves which are produced are much flatter and longer than the curves produced by traditional pulmonary artery thermodilution techniques. The PiCCO results, unlike those produced by a pulmonary artery, are not affected by the respiratory cycle.

How is thoracic impedance used to measure cardiac output?

Two different electrodes are placed on the neck and lower thorax. A low amplitude high-frequency AC is introduced between the two electrodes. The electrical impedance between these two electrodes can be measured and represents the thoracic impedance. Thoracic impedance is affected by pulsatile blood flow and ventilation. By only looking at the pulsatile changes in the thoracic impedance the stroke volume can be calculated. This leads to measurement of the cardiac output by multiplying the stroke volume by the heart rate.

Chapter

3.8

Electricity

3.8.1. Electricity – Emily K Johnson

Questions on electricity could be asked in the OSCE or structured oral examination. You may be shown pictures of electrical symbols that you will be asked to identify and explain the principles behind how they work. You should therefore be familiar with all the commonly used electrical symbols and be able to identify and draw them. Such questions may lead to other topics such as diathermy or defibrillators, which are covered in other chapters.

What do you understand by the concept of electric charge?

You may be asked about the basic electrical principles and you need to understand these to pass.

A charged body can display either a positive or negative charge. This results from electron transfer with the electron being responsible for the negative charge and the atomic nuclei being responsible for the positive charge. Therefore excess electrons results in a negative charge and a deficit of electrons results in a positive charge.

Charge is the quantity of electricity and is measured in coulombs. One coulomb is the quantity of electric charge that passes a point when the current of 1 ampere flows for a period of 1 second.

How does this relate to electric current?

Electric current is the rate of passage of electrons through a substance, that is the rate of passage of electric charge. It is therefore measured in coulombs per second, which is the ampere. One ampere is equal to 1 coulomb per second.

Electric current can be classified into direct current (DC) and alternating current (AC). DC describes the flow of current in one direction only, whereas AC describes the direction of flow changing back and forth. See Figure 3.8.1a.

You should be able to draw diagrams to illustrate the difference between direct and alternating current. Learn them and practice drawing them.

What sources of DC do you know?

Batteries and thermocouples supply DC.

Dr Podcast Scripts for the Primary FRCA, ed. Rebecca A. Leslie, Emily K. Johnson and Alexander P. L. Goodwin.   Published by Cambridge University Press. © R. A. Leslie, E. K. Johnson and A. P. L. Goodwin 2011.

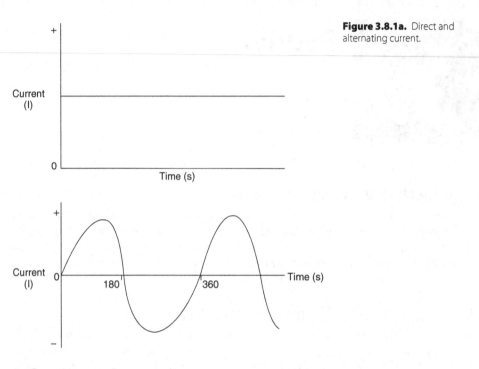

Figure 3.8.1a. Direct and alternating current.

Define amperes?

Amperes are the units of current measurement in the SI system. One ampere represents the flow of 6.24×10^{18} electrons per second. One ampere is also equal to 1 coulomb per second.

What are the features of the mains electricity supply?

The UK mains current is AC with a frequency of 50 Hz and a root mean square voltage of 240 V. The peak voltage is 340 V.

What materials are good conductors and why?

Conductors are readily able to conduct electrons from one atom to another and therefore an electric current passes through the material. They are usually metals as the outer shell electrons are loosely bound and move readily under the influence of a potential difference. Carbon, saline and body fluids are also good conductors.

Insulators are the opposite of conductors and have tightly bound electrons in their outer shell so they are unable to move and form an electric current.

What are semiconductors and when do we use them?

Semiconductors are materials with conductivity between that of conductors and insulators. They have outer shell electrons bound reasonably tightly but they are able to escape and conduct with some extra energy. This principle gives semiconductors a useful role in many devices such as thermistors, transistors and diodes. They are used in thermistors when heat is the source of extra energy, the more heat the more electrons escape so the more electricity is conducted.

What is Ohm's law?

Ohm's law describes the relationship between potential difference, current and resistance. It states that at a constant temperature, current passing through a conductor is directly proportional to the potential difference and inversely proportional to the resistance.

$$\text{Current (I)} = \frac{\text{Voltage (V)}}{\text{Resistance (R)}}.$$

There is another law referring to flow of a fluid that is analogous to Ohm's law. Do you know what this is?

Yes. Poiseuille's law that states that in laminar flow, the flow of fluid is directly proportional to the pressure difference and inversely proportional to the resistance to flow. Therefore electrical resistance behaves the same way as resistance to flow.

Can you explain a little more about the concepts of potential difference and resistance?

As described by Ohm's law the resistance is equal to the potential difference or voltage over the current in amperes. When a potential difference between two points exists then current flows. The resistance to the movement of electrons or ions through a material is caused by the collision of electrons, resulting in heat energy being dispersed to the surrounding molecules. The unit of resistance is called the ohm.

Potential difference is measured in volts. One volt is the potential difference which produces a current of 1 ampere in a conductor when the power dissipated between the two points is 1 watt.

$$\text{Voltage (V)} = \frac{\text{Power (W)}}{\text{Current (A)}}.$$

What factors may increase electrical resistance?

Electrical resistance in a conductor will rise with increased temperature but the inverse applies to semiconductors. Resistance will increase if a wire is stretched and becomes longer and thinner. This is the principle used in a strain gauge when the resulting changes in current flow are amplified and displayed. For example in pressure transducers used for monitoring invasive blood pressure.

What is a Wheatstone bridge and can you draw one?

Practice drawing the Wheatstone bridge circuit (Figure 3.8.1b).

A Wheatstone bridge is a circuit used to monitor changes in resistance. It consists of a set of four resistors, a source of electrical potential and a galvanometer. The bridge should be balanced out and when the two arms of the bridge are equal no current flows through the galvanometer. Two of the resistances are fixed and one is variable with the fourth being unknown. One branch of the bridge contains the unknown and variable resistor and the other branch the two of known resistance. They are all balanced until the galvanometer reads zero. Any deflection thereafter is from the unknown resistor and the signal can be amplified and recorded.

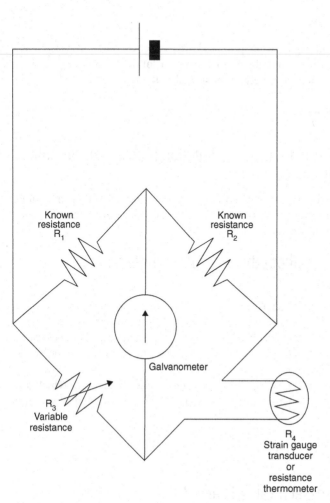

Figure 3.8.1b. Wheatstone bridge circuit.

What is capacitance?

A question on capacitance may well lead to further questions on the principles of the defibrillator.

Capacitance is the ability to hold electric charge and is measured in farads. A capacitor has 1 farad of capacitance if a potential difference of 1 volt is present across its plates when they hold a charge of 1 coulomb.

A capacitor consists of two plates separated by an insulator, the insulator is known as the dielectric. It will allow the passage of AC as it is continually charging and discharging with the reversing flow of current. This property of AC allows it to pass across an air gap and interfere with biological electrical signals. DC charges up the plates but fades away as the capacitor becomes fully charged. Capacitors are used in defibrillator circuits to store charge.

What factors improve the ability of a capacitor to store charge?

The factors influencing the ability of a capacitor to store charge are the area of the plates, with a larger area indicating a better capacity for storage. The distance between the plates also increases the amount of charge that can be stored as do the properties of the particular insulating material used.

What is inductance?

Inductance is the capacity for an electromotive force to be induced in a circuit by changing the current flowing in that circuit or a neighbouring circuit. Every wire with AC flowing down it is surrounded by a magnetic field, and this induces an electromotive force proportional to the rate of change of the current. The induction is caused by the opening and closing of a DC circuit or the continuous changing directions of an AC circuit.

An inductor is a coil of wire and is used in many electrical circuits including defibrillator and transformers. Inductance is a source of interference in biological electrical signals.

The unit of inductance is the Henry, and the symbol is an L.

Why is an inductor used in the defibrillator circuit?

The inductor is necessary in a defibrillator circuit because the current and charge from the discharging capacitor decay rapidly and so the inductors are useful to prolong the duration of current flow.

What is impedance?

Impedance is the sum of the capacitance, inductance and the resistance of an alternating current in an electrical circuit. In other words it is the opposition to flow of the current in AC circuits.

It is similar to resistance and is measured in ohms but it is dependent on current frequency and is represented by the letter Z. An example of the use of impedance is in the isolating capacitor. This is present in some diathermy circuits and offers high impedance against the dangerous mains frequency so protecting the patient against electrocution.

3.8.2. Electrical safety – Joy M Sanders

What is electrical current?

Electrical current is the flow of electrons through a conductor past a given point per unit time. It is measured in amperes.

What is potential difference?

When a current of 1 ampere is carried along a conductor, such that 1 watt of power is dissipated between the two points, the potential difference between those points is 1 volt (V).

What is resistance?

This is the opposition to a flow of DC along a conductor. It is not frequency dependent and is measured in ohms.

Can you define Ohm's law?

Ohm's law states that the current (I) flowing through a resistance (R) is proportional to the potential difference (V) across it.

$V = IR$.

What is impedance?

The impedance is an equivalent concept to resistance, and is the opposition to current flow in an AC circuit. Unlike resistance, impedance does vary with the frequency of the current. Conductors have low impedance and insulators have high impedance. High-frequency AC current passes more easily through capacitors, whereas low-frequency current passes more easily through inductors. Impedance is measured, like resistance, in ohms but has the symbol z.

What are the sources of electrical interference in biological signals?

Electrical interference can be due to external or internal causes.

External causes

This is mainly due to the AC mains current, which may be responsible for capacitive coupling. Any electrical device powered by AC current lying close to a patient can act as one plate of a capacitor, with the patient acting as the other plate. The circuit is completed because both plates are connected to earth. The alternating positive and negative current in the live lead causes a similarly alternating charge on the other plate, which is seen as a 50-Hz signal on the recording electrodes (e.g., ECG). This can be resolved by either increasing the distance between the patient and the live conductor or by shielding the two plates of the capacitor with an earthed screen. This reduces the effect of the capacitive coupling, by discharging the charge from the live plate to earth. Electrode leads are screened by having a wire mesh covering which is connected to earth, so interference currents are induced here and not in the signal leads. The screening layer may also be covered with a second layer of insulation.

One method of removing this interference is to use a differential operational amplifier. A differential amplifier measures the difference between the potential from two inputs. Therefore, if there is interference common to both input terminals (e.g., mains frequency 50 Hz), it is eliminated as it is only the difference that is amplified. This is termed common mode rejection.

Internal causes

This is due to the presence of other electrical activity, from the patient. The most common reason for this is skeletal muscle activity, for example caused by movement or shivering. It is important to try to maximise the signal that is measured by reducing movement and keeping the patient warm. Placement of electrodes over bony prominences will also reduce artefact.

What methods exist for preventing electrocution in theatre?

General measures include the following:

- The use of appropriate equipment in good working order with proper maintenance
- Ensuring that electrical equipment, plugs, etc. are not placed on the floor where solutions may fall on them
- Ensuring correct humidity in theatre
- Wearing suitable footwear to optimise impedance
- The use of anti-static flooring.

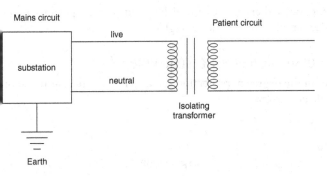

Figure 3.8.2a. Isolated (floating) patient circuit.

Those involving the mains supply include the following:

- Isolation transformers
  - These can supply all outlets of a theatre complex and can also be used in single pieces of equipment. The theory is that patients are not connected directly to earth via electrodes (e.g. in ECG) and plates (e.g. in diathermy) but via transformers within each piece of equipment. Current cannot therefore reach earth via the patient if contact with a live supply occurs.
  - However, faults in one piece of equipment may interfere with the power supply to other pieces of equipment. Problems can also arise if several pieces of equipment each with small leakage currents are used together, as when combined this can be enough to interrupt the power.

- Earth leakage circuit breaker (ELCB)
  - These measure the earth current directly. They detect even a small current to earth (which may be as small as 30 mA) and if present, break the circuit, causing an alarm to sound.

- Residual current devices
  - These detect any imbalances of current and any differences in magnetic flux between the neutral and live lines. If imbalance occurs, they break the circuit.

- Leakage current monitors
  - Line isolation monitors continuously monitor the impedance from all lines to the ground and indicate the potential for current to flow. If this potential is too high, current flows to the ground and the circuit breaks or an alarm is sounded. Leakage current monitors are sensitive to only a few mAs.

Those involving the patient include the following:

- The use of isolated "floating" circuits with no earth connection to the patient (see Figure 3.8.2a)
- Isolating electrical components that are in direct contact with the patient, for example, using isolating transformers or battery powered equipment
- Ensuring that the patient is not in contact with metal conductors
- Ensuring that the diathermy electrode plates are properly and uniformly applied to the patient

- Using isolating capacitors in the diathermy circuit, which provide high impedance to the low mains frequency (50 Hz) and low impedance to high diathermy frequency (1 MHz).

What are the main types of medical electrical equipment?

Equipment is classified based on the degree of protection against electrocution or based on the maximum permissible leakage current.

Table 3.8.2a. Classification of electrical equipment

Based on the degree of protection:		
Class	**Symbol**	**Explanation**
I	No symbol	Class I equipment only offers basic protection. Any conducting part that can be touched by the user (for example, the metal casing) must be connected to the earth wire via the plug, and must be insulated from the live supply. There are fuses on the live and neutral supply in the equipment, as well as a third fuse on the live wire in the mains plug. If a fault occurs, this fuse melts and disconnects the electrical circuit therefore providing protection against electric shock. Current will be conducted through the low resistance earth wire, causing the fuse to blow and removal of the source current (or "leakage current").
II		This equipment has double or reinforced insulation that protects all the accessible parts. An earth wire is not required. The power cable only has live and neutral conductors and only one fuse.
III	No symbol	This equipment does not need potentials greater than 24 V AC or 50 V DC. The voltage used is known as safety extra low voltage (SELV). There is no risk of gross electric shock but microshock can still occur as leakage currents may flow to earth if insulation of live circuits is disrupted. This equipment may have an internal power source (a battery) or may be connected to the mains supply by a step down transformer.
Based on maximum permissible leakage currents:		
B		This can be from Class I, II or III, but maximum leakage current must not exceed 100 μA. It can come into contact with the **b**ody, but is not considered safe for direct connection to the heart.
		This equipment may be defibrillator protected.

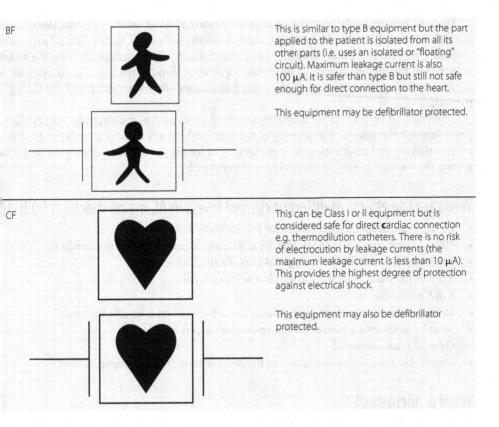

BF
This is similar to type B equipment but the part applied to the patient is isolated from all its other parts (i.e. uses an isolated or "floating" circuit). Maximum leakage current is also 100 μA. It is safer than type B but still not safe enough for direct connection to the heart.

This equipment may be defibrillator protected.

CF
This can be Class I or II equipment but is considered safe for direct cardiac connection e.g. thermodilution catheters. There is no risk of electrocution by leakage currents (the maximum leakage current is less than 10 μA). This provides the highest degree of protection against electrical shock.

This equipment may also be defibrillator protected.

What factors determine the extent of injury following an electric shock?

An electric shock can occur whenever a person completes an electric circuit. For current to flow, the individual must be in contact with the circuit at two points with a potential difference between the points.

The extent of the injury is determined by the amount of current, the type of current, the frequency of the current, the current density, the current pathway and the duration of application.

In the UK, mains supplies are maintained at a voltage of approximately 240 V. Ohm's law states that current flow is inversely proportional to impedance. Therefore, high impedance will reduce the current flow and low impedance will allow an increase in current flow. The main source of impedance is the skin resistance, which can vary from a few thousand ohms per square cm to one million ohms per square cm. Impedance is highest when the skin is dry and lowest when it is wet, encouraging the flow of current.

Electric shock can occur with both AC and DC. The DC required to cause ventricular fibrillation (VF) (500 mA) is considerably higher than the AC (100 mA). The current frequency is also important, with 50 Hz (the frequency of AC in the UK) being the most lethal frequency. At this frequency, high voltages can be generated which can be transmitted along power lines and readily transformed. However, ion flux across all cell membranes will be disrupted, forcing ions in both directions. The higher the frequency, the less dangerous it becomes, and above 100 Hz there is no fibrillatory potential at all.

Current density is the amount of current flowing divided by the cross-sectional area through which it flows. In the body, the current usually diffuses in all directions. Large currents or small contact areas result in high current density. The greatest effect on the heart is seen with the highest current density passing directly through the heart. Consequently, a current travelling from one arm to the other has a larger effect than one travelling through the feet.

In electrocution there is additional thermal injury, caused as the electrical energy dissipates through the tissues. The severity of the electrical burn is directly proportional to the current density and its duration of application. The longer the duration of current flow, the greater the damage caused to tissues in the current path.

What are the effects at different current levels in AC mains shock (at 50 Hz)?

- 10 μA is the absolute safety value for connections to the heart
- 100 μA can cause microshock and VF if directly connected to the myocardium
- 1 mA is the threshold for feeling and causes a tingling sensation
- 5 mA is the maximum safe current but will cause pain
- 8 mA causes burns
- 15 mA causes tonic contraction of muscles and the victim is unable to "let go"
- 50 mA causes severe pain and even respiratory arrest
- Over 100 mA causes VF
- Over 5 A causes tonic contraction of the myocardium (used in defibrillation).

What is microshock?

Under normal circumstances, gross electric shock caused by energy applied to the surface of the body requires currents of around 100 mA. However, currents as small as 50–100 μA are sufficient to cause VF if delivered directly to the heart. This effect is known as microshock and will only occur if specific circumstances arise. It requires electrical contact applied directly over a small area of ventricle (i.e. a high current density) which can be earthed through the patient. Microshock can occur if an intra-cardiac catheter is faulty, or if a staff member holding an intra-cardiac device is simultaneously touching a leaking source and therefore completing an electric circuit. Such potential sources of microshock include central venous catheters, pulmonary artery catheters, pacing wires and oesophageal temperature probes (in the lower third of the oesophagus). Avoiding the use of conducting solutions like saline in intra-cardiac lines will reduce the risk.

Tell me more about anti-static precautions

Anti-static measures are used in operating theatres to prevent build-up of static electricity with the potential for sparks, fires and explosions. Materials and surfaces should have appropriately low electrical impedance that permits the leakage of charge to earth but not so low as to cause electrocution or electrical burns.

Sparks are more likely to occur if the theatre is cold and dry, therefore relative humidity should be kept greater than 50% and room temperature should exceed 20°C. Materials such as wool, nylon and silk should be avoided as they may create static charge. Cotton blankets and clothing are ideal. Anti-static rubber containing carbon should be used for such things as tubing. It is black in colour with yellow labels and has a resistance of 100 000–10 000 000 ohms/cm.

Anti-static precautions also involve the use of a terrazzo floor, which consists of stone pieces imbedded in cement and then polished. The resistance should be 20 000–5 000 000 ohms between two points 60 cm apart. This ensures that the impedance to the floor is not so low that high currents may flow to it, but is not so high that sparks may find another pathway to earth.

In addition, trolleys and other equipment should have conducting wheels and staff should wear anti-static shoes.

However, the need for expensive anti-static flooring and other precautions is questionable. Although fires may still occur with substances such as alcohol skin preparation, they are usually a result of a high energy source such as laser or diathermy rather than by static electricity per se.

Equipment

3.9

3.9.1. Defibrillators – Natasha A Joshi

What is capacitance?

Start with a short and snappy broad definition. Remember to define the SI units and write down the equation for capacitance. This will convey lots of information in a short space of time, and demonstrate understanding.

Capacitance is a measure of the ability of an object to store electrical charge. It is defined as the charge stored by an object per voltage difference across it. The SI unit of capacitance is the farad. One farad is the capacity to store 1 coulomb of charge, when a potential difference of 1 volt is applied.

Capacitance (Farads) = Charge (Coulombs)/Potential Difference (Volts).

What is a capacitor? Give an example of its importance in clinical practice

A capacitor is an electrical component, made up of two conducting plates that are separated by an insulator.

At this point you should draw the electrical symbol (Figure 3.9.1a).

A capacitor will become charged when a potential difference exists across it, but it will not allow DC to flow. The charge stored by a capacitor may then be discharged. AC induces repeated charging and discharging of a capacitor. In this case, as a potential difference always exists current will flow across the capacitor.

In clinical practice, a capacitor is an essential electrical component of the defibrillator. It allows charge to be stored and then released in a controlled fashion, providing optimum conditions for defibrillation of the myocardium.

What factors improve the ability of a capacitor to store charge?

The amount of energy stored by a capacitor depends on its capacitance, the charge and the potential difference that exists. If the potential difference across a capacitor is increased, the energy required to store the same amount of charge in that capacitor will also be increased.

Dr Podcast Scripts for the Primary FRCA, ed. Rebecca A. Leslie, Emily K. Johnson and Alexander P. L. Goodwin.   Published by Cambridge University Press. © R. A. Leslie, E. K. Johnson and A. P. L. Goodwin 2011.

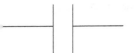

Figure 3.9.1a.
Electrical symbol for
capacitor.

Figure 3.9.1b.
Electrical symbol for
inductor.

How do you calculate the stored energy in a capacitor?

Stored energy may be calculated from the equation:

$$E = \tfrac{1}{2} \times QV$$

where E represents energy, Q represents the charge in coulombs, and V represents the potential difference, in volts.

Can you give an example of interference caused by capacitance in the operating theatre environment?

Capacitance may cause interference on the ECG trace due to alternating current passing from the operating theatre light to the patient. This is because the light acts as one plate of the capacitor, and the patient acts as the other. The air gap between the two is the insulator. A small amount of 50 Hz AC passes from the lamp to the patient, resulting in interference seen on the ECG.

Within a capacitor electrons cannot be conducted directly across the insulator from one conducting plate to the other. Initially when DC is applied to an uncharged capacitor current will flow to charge up the capacitor plates. The flow of current will then stop as the capacitor becomes fully charged. When AC is applied to the capacitor, there will be a continuous flow of current as the capacitor is being continuously charged and discharged.

What is inductance?

Inductance is defined as the capacity for an electromotive force to be induced in an electrical circuit. It achieves this by changing the current flowing in the circuit, or in a neighbouring one.

Inductance is therefore based on electromagnetic effects and can also lead to interference in biological electrical signals.

What is an inductor? Give an example of its importance in clinical practice

An inductor is an electrical component that induces an electromotive force in an electrical circuit. It achieves this by changing the current flowing in the circuit. It is typically a coil of wire, as indicated by its electrical symbol (Figure 3.9.1b).

An inductor is an essential electrical component of a defibrillator. It ensures that the electrical pulse delivered to the patient has the optimum shape and duration. When the defibrillator is discharged, the inductor absorbs some of the energy stored in the capacitor, so that not all of the stored energy is delivered to the patient.

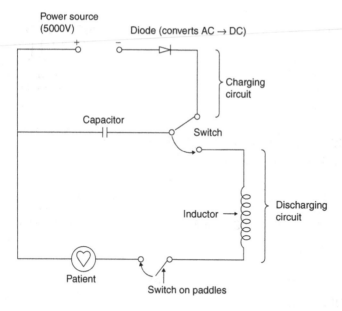

Figure 3.9.1c. Defibrillator.

What is a defibrillator? How does it work?

A defibrillator is a piece of electrical equipment that is used in the treatment of ventricular fibrillation and for electrical cardioversion. It is a device that enables electrical charge to be stored, and then delivered to the patient in a controlled fashion.

The defibrillator is essentially made up of two separate circuits; one is for charging, and the other is for discharging. There is a switch to flip between the two circuits. There is another switch in the discharging circuit (on the paddles) to initiate delivery of the charge.

It is very helpful to draw a diagram of the basic electrical circuit found in a defibrillator. This will convey the information more concisely and illustrate understanding, see Figure 3.9.1c.

The charging circuit contains a power source (either from mains electricity or a battery), a rectifier (or diode) to convert AC into DC and a capacitor, to store the electrical charge. The potential difference supplied from the power source to the circuit is 5000 volts DC. Once the capacitor is fully charged, a switch then moves to complete the discharging circuit.

The discharging circuit contains the capacitor, an inductor and another switch (often on the paddles). The patient completes the circuit when the two paddles are applied to the chest. Only when the paddle switch is activated, will the stored charge be released from the capacitor. This charge then passes through an inductor, which functions to oppose a sudden change in current flow and slows down the rapid discharge from the capacitor. The inductor therefore ensures that the electrical pulse delivered to the patient has the optimum shape and duration to reduce the likelihood of burns and for effective defibrillation. The inductor absorbs some of the electrical charge, so the amount of delivered charge is always less than the stored charge.

How do monophasic differ from biphasic defibrillators?

A monophasic defibrillator produces a single pulse of current, known as a monophasic waveform, that travels in one direction through the chest. A biphasic defibrillator produces two

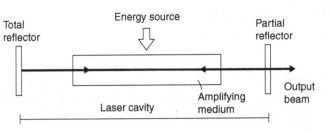

Figure 3.9.2a. Principles of LASER.

consecutive pulses of current, where current travels first in one direction, and then in the other through the chest.

Research has demonstrated that biphasic defibrillators achieve successful defibrillation of the myocardium at a lower energy threshold than monophasic ones.

3.9.2. Lasers and diathermy – Emily K Johnson

What does LASER stand for?

Laser stands for Light Amplification and Stimulated Emission of Radiation

How do lasers work?

A basic diagram may help you keep your answer concise and clear (Figure 3.9.2a).
Lasers have three basic components:

- An excitation energy source such as a flash lamp, a continuous light source, a diode or another laser
- A lasing medium, which could be gas, liquid or solid
- An optical resonator and outlet coupler.

The lasing medium gives the laser its name, for example, a carbon dioxide laser. The medium contains unexcited molecules, otherwise known as molecules in their "ground state". The excitation energy source is used to excite these molecules. Some of the excited molecules then spontaneously decay back to their ground state and thereby release a photon in a random direction, this is known as random emission. The photon is reflected within the optical resonator back into the lasing medium where it may collide with another excited atom. Such a collision causes the excited atom to decay back to its ground state releasing two photons. These two photons are then parallel, in step with each other or coherent and of the same wavelength or monochromatic. This process emitting parallel, coherent monochromatic light energy is known as stimulated emission. When the lasing medium contains molecules mostly in their excited state a cascade occurs leading to amplification of light energy.

The laser energy is then delivered to a target area by a delivery system such as a glass fibre, a fibreoptic cable or metal tubing containing mirrors to reflect the light.

When the light energy strikes the tissues it is reflected, scattered, transmitted to deeper tissues or absorbed. It is when absorbed light is converted to heat that a clinical effect is produced. Different tissue types absorb light of different wavelengths which is determined by their chemical structure. Therefore lasers at particular wavelengths will target specific tissues and it is the wavelengths that define lasers.

What different types of lasers do you know?

Learn some common examples, their wavelengths and uses.

The carbon dioxide laser

This has a long wavelength of 10 600 nm which is in the infrared spectrum and is preferentially absorbed by water. It penetrates to a shallow depth so tissue damage can be observed. An example of its use would be in resecting tumours of the airway, as it is as effective as a scalpel, and in achieving haemostasis.

The Nd-YAG (neodymium: yttrium-aluminium-garnet) laser

This has a wavelength of 1064 or 1320 nm which is in the near infrared spectrum. It has good tissue penetration and is transmitted through clear fluids and absorbed by dark matter. It is therefore good for use in cutting and coagulation of tissues in vascular malformations and ophthalmic surgery and black tattoo removal.

The pulsed dye laser

This has a wavelength of 577–585 nm. This targets red blood cells and is therefore useful for treating port wine skin lesions while causing minimal scarring to the dermis where the energy is dissipated.

The argon laser

This has a wavelength of 488–514 nm which is in the blue green spectrum. It is used in retinal surgery.

There are many other types of lasers such as the Er:YAG, Ho:YAG, ruby, KTP lasers.

What are the risks of using lasers?

There are general risks and specific anaesthetic risks.

The general risks are electrocution or burns from power supplies, burns to skin, clothes or other objects and eye injury. The parallel output beam of most lasers is focused using a lens. This results in a high power density at the point of focus but provides a safety mechanism as the beam diverges beyond this point so reducing the power density. The lens of the eye can refocus stray light onto the retina resulting in painless retinal burns, which leave a permanent blind spot in the visual field.

The specific anaesthetic risks are in upper airway surgery when the tracheal tube can be ignited and an airway fire ensues.

What safety precautions should be taken when using lasers?

A designated laser safety officer should be present at all times when lasers are in use and an illuminating sign should be displayed outside the theatre.

Eye protection must be worn when lasers are in use. Different wavelengths require different types of protection so goggles must be appropriate for the wavelength of the laser in use. Side shields should be present on the goggles.

The patient's eyes must also be appropriately protected.

The patient's skin should be covered with non-combustible drapes and tissue adjacent to the site of surgery should be protected with damp swabs. Skin preps should be non-flammable.

Medical instruments used alongside lasers should have matt rather than shiny surfaces to reduce the risks of reflection.

Nitrous oxide and oxygen support combustion so inspired oxygen concentrations of less than 30% are recommended in either nitrogen or helium. Plastic and rubber materials can be ignited by laser so special laser-resistant endotracheal tubes made of flexible stainless steel are available. These have twin cuffs that are filled with saline not air. Methylene blue can be added to the saline so puncture is obvious.

How does diathermy work?

Define and classify.
Diathermy is a piece of electrosurgical equipment used to cut, destroy and coagulate tissues during surgery. It has two forms, monopolar and bipolar diathermy. They both work on the principle of passing an electrical current through tissues and the heating effect causes the cutting or coagulation required.

Can you explain the basic electrical principles behind this and why patients are not electrocuted by diathermy?

When a voltage is applied across a conductor a current flows. In the use of diathermy a voltage is supplied via electrodes across the body, which becomes part of the circuit, and current flows through it. This current either heats or causes other physiological effects which depend on the frequency of the driving voltage. DC or low-frequency AC such as the UK mains supply, which is at 50 Hz, have effects proportional to the size of the current. For example, low currents cause tingling and pain and high currents cause muscle stimulation and ventricular fibrillation.

High-frequency voltages have increased heating effects and decreased stimulation. Frequencies above 100 kHz have entirely heating properties and no stimulation and this effect in the body is called diathermy. For surgical diathermy an AC with a frequency of 0.5–1 MHz is used. There are no physiological effects on skeletal and cardiac muscle at such high frequencies and electrocution does not occur. How the heating effect is used depends on the electrodes and the current density.

Define current density, and explain why it is important in diathermy

The current density is the current per unit area. If the current flows in a large material the heating effect will be minimal or absent but if the same current flows in a small material the heating effect will be large. In other words the resistance of the material is proportional to its size, so small material has a large resistance. The heating power is the product of current squared and resistance which shows for the same current material with a high resistance will have a greater heating power.

In surgical diathermy when one or both electrodes are very small pointed surgical instruments they will have a high current density so can be used to cut or coagulate tissue accurately. This is an active or live electrode and may have a heating power of up to 200 W with a current density of 10 A/cm^2. In monopolar diathermy there is one live electrode and the other is a neutral plate which has a much larger surface area and therefore lower current density so no heating occurs.

What are the different electrode systems?

There are monopolar and bipolar diathermy systems.

Monopolar diathermy has two connections to the patient, an active cutting or coagulation electrode and a neutral plate. Current passes through both but the current density at the active electrode is very high and so high temperatures are generated. At the neutral plate the current density is dispersed over a larger area and so heating does not occur. The patient forms a major part of the circuit. The neutral plate and therefore the patient are kept at earth potential reducing the risk of stray capacitance; however modern diathermy machines incorporate isolating capacitors to reduce this problem. A floating or earth-free circuit can also be used to prevent this problem.

Bipolar diathermy consists of two small electrodes both with high current densities and the body does not form a major part of the circuit. The electrodes are normally incorporated in a pair of forceps. This type of diathermy has good coagulation properties but not such good cutting ability and low power is used which limits its coagulation abilities to small vessels. The circuit is not earthed.

Explain the different effects of diathermy and how these are achieved

Diathermy can be used for its cutting or coagulation effects.

Cutting is achieved by a fine arc between a very small active electrode and the tissues. It produces a rapid heating of tissue over a small area. The waveform for cutting diathermy is a continuous, high-frequency sine wave at a voltage of 250 to 3000 volts and a frequency typically around 0.5 MHz.

Diagrams of the different waveforms would help to illustrate your answer. Learn the diagrams for the cutting, coagulation and blended modes of diathermy (Figure 3.9.2b).

Coagulation is achieved by spray and dessication. Spray coagulation results from arcing from the electrode tip charring surrounding tissues. Usually the electrode is a spatula or a ball. Higher voltages are required to produce arcing between a blunt electrode and the tissues, voltages of up to 9 kV are used. Damped or pulsed waveforms are used for coagulation typically at frequencies of 1.0 to 1.5 MHz. The waveform can be active for as little as 6% of the complete cycle. Dessication or contact coagulation is when the tissues are heated by contact between the active electrode and the tissues. Tissue temperature increases and intra-cellular water evaporates and tissues become dried out. Waveform isn't critical, and lower voltages and heating power are used.

Blended modes of diathermy are used to provide a mixture of cutting and coagulation. The waves can be pulsed, 50% on and 50% off, or 25% on and 75% off or other combinations. Less active waveforms result in better coagulation, more active waveforms are better for cutting.

What are the potential hazards of diathermy?

Start your answer by classifying the hazards.

There are electrical problems, problems of diathermy interference and problems with diathermy smoke and tissue damage.

Old diathermy machines used to have the neutral plate at earth potential, but earthing the patient is not advisable for electrical safety reasons. Modern diathermy machines have circuits that are completely isolated by either an isolating capacitor or they have floating

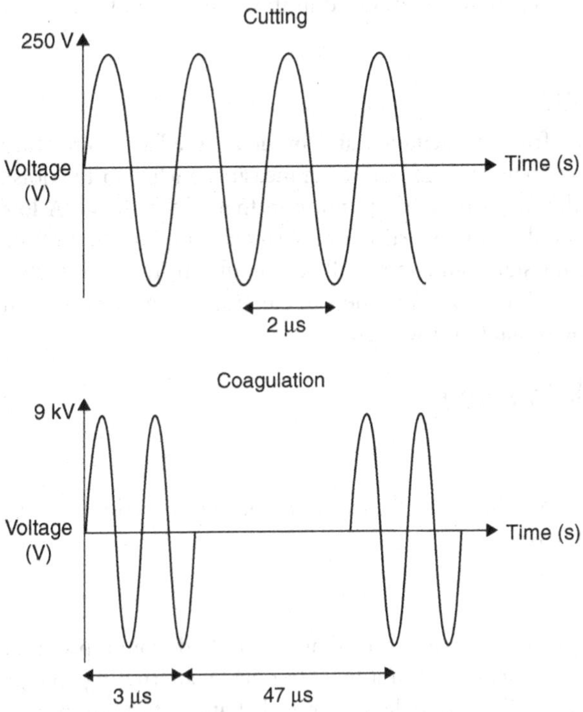

Figure 3.9.2b. Diathermy waveforms.

circuits. There is still the problem of stray capacitance, which is when small currents may pass between two parallel plates of a capacitor at higher frequencies and stray circuits form causing burns. This will occur if there is a poor connection with the neutral plate and the current takes the easiest route. Burns may also occur where the neutral plate has a poor connection with the patient so increasing current density at the points of contact. The neutral plate must therefore be securely attached and no other objects should be touching the patient when diathermy is in use. Lower frequencies also help reduce this risk, so 500 kHz is now used instead of up to 2 MHz.

Radiowaves are used in diathermy so sensitive monitors can receive such signals and interference occurs. Interference can also cause problems with cardiac pacemaker function so the neutral plate should be positioned far away from the pacemaker or only short bursts of monopolar diathermy used.

Diathermy smoke has become a major pollutant of the operating theatre environment causing potential hazard to health. It has been shown to cause inflammatory changes to the respiratory tract and may contain viable cells resulting in dissemination of disease. Surgical masks are not adequate protection so suctioning devices are recommended.

Diathermy should not be used on delicate end arteries or it can lead to ischaemia and infarction.

How can diathermy interference be avoided?

Interference can be avoided by positioning monitors as far away from diathermy as possible and by the use of electrical filters. Patient monitoring leads are covered by a sheath of woven metal which is earthed so interference currents are induced in this filter and not the signal leads.

What is the signal-to-noise ratio?

Interference in electrical waveforms from capacitance and inductance effect from other sources is known as "noise". The signal to noise ratio is a way of measuring whether the noise is a practical problem as it relates the magnitude of the noise to that of the signal. A low signal to noise ratio may present a problem in distortion of the signal. Amplification of the waveform will not improve things as the signal and noise will be amplified by the same factor. Elimination of the source of the noise, differential amplifiers or electronic filters can be used in such circumstances to improve the signal to noise ratio.

3.9.3 Ultrasound – Emily K Johnson

What is ultrasound?

Ultrasound is an imaging technique that is based on the transmission and reflection of high-frequency ultrasonic sound waves in tissues.

How does ultrasound work?

Ultrasound waves are high-frequency, mechanical waves that are emitted from a probe in pulses. The waves are generated by the application of a high-frequency alternating voltage to two sides of a piezoelectric transducer. The piezoelectric crystal changes dimensions and emits ultrasonic radiation at the exact frequency of the applied voltage. The waves are transmitted through the tissue medium and get reflected back at tissue interfaces. The probe detects the returning signal and the piezoelectric transducer performs the reverse procedure, transforming ultrasonic waves back into an electrical signal from which an image is produced on a monitor.

Using the wave propagation speed of sound in tissues (1540 m/s at a temperature of 37°C), the delay in the time between signal going out and reflection signal returning can be interpreted as the distance of the tissue interface from the probe.

The image is then formed by dots on the monitor representing each reflected wave. The strength of the reflected wave is represented by the brightness of the dot, and the position of the dot represents the depth from where the echo was reflected. All the dots combine to create an image which shows the strong reflections from solid structures such as gallstones or bone as white dots, the weaker reflections from most solid organs or thick fluids as grey dots and the absence of reflections from fluids such as blood or urine as black dots.

What is the frequency of ultrasound?

Ultrasound waves have a frequency above 20 000 Hz or 20 kHz. Medical ultrasound uses frequencies between 2.5 MHz and 15 MHz. This is well above the frequency threshold for human hearing, which is between 20 and 20 000 Hz.

What are the effects of using different frequencies for ultrasound?

If the frequency of the ultrasound waves is increased the resolution of the image is improved but the tissue penetration is diminished. Therefore to image deep structures the frequency should be lower but the resolution will not be as good. It is advisable to use the highest possible frequency transducer that will reach the required depth.

What do you understand by "half-power distance"?

"Half-power distance" is the depth at which the sound is reduced by half. For water this depth is 3,800 mm, and for air and lung it is less than 1 mm. Sound is attenuated by bone at a depth of 2 to 7 mm and by muscle at a depth of 6 to 10 mm.

What is a transducer?

Define and classify.
A transducer is a device that converts energy from one form to another. They can be divided into active and passive transducers.

Active transducers involve the generation of potentials and include electromagnetic induction, photoelectric cells and the piezoelectric effect.

Passive transducers involve changes in resistance, inductance and capacitance.

What is the piezoelectric effect?

The piezoelectric effect is when an electric potential is applied across a quartz crystal and the crystal changes its dimensions slightly. It is this characteristic of a transducer that changes energy from electrical to mechanical energy and vice versa. Ultrasonic transducers use lead zirconate titanates.

What is the Doppler effect?

The Doppler effect is the increase in the frequency of a signal when the source of the signal approaches the observer and a decrease in the signal frequency as the source moves away. A good example is a police car siren, as the car moves towards you the wavelength of the sound waves decreases and its frequency increases, causing a higher pitch. If the car were moving away then the wavelength would increase, the frequency decrease and the pitch lower.

How is the Doppler effect used clinically?

Clinically the Doppler effect is used in ultrasound to determine velocities and flow rates of moving substances. For example to measure blood flow the ultrasound beam can be directed along the path of flow. The sound waves reflect off the red blood cell surfaces and the reflected frequencies are analysed. From this information the velocity of the blood flow can be determined. The Doppler shift can be calculated by the ultrasound machine using a pre-programmed equation:
Write out the Doppler equation and talk it through.

$$Fd = \frac{2Ft \ V \ Cos\theta}{C}$$

- Fd is the Doppler frequency shift
- Ft is the transmitted Doppler frequency
- V is the speed of blood flow
- $Cos\theta$ is the cosine of the blood flow to the beam angle
- C is the speed of sound in tissue.

Doppler is used in this way as a non-invasive estimation of cardiac output by measurement of the velocity of blood in the aortic arch and relating it to vessel diameter. It is also used to measure blood flow in carotid arteries and vessels of the lower limbs following vascular surgery. Transcranial Doppler ultrasonography is used to measure the flow of blood through large cerebral arteries.

What is colour Doppler?

Colour Doppler uses the Doppler principles to generate a colour image which is superimposed onto the black and white image. Different colours are used to demonstrate directions of flow. Commonly red denotes flow towards the probe and blue is flow away from the probe. Turbulent flow may be represented by a mixture of the colours and green can be seen when flow exceeds a certain limit. Therefore information about direction and velocity is obtained.

What clinical uses of ultrasound are you familiar with?

Ultrasound has many clinical uses in anaesthesia and intensive care. It can be used to scan the abdomen and thorax of patients, to identify and aid drainage of fluid collections. Ultrasound is used as an aid to central venous cannulation to help correct placement and avoid complications. It is recommended in NICE guidelines for this purpose. Cranial scanning is also used in neonates to detect haemorrhage and midline shift.

Echocardiography is a frequent pre-operative assessment of a patient's cardiac function. It can be performed transthoracically to give information about valvular and ventricular function, and transoesophageally for more detailed information as this provides better defined images of the heart. Transoesophageal echocardiography is used particularly for the investigation of valvular heart disease, bacterial endocarditis, thrombus identification and congenital heart disease. It can be used acutely to investigate left ventricular pre-load and function and can detect ventricular dysfunction, ischaemia and air embolism.

What are the limitations of the use of ultrasound?

Ultrasound waves are unable to penetrate very far into bone or gas filled structures therefore imaging of bone or lungs is not possible.

The Doppler ultrasound probes can be difficult to calibrate due to changing vessel calibres and non-uniform flow profiles within the vessel. Therefore the Doppler estimations of cardiac output may not be precise but act as a guide and trends can be useful in monitoring.

Oesophageal probes must be avoided in patients with oesophageal strictures or tumours and used with caution in patients with oesophageal varices. Such oesophageal probes also carry the risk of oesophageal perforations and bleeding.

Index

Printed in the United States
By Bookmasters